An Introduction to
Theory and Reasoning in Nursing

3rd Edition

An Introduction to
Theory and Reasoning in Nursing

3rd Edition

Betty M. Johnson, PhD, RN
Professor Emeritus and Former Chair
Department of Nursing
The University of Virginia's College at Wise
Wise, Virginia

Pamela B. Webber, PhD, FNP
Professor
Division of Nursing
Shenandoah University
Winchester, Virginia

Wolters Kluwer | Lippincott Williams & Wilkins
Health

Philadelphia • Baltimore • New York • London
Buenos Aires • Hong Kong • Sydney • Tokyo

Acquisitions Editor: Jean Rodenberger
Development Editors: Helen Kogut
Director of Nursing Production: Helen Ewan
Managing Editor / Production: Erika Kors
Art Director, Design: Holly McLaughlin
Art Director, Illustration: Brett MacNaughton
Manufacturing Coordinator: Karin Duffield
Production Services / Compositor: Aptara, Inc.

3rd Edition

9 8 7 6 5 4 3 2 1

Printed in China

Library of Congress Cataloging-in-Publication Data

Johnson, Betty M.
  An introduction to theory and reasoning in nursing / Betty M. Johnson, Pamela B. Webber. — 3rd ed.
     p. ; cm.
  Includes bibliographical references and index.
  ISBN 978-0-7817-9103-8 (alk. paper)
  1. Nursing—Philosophy. 2. Reasoning. I. Webber, Pamela Bayliss. II. Title.
  [DNLM: 1. Nursing Theory. 2. Philosophy, Nursing. WY 86 J66i 2010]
  RT84.5.J637 2010
  610.73'01—dc22

                                      2008052932

RRS0812

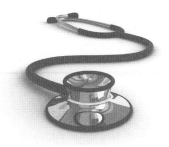

One might think that by the time a book reaches a successful 3rd edition that the writing gets easier and requires less time. It doesn't. If anything, the amount of intellectual energy needed and the time commitment increases and makes busy lives even more complicated. This work simply could not have been accomplished without the ongoing and loving support of our families and their willingness to commit their time and energy to support us. Therefore, we once again dedicate this work to:

Jeff Webber
Michael Webber
Sarah Webber
Cindy Webber

Janet Johnson
Lucille Johnson
Debra and Eric Nelson
Jon and Diana Johnson
Suzi Johnson
and Tim, Jessica, Aren, Ryne, Kelsey, Karl, and Kyle

Contributors

Barbara E. Chandler, PhD, OTR/L, FAOTA
Therapy Supervisor, Home Care Services
Haywood Regional Medical Center
Clyde, North Carolina

Sean Clarke, RN, PhD, FAAN
RBC Chair in Cardiovascular Nursing
University of Toronto
Lawrence S. Bloomberg Faculty of Nursing
Toronto, Ontario, Canada

Elizabeth T. Courts, MSN, APRN, BC, FNP
Assistant Professor
Shenandoah University
Winchester, Virginia

Lon H. McPherson, MD
Senior Vice President of Medical Affairs
Chief Quality Officer
Munroe Medical Center
Ocala, Florida

Caren Werlinger, BS, PT
President
Physical Evaluation and Rehabilitation Center
Winchester, Virginia

Reviewers

Lynn Aquadro, PhD, CRNP, MSN, RN
Associate Professor of Nursing
University of North Alabama
Florence, Alabama

Jean Chow, RN, MN, PhD
Assistant Professor
University of Calgary
Calgary, Alberta

Thomas L. Christenberry, PhD, RN
Assistant Professor of Nursing
Vanderbilt University School of Nursing
Nashville, Tennessee

Lenore Duquette, RN, BScN, MEd, EdD
Faculty Member
Humber ITAL
Toronto, Ontario

Sarah C. Fogel, PhD, RN
Assistant Professor
Vanderbilt University School of Nursing
Nashville, Tennessee

Kay Foland, PhD, MSN, BS, RN, APRN, BC, CNP
Associate Professor
South Dakota State University College of Nursing West River
Department
Rapid City, South Dakota

Carol D. Gaskamp PhD, RN, CNE
Assistant Professor in Clinical Nursing
University of Texas at Austin School of Nursing
Austin, Texas

Margaret M. Lowenthal, RN, MSN, CCRN, CRNP
Assistant Professor
LaSalle University
Philadelphia, Pennsylvania

Cheryl Slaughter Smith, PhD, RN
Associate Professor of Nursing
Arkansas Tech University
Russellville, Arkansas

Foreword

Consciously or unconsciously, nurses use theory, reasoning, and evidence every day. Theories provide frameworks for the phenomena that nurses observe while caring for patients, families, and communities. Theories guide nurses toward the identification of key concepts, ideas, values, beliefs, meanings, and intentions that must be considered for thorough assessment, planning, implementation, evaluation, and effectiveness. *An Introduction to Theory and Reasoning in Nursing* clearly defines terms and provides opportunities for application from the work of Florence Nightingale to the theorists of the 21st century. Clinical reasoning, with theoretical underpinnings, guides nurses in making sense across clinical settings. This book fills a major gap in the literature by presenting a detailed discussion of the relationship between theory, research, and reasoning in nursing. This edition emphasizes information needed across the novice to expert continuum.

The third edition of *An Introduction to Theory and Reasoning in Nursing* is best read in sequence, although each chapter can stand alone. Students will be able to explore and appreciate nursing theories and their use in nursing practice. Educators will find that the book assists students in their comprehension of the connection between theory and clinical reasoning. Faculty will be able to more effectively frame and ground their teaching/learning methods, their scholarship, and their practice in nursing theory.

Summaries of each theorist are supported with notations related to key concepts or variables. The criterion-based critique (C-BaC) model is extremely useful for evaluation of theories and research efforts. Nursing stories provide examples of theory application. For some readers, a favorite theorist will emerge. For most, a goodness of fit with a theory or theorist will be guided by the questions and passions of the time, place, culture, population, societal trends, and world view.

The thoughtful sharing and deep understanding of Drs. Johnson and Webber in this current edition of *An Introduction to Theory and Reasoning in Nursing* fills a significant gap in our literature. Their appreciation of the art and science of nursing is evident throughout the text. The interdisciplinary component illustrates the real work of practice. The authors support reflection and inquiry as they guide students toward making sense of their experiences, linking concepts, asking questions, comparing and contrasting, testing hypotheses, and generating evidence for best practice, safe passage, and optimal healthcare system design and delivery.

Julie C. Novak, DNSc, RN, CPNP, FAANP
Purdue University School of Nursing
Director, Doctor of Nursing Practice Program
Director, Purdue School of Nursing Clinics

Preface

Welcome to the world of theory, research, reasoning, and nursing! As an undergraduate nursing student you will become a knowledgeable, competent, and caring professional who serves others in need of nursing and health care. To meet this goal, you need to develop knowledge, skills, values, meanings, and experiences that are inherent in nursing. In addition, you will develop reasoning skills to help integrate these essential components into your nursing practice. This text, *An Introduction to Theory and Reasoning in Nursing*, is designed to help you do these things.

Each chapter of the third edition was reviewed and updated to ensure its continuing relevance to the changes in nursing and research.

The Journey

Have you ever been driving and not had a clue where you were going? More than likely when you get lost traveling you simply pick up a map and determine the most desirable route to your destination. The same approach will be helpful when studying theory, research, and reasoning. When you begin a course of study, it is important for you to know where you are supposed to go and use a guide or map to help you get there. Knowing where you are going and having a guide to get will help you to understand your journey through the following chapters and help meet the ultimate goal of establishing a firm foundation in theory, research, and reasoning to support your nursing practice.

Organization of the Text

Chapter 1 introduces you to some common activities you may encounter in everyday life that have a theoretical basis. For example, if you have ever ridden on a roller coaster, you will understand the discussion about the "theory of the thrill," and if you have ever been influenced to buy something in a shopping mall because of where it is placed in your line of sight, you will understand a significant component of marketing theory. These examples will provide you with some insight into how theory supports much of what you do in life and in nursing.

Chapter 2 introduces you to the unique language, meanings, and structure associated with theory. You will see how meanings of words are developed and built on to provide expanded meanings with greater application. You will also see how the meanings of these words interrelate in such a manner that they provide structure for theory, research, and reasoning.

Chapter 3 explores types of theory, the essential and interdependent relationships among theory, research, reasoning, and how they are operationalized within nursing practice.

Chapter 4 identifies components and processes associated with reasoning, and factors that influence reasoning, and demonstrates how they are used within nursing practice. In addition, it introduces you to how theory, knowledge, and research are applied in nursing through reasoning.

Chapter 5 presents the historical foundations of theory and knowledge development in nursing by exploring some of the universally accepted support theories from the arts, sciences, and humanities that helped established the early basis of nursing theory and practice and continue to influence the development of nursing theory today.

Chapter 6 chronicles the emergence of nursing theory and includes significant factors contributing to the development of professional nursing, such as Florence Nightingale; changes in nursing education and practice; legislative actions; and societal trends. As you become acquainted with these historical happenings you will discover the impact they had on nursings theoretical development.

Chapter 7 introduces you to many of the nursing theorists and theories that have influenced the development of nursing knowledge in the 20th and 21st centuries. You will learn about the theorists as individuals and how their theories have influenced nursing education, practice, and research.

Chapter 8 describes an easy method of critiquing theory using a criterion-based (C-BaC) model. Using specific criteria to evaluate theory allows you to determine the usefulness of a particular theory to you and in your practice. Theory is valuable only when you understand what it means and are able to apply it to practice.

Chapter 9 introduces you to the research process, some of the most significant philosophies that have influenced how research is conducted, and some of the issues that influence research in nursing today. In addition, the C-BaC model presented in Chapter 8 is used to demonstrate how you can effectively evaluate research for inclusion into your practice.

Chapter 10 illustrates how practice and theory are connected through the use of observation, questioning, comparing, and contrasting. Recognizing and using a theoretical base enables you to find answers to questions, solve problems, and address phenomena in nursing practice, which will ultimately make you a more effective practitioner.

Chapter 11 is unique to this text in that it introduces you to multidisciplinary theory and how that theory is applied in practice with nursing. A team of experts from nursing, medicine, occupational therapy, and physical therapy come together to introduce their theoretical base and essential reasoning processes in caring for an elderly Japanese man who has experienced a stroke.

Chapter 12 discusses the continued development of nursing as a profession, a discipline, and a science, and projects effects that theory may have on this development.

Text Features

The text includes carefully designed features that enable you to "put the pieces together" and move from "Why do I have to take theory?" to "Theory is essential to my practice." Recurring features include:

- **Chapter Intent**: Chapter overviews help you focus on what you should learn and how it can be applied to practice.
- **Key Words/Concepts**: Lists of key words and concepts provide a ready reference for you. The terms first appear in boldface type to draw your attention to them and are defined as they are used. Many of these terms also appear in the glossary.
- **Chapter Outlines**: Chapter outlines give you the organization and arrangement of content and will help you locate specific sections for review.
- **Chapter Introductions**: Chapter introductions provide the background of the chapter content as well as the relationships it might have with theory, knowledge, research, reasoning, and practice.
- **Nursing Stories**: Special boxes highlight stories that illustrate the use of theory and reasoning. The stories will be helpful when analyzing theoretical concepts and their relationships to actual practice.
- **Boxes, Tables, and Figures**: Numerous boxes, tables, and displays summarize important information in an easy-to-understand format that will assist you to make more effective use of information as you proceed through the book.

- **Theorist Boxes**: New to this edition, photos of theorists (when available) and a brief synopsis of their lives appear in special boxes in Chapter 7 to help these people and their theories come alive.
- **Summaries of Individual Support Theories and Nursing Theories**: Chapters 5 and 7 include summary boxes that identify phenomena, internal concepts or variables, propositions, external variables, assumptions, and, when relevant, facts, principles, and laws derived from theories used in nursing.
- **Chapter Summaries**: Chapter summaries provide brief comments about the content of the chapter and how it helps meet the goals of the book and chapter.
- **Learning Activities**: These exercises can be used in class or as preparation for class. They can also stimulate students and faculty to formulate questions and other activities that will assist in learning about theory, research, and reasoning and their application to nursing practice.
- **References**: A list of references used in each chapter enables you to expand your reading of specific topics.
- **Appendix Internet Guide**: Internet addresses help you become acquainted with theorists and their theories as well as what scholars are talking about related to the influence of theories in nursing education, practice, and research.
- **Glossary**: Includes definitions from the book.

Betty Johnson and Pam Webber

Acknowledgments

The authors would like to thank the anonymous reviewers of the second edition of *An Introduction to Theory and Reasoning in Nursing*. By their comments, they recognized the value of an introductory textbook in nursing theory and reasoning, but also made suggestions to enhance the value of the text to both undergraduate and graduate students.

The completion of the third edition of the text is dependent in large part on the patience and persistence of everyone with whom we worked at Lippincott Williams & Wilkins, especially Brandi Spade, Helen Kogut, and Jean Rodenberger, as well as others who played various but important parts in the final product.

A special thanks also goes to the undergraduate and graduate nursing students at Shenandoah University who, once again, played an important role in critiquing chapters for clarity and ease of reading, offering suggestions for stories, and, most importantly, for their encouragement and support. Quite simply, students are the reason for this book.

The thoughtful evaluation of chapters or parts of chapters by Dr. Bruce Leonard, Dr. Betty Wendt Mayer, Sally Thorne, and Mary B. Delashmutt also helped enhance the effectiveness of this text and is greatly appreciated.

Last, but not least, we would like to thank Margaret Wilson, Library Coordinator at the Sigma Theta Tau Virginia Henderson International Nursing Library in Indianapolis, Indiana, and Denise Blake, Health Professions Librarian at Shenandoah University, for their time and expert assistance.

Contents

An Introduction

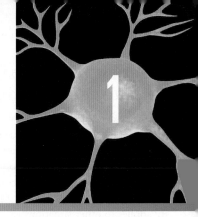

1

Intent: Your everyday life is affected by theory, reasoning, and research, and this chapter will help you understand how to use them in your nursing practice.

Key Words/Concepts

acceleration	inertia	reasoning
evidence	knowledge	research
gravity	phenomenon(a)	theory

Introduction

As a college student, you may view courses as either theoretical or practical in nature. If you assume that theory is applicable in the classroom rather than the laboratory, you are partially correct, but you will also learn that **theory** is useful in the practice of nursing. A significant amount of the subject matter you study for class is based on theory and **knowledge.** When you ask a professor why certain things happen, he or she will rely on theory for many answers, even though the word theory may not be mentioned. Theory and knowledge provide the foundation for some of the psychomotor and **reasoning** skills you use in the laboratory and also help increase your understanding about objects, events, and relationships in patient care settings.

As you learn about theory, reasoning, and **research,** you will recognize that what you learn about nursing and health care relates to theory, although you might not be able to identify a specific theory. By the time you finish reviewing and studying this book, you will understand what theory and research are, how they support reasoning, and the relationships between theory, reasoning, and nursing practice.

Before you begin to examine theory, reasoning, and research, let's explore some familiar activities and events in everyday life. This will prepare you to consider questions about relationships between knowledge, theory, and research. By the time you reach the end of the chapter, you may begin to identify relationships between what occurs in your everyday life and your professional nursing life. Although this chapter includes little that is specifically about theory, reasoning, and research, the explanation of some common activities will help you understand these concepts for future reference.

Theory, Reasoning, and Research in Everyday Life

Theory and research are perceived by many to be abstract concepts; however, they will become more concrete when you examine their roles in everyday activities and events. You seldom hear the word theory used in conversation. For example, as a young child, you may have asked your parents why apples and leaves fall off trees. You may not have understood what they said as they explained Sir Isaac Newton's theory of **gravity,** but you learned something about its effect from their explanation. Later, when you studied Newton's theory in school, you became aware of how gravity applies to other situations as well. For example, you came to understand why it is more difficult to pedal your bicycle up a long hill compared to the ease of coasting down the hill. You may seldom think about gravity these days, but you might use your reasoning skills when you face tasks such as moving into a university residence hall or a new apartment. And you might think about it when you need to assist a patient into bed. When you see how small your dorm room is, you might get a measuring tape to collect data about the space before deciding to add a favorite chair to the room. You might not call that research, but you are using related intellectual skills.

Frequently, you use theory, research, and reasoning without realizing that you are doing so. You can drive a car, repair an electrical switch, follow a recipe, or even surf the Internet without knowing what makes the car go, how electricity causes light, why cakes rise in the oven, or how images from around the world enter your computer. You can rely on scientists to develop the technology and only concern yourself with learning how to use it.

Have you recently read or heard about discoveries in fields such as engineering, chemistry, and biology? Although reporters seldom mention theory or research associated with these discoveries, you might want to think about what it took to make the discovery. Reports about the Human Genome Project, for example, are related to scientific advances in biological and genetic theory. When scientists describe how genomes are essential to mapping out DNA, they may not explain the theory on which it is based.

You may experience a similar situation when you read or hear about breakthroughs in health care. Think about a recent breakthrough and try to relate the information to what you already know. You may be able to find an article in a scientific journal and exercise your reasoning skills to make judgments about the meaning and significance of the breakthrough to you.

The following are examples of how theory, reasoning, and research are applied to everyday activities and objects, such as roller coaster rides, college campuses, and shopping malls. As you read and think about these activities, try to draw parallels between the examples.

The Theory of the Thrill

Have you ever taken a ride on a roller coaster, with its gut-wrenching drops, disorienting speed, and upside-down loops? Videos of people riding a coaster show them screaming and crying, many with their hands up in the air in excitement. The rides may be frightening, but many riders return again and again to experience the thrill. Maybe you have wondered why riders do not fall out of the cars as they race up and down steep inclines, sometimes completely upside down. Riders wear safety harnesses and lap bars, but experts tell us that even if you are not strapped in, it is unlikely you will fall out of most coasters.

According to Wright (1997), an expert on the physics of roller coasters, two natural **phenomena,** inertia and acceleration, that are related to the theory of gravity keep you in your seat and give you the sensation of flying, tumbling through the air, and weightlessness. **Inertia** is the tendency of an object to keep moving in the direction that it is already moving. **Acceleration** is any change in speed or direction of an object, not just an increase in speed, as we commonly define it.

Theory associated with gravity, inertia, and acceleration is evident not only in roller coaster rides, but also when you drive a car. When you brake the car suddenly, you keep moving, even though the car slows down. Seat belts and air bags prevent you from colliding with the dashboard when the driver brakes or suddenly slows the car down, stops, or changes direction. This is similar to a roller coaster ride, during which gravity, inertia, and acceleration keep you moving in the direction of the coaster car and give you the thrill. You might feel safer in a car, because you ride it more often, but the next time you drive or ride in a car, think about inertia and acceleration. We might wonder where the inventor of the coaster got the idea before one was built. Recently a roller coaster stopped in midair and the riders spent several hours before technicians were able to bring it down to earth. How many riders do you think asked themselves why they had taken the ride? How many vowed they would never ride another coaster? How many got right back in one again, just to experience the thrill? In many cases, just because you are familiar with the theory behind the roller coaster does not mean that you want to experience the thrill.

The College Campus: Why Does It Look the Way It Does?

As a student in a university or college (hereafter referred to as college), you know something about how a college campus is arranged. After arriving at college, you quickly learn your way around the campus but may wonder about the location and arrangement of specific buildings. You might wonder why the library is not closer to the residences and why classes are spread around in various buildings. What if you were asked to develop a theory for designing a college campus? Where would you start?

Architects, planners, and engineers who design college campuses depend on a specific body of knowledge about the organization and arrangement of educational institutions. They study how a college functions, how it looks, and the kind of feelings it gives to students and their parents. Although some college campuses appear to be arranged haphazardly, if you investigate, you may find that most have a master plan with a central theme that guides the growth of the institution. Following the plan ensures that a campus is convenient, attractive, and unified. The plan reflects the beliefs of various groups, such as the college governing board, administration, and faculty. In some cases, even the student body is involved. The master plan may identify sites for future buildings, such as classrooms, office buildings, and student residences, and may designate space for athletics and parking.

The next time you walk through the campus, ask yourself why the student center and the financial aid office are located where they are, why the cafeteria is not closer to the classroom buildings, and the reasoning behind the placement of parking lots. You may notice that there are similarities in the type of material used for constructing buildings, such as brick, stone, or wood, as well as other characteristics, such as the kind of windows, roofs, and entrances. If there are buildings that do not conform to the master plan, you may wish to explore the reasoning behind the differences. If you have attended classes on more than one campus, you might have different questions. Why is one campus so quiet and distinguished, while another seems lively and energetic? Why are buildings on one campus traditional in appearance and very modern on another? On larger campuses, you may notice that the appearance and feeling of the campus change as you move from one area to another. For example, what are the similarities and differences between the health science center and the business school or the liberal arts building and the library?

Suppose you attended a small, rural college with expansive green lawns between buildings, benches along tree-lined walkways, shaded parking areas, and recreational space near student residences. After 2 years, you transfer to a large urban university located among the skyscrapers in a large metropolitan area. You may wonder whether this is really a campus, how to identify the boundaries of the campus, and whether students can learn as effectively in such an environment.

There are many types of campuses, but many have similar properties, objects, and events that distinguish it from other types of institutions, such as parks, housing subdivisions, and shopping malls. Almost every campus has buildings of classrooms, laboratories, and offices; a catalog of courses; and students, professors, and staff. There may be student and faculty residences, libraries, parking areas, a security department, and athletic facilities. Frequently, buildings of a certain type are clustered; for example, student residences may be located together and adjacent to the cafeteria. On a larger campus, there may be several areas devoted to student residences surrounding academic sections of the campus. The college library may be located centrally on the campus; however, in large institutions with numerous libraries, libraries will be located near buildings housing specific disciplines. A campus may be viewed as open to the community, accessible to the disabled, friendly or inhospitable, and spacious or crowded. As you observe your college campus or visit other campuses, you may notice that each campus has a distinct personality.

These factors and others could contribute to developing a theory for designing a college campus. If you were an architect and asked to design a college campus, what characteristics would you consider important to carry throughout the campus, and how would you improve the structure and functionality of the campus? How many campuses would you visit to collect data before you decided the most effective way to stimulate intellectual thinking? While you were exploring what college to enroll in, what helped you most in making up your mind? What reasons did you use to help choose your campus, and how did you come to your decision? If you used other characteristics than these to make your decision, ask yourself questions that might be related to research and reasoning skills. One last thought: How would you perceive the campus, if you were enrolled in a distance learning course and didn't even come to the campus?

Shopping Malls: Building Stores and Arranging Stock

Now shift your attention from a theory of designing college campuses to a theory of designing shopping malls. Think about the shopping malls you visit. What physical and behavioral characteristics do they display? How are they similar to or different from each other? What characteristics, if any, do they share with college campuses? What purposes do shopping malls serve other than selling merchandise and food? How are these purposes guided by theory? If you moved from another city to attend college, what did you look for in a shopping mall, if you just wanted to "hang out"?

Basic premises used in building shopping malls include recruiting several large well-known department stores, locating them at strategic points within the mall, and then filling the areas between them with a variety of specialty shops. What is the value of using this plan? What research would be helpful in planning? Why are the larger stores placed in strategic areas? Is there a reason for the arrangement of the smaller stores? How do the arrangements and characteristics of a mall reflect what people value, such as convenient parking, protected walkways, food courts, and a play area for children? If you have visited shopping malls in various parts of the country, have you noticed any differences between malls?

You are probably familiar with today's large enclosed malls, but earlier malls, known as strip malls, are still evident in some neighborhoods. Strip malls are composed of a group of stores along one or more blocks, sometimes on both sides of the street, and away from the center of the city. In some, parking is limited to the space in front of the store. Although we still have strip malls, what events stimulated the development of the large indoor malls that are so popular? How do large regional discount malls resemble and differ from the neighborhood malls? What characteristics do all malls have in common?

The next time you are in a large shopping mall or a small strip mall, observe the events, objects, and climate of the mall, including activities sponsored by the mall and characteristics of the shoppers. Notice things you expect to see there, but also look for unusual things as well. Think about the theory and reasoning that went into the planning, development, and building of the mall. Also think about the addition of dental offices, urgent care units, and other services that might be added to shopping malls in the future.

While you are exploring theory in everyday life, begin to think about how theory might be used in nursing practice. Start with simple, concrete ideas, and then proceed to ideas that are more complex and abstract.

Summary

You now know how theory, research, and reasoning are related to common events, objects, and relationships in your everyday life. Theory, research, and reasoning apply to your nursing education and practice as well. This book will help you recognize, understand, and use theory, research, and reasoning in your daily nursing practice. If your ideas about theory, research, and reasoning become a little blurred, regain your perspective by returning to the theoretical world of roller coasters, campuses, and shopping malls.

Learning Activities

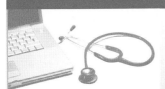

1. Nurses are increasingly interested in **evidence** that supports their practice. The Agency for Healthcare Research and Quality, part of the U.S. Department of Health and Human Services, published a book early in 2008 targeting nurses, especially in schools of nursing (Hughes, 2008). Nurses can obtain the book without cost through the agency. Since the book has 90 authors and 900 pages, you may wish to look at it section by section on the Internet. To get you started, you might examine Section I: Patient Safety and Quality, specifically the section on Clinical Reasoning, Decision Making and Action: Thinking Critically and Clinically, by Patricia E. Benner, Molly Sutphen, and Rhonda Hughes.

2. PubMed is another site that focuses on health care, but this one is primarily for the physician. As you look at this Internet site, you may begin by making comparisons between Hughes (2008) and PubMed.

References

Hughes, R. G. (2008). *Patient safety and quality: An evidence based handbook for nurses*. Washington, DC: Agency for Healthcare Research and Quality. www.ahrq.gov

PubMed. www.nchi.nlmc.nih.gov/pubmed

Wright, D. (1997, August 13). *The theory behind the thrill*. Washington Post, pp. H1, H4.

Language, Meaning, and Structure

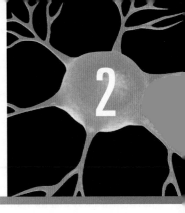

2

Intent: This chapter introduces you to how words and meanings are developed. In addition, it introduces you to the specific words and meanings that are considered fundamental building blocks of theory, research, and reasoning. The dependent and progressive relationships among these building blocks will also be discussed in relation to their structure, organization, and the role they play in knowledge development and nursing practice.

Key Words/Concepts		
assumption	idea	philosophy
axiom	independent variable	principle
concept	knowledge	proposition
conceptual definition	law	qualitative
construct	meanings	quantitative
dependent variable	metaparadigm	reasoning
epistemology	metatheory	research
established theory	middle-range theory	speculative theory
fact	model	theorem
grand theory	operational definition	theory
hermeneutics	paradigm	triangulation
hypothesis	phenomenon(a)	variable

Chapter Outline

Introduction

Before you begin to study theory, research, and reasoning, you must first be introduced to the language (words and meanings) that is unique to them. Simply memorizing definitions of words associated with these topics is not sufficient. For them to be meaningful and useful, you will need to draw words and meanings from within your existing language and expand them to include words and meanings associated with theory, research, and reasoning.

The study of words and **meanings** dates back to the days of Greek mythology and Hermes, the messenger of the gods. Hermes was charged with interpreting messages from Zeus and the other gods in such a way that the mortals on Earth understood them. Today, it is this mythology that gives rise to **hermeneutics** (her·me·nu·tiks), which is the science of interpreting words and their evolving meanings. Hermeneutics allows us to understand and use expanded meanings of words in different situations and combinations. This expandability in establishing meaning is an important tool because it enhances your ability to grow and develop enhanced language and intellectual skills while ensuring that the words remain rooted in their original meaning. For example, as a child, you learned words and meanings associated with counting from one (1) to ten (10). As an adult, you build on these basic meanings when using math to manage your finances. As a nursing student, you use these basic meanings when learning to calculate drug dosages and intravenous fluid drip rates. Even mathematicians capable of solving complex formulas have to use these basic words and meanings to do higher-level work. In other words, basic words and meanings associated with counting from 1 to 10 provide the foundation, which is then expanded based on your need and capability.

Most people assign meanings to words based on how those words are used within their families, schools, cultures, societies, and experiences. For instance, toddlers learn the word hot; however, they do not understand the meaning of hot until they touch something hot, such as an oven, and begin to associate the word hot with that feeling and their mothers yelling, "No! Hot!" Over time, the word hot takes on expanded meaning by being associated with other things that cause the same or similar feelings. Examples of the expanded meaning of hot include the description of the temperature outside, a hot day; a fast car, a hot rod; and a type of social dating, a hot date. Nurses even use this expanded meaning when describing a patient's elevated temperature, hot with fever. Hence, the word hot has taken on expanded meanings and broader applications. In addition to expanding the meaning of hot by using it in these contexts, its use in combination with other words, such as day, rod, date, and fever, creates new, shared meanings that are larger than the meanings of the two separate words. Although meanings and relationships among these words vary somewhat from the original, they still have commonalities with their root words and meanings. It is the root commonalities of words and their meanings that help us build, remember, and use new or expanded meanings. Perhaps the old adage about the whole being greater than the sum of its parts applies to meanings created by expanding and combining words. The words and meanings associated with theory, research, and reasoning are expanded in much the same way.

Theory, Knowledge, Research, and Reasoning: What Are They and Why Are They Important?

Theory

The word **theory** is an excellent example of how a word and its meaning can be expanded over time. The word theory originates from the Greek word *theoria*, which means to speculate;

however, the meaning of theory has evolved to also mean organized information that is intended to explain phenomena. If you combine these two definitions, then you could safely assume that theory involves explanations based on speculation. For example, scientists speculate that a large meteor hit the earth and caused the extinction of the dinosaurs. They do not know this for a fact but continue to search for clues that would confirm or deny this **speculative theory.** Over time, the meaning of theory has continued to expand beyond just speculative explanation to include explanation through facts, principles, and laws. This type of theory is viewed as **established theory.** Speculative and established theory will be discussed in more depth in Chapter 3.

The majority of what you study in school is theory; however, it is seldom called theory. You read theory in textbooks, you hear theory in classrooms, and you practice using theory in clinical settings. When you are taking a biology class, you are studying biological theory; when you are taking a psychology class, you are studying psychological theory; when you learn about drugs, you are studying pharmacological theory; and when you learn about nursing, you are studying nursing theory. As a nurse, you will draw on the theory of all of these disciplines and more to answer questions, solve problems, and explore phenomena relating to nursing practice. It is important to remember that theory is not something intangible that you study in a single theory class. It is the foundation of every class you take and is the essential component of what you know and understand. Quite simply, theory is the foundation of what you do in nursing. Examples of theories that have contributed to nursing's theoretical base include systems theory, which began with biologist Ludwig von Bertalanffy's work on general and open system theories (1968); stress adaptation theory, which began with Hans Selye's work on the physiological effects of stress (1956); change theory, which became popular with Kurt Lewin's force field analysis theory (1951); and self-care theory, which became popular with Dorothea Orem's theory of self-care (1971).

There are different classifications of theory based on scope and practical applicability. For example, theory that is more abstract and broad in scope is often referred to as **grand theory** or **metatheory.** Theory that is more narrow in scope and addresses specific practice-based issues is commonly referred to as **middle-range theory.** Grand and middle-range theories will be addressed in more detail in Chapter 7.

Frequently, disciplines take ownership of theory that they consider unique to them. For example, a nurse may use terms such as nursing theory and nursing research, and a physician may use terms such as medical theory and medical research. However, discipline-specific theory is often shared among health care professionals when answers to questions, solutions to problems, or explanations of phenomena fall into another discipline's theoretical base. For example, theory related to administering a medication by injection includes specific medical theory related to the selection and prescribing of the drug, while also including specific nursing theory about how to administer the injection safely with minimal pain and maximum absorption. In addition, medicine and nursing share theory related to the action, dosage, potential adverse drug reactions, and efficacy of the drug. Sharing of interdisciplinary theory is demonstrated in Figure 2.1. As beneficial as interdisciplinary sharing of theory is to practice, Meleis (2007, p. 458) cautions that in this day of blurring disciplinary boundaries, nursing, as a discipline, needs to keep its epistemological focus on its goal of advancing nursing.

Knowledge

The word **knowledge** is derived from the Old English term *cnawan*, which means to recognize or identify (McKean, 2005). Today it means what is identified and understood through the

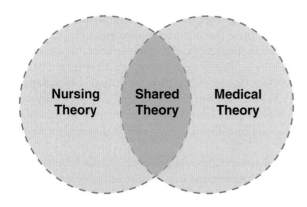

Figure 2.1 Shared theory.

integration of education and experience. Knowledge, although not synonymous with theory, is dependent upon theory and research to provide an ongoing, cumulative, and organized body of current information that can be used to answer questions, solve problems, explore phenomena, and generate new theory.

Epistemology (e·pis·te·mol·o·gy) is a Greek word that means the study of knowledge, or more specifically, the study of the scope, methods, and validity of knowledge (McKean, 2005). Although epistemology is not a word you use every day, it is important to understand its essential meaning and the effect it has on theory development and nursing practice. It is necessary to study knowledge, especially discipline-specific knowledge, to ensure that the integrity of that knowledge is maintained and its development is strategic in its intent to advance the discipline. For example, if nursing is to grow and develop in a way that is beneficial to itself and society, it must continually develop a knowledge base that is effective, accurate, and reliable. In essence, epistemology provides us with a measuring stick to determine the relevance and quality of knowledge that has been and is being developed. For example, you may read in the literature or hear a faculty member say, "the epistemological significance of this study to nursing is. . . ." This statement represents an intellectual judgment with regard to the significance or value of information to the totality of nursing knowledge. The value of theory is dependent not only on what is being studied and its relationship with established theory, but also on how it is being studied and its actual and potential contribution to nursing's body of knowledge.

Philosophies, Paradigms, and Models

In addition to theory, knowledge also encompasses **philosophies,** which are significant to nursing because of the nature of what nurses think about, study, and do. Philosophies are broad, connected statements about beliefs and values and have the potential to guide thinking and behavior of individuals, disciplines, and societies. Philosophies may include theoretical components and personal views and opinions. This integration of philosophy and theory has sometimes led to confusion in trying to differentiate one from the other. For example, Florence Nightingale's work concerning what nursing is and is not (1859, 1992) and Patricia Benner's work on competency development in nursing practice (1984, 2000; Benner & Wrubel, 1989; Benner, Tanner, & Chesla, 1996) have each been called a theory and a philosophy, because they both have the elements of theory as well as personal views and opinions. However, the fact remains that their work is rich enough to offer specific nursing knowledge that helps answer questions, solve problems, explore phenomena, and generate new theory. As a result, both are considered usable theory with philosophical overtones.

Another term used in theory and research is **paradigm.** Powers and Knapp (2006, p. 121) define paradigm as patterns or systems of beliefs (or worldviews) about science and knowledge within and across disciplines, whereas McKean (2005) defines paradigm as a model or pattern. From these two definitions you could conclude that a paradigm is a pattern of beliefs that can be represented in model form; however, though the terms paradigm, model, and pattern work well together, they are not synonyms and should not be treated as such, because of the potential for confusion. For example, in the late 20th century, nursing used the concepts of person, society, environment, health, and nursing as a paradigm or **metaparadigm** for all of nursing (Fawcett, 2004). Over time, the profession began to realize two things about this paradigm. The first was that it used nursing, in part, to define itself, which was a tautological mistake (Chinn & Kramer, 2008; Meleis, 1997;), and the second was that it did not represent a governing paradigm for nursing at all, but was simply a model demonstrating who and what nursing interacted with (Webber, 2002). Nursing's misuse of these combined concepts as a metaparadigm most likely represents a simple misstep in our epistemological development that has actually helped nursing scientists clarify what nursing is and is not. To date, a new, more accurate paradigm for nursing has yet to emerge, which, again, may simply reflect our epistemological development to date.

Models, which are visual representations or diagrams that demonstrate theoretical relationships, are also used to guide thinking and behavior. Most people have previously assigned meaning to the word model based on their experience with the word. For example, phrases such as model car, fashion model, and model home are common in Western society. By associating this definition of model with other words, you can assume that a model car diagrams the relationship with full-size cars, a fashion model diagrams the relationship between the human body and clothes, and a model home diagrams the relationship with other homes. Models are also used to provide visual representations of key components of theories and other intellectual work. For example, Abraham Maslow (1954) used a pyramid-shaped model of basic human needs to demonstrate the relationship among the key concepts of his theory of human motivation and hierarchy of basic human needs (refer to Chapter 5), and Madeline Leininger (1985) used a model of a sunrise to describe her theory of culture care diversity in nursing (refer to Chapter 7). Nursing students and practicing nurses use models in much the same way. For example, there are model patients that students practice nursing skills on called Sim-Man (Laerdal, 2008), and these model patients are often located in model hospital rooms that have been set up in learning laboratories within schools of nursing. While these examples of models are three dimensional, some models are simply words and lines on paper (or computer). Nurses use a variety of paper and computer models to help guide their practice, such as model care plans to guide patient care, scheduling models to guide how a particular unit is staffed, and competency models to guide the development of clinical proficiency.

Historically, some nursing authors have spent decades debating what constitutes philosophies, theories, and models, which Meleis (2007, p. 151) contends is "splitting hairs" over an issue of semantics. Ultimately, the outcome has been confusion about these terms in the novice and experienced alike. "This confusion may have contributed to the slow progress, and, at times, stilted theory development in nursing and has led to . . . a preoccupation with method and process rather than content and consequences" (Meleis, 2007, p. 151). The reality is that if theory is intended to explain and models are intended to demonstrate relationships, then models are simply theory in picture form. Therefore, use of models may ultimately enhance understanding of the theory.

Even as a student, you can develop and use models to help answer questions, solve problems, or simply understand complex material. As you read this and other chapters, make note of how a variety of models are used to visually demonstrate the text being presented.

Research

The term **research** is derived from the 16th century French word *recherche*, which means to search (McKean, 2005). Today the meaning of the term has been expanded to mean diligent and systematic inquiry or investigation. However, it may also be used to describe (1) the actual process of systematic inquiry, such as when you research the answer to a question; (2) the outcomes of systematic inquiry, such as when you hear a faculty member say "research revealed that . . ."; or (3) the study of the process of systematic inquiry, which is demonstrated by the fact that you take a research course within your nursing curriculum.

Research is used to investigate speculative theory, refine and test the reliability and validity of established theory, and, ultimately, generate new theory. In other words, research is the way theory perpetuates itself. Theory developed through research sent men and women into space, and theory developed through research will solve many of today's problems, such as global warming, acquired immunodeficiency syndrome (AIDS), sudden acute respiratory syndrome (SARS), avian flu, and the common cold. In nursing, theory developed through research will lead the profession in developing the most effective approaches to facilitating health and well-being. The development of new theory is the most important outcome of research. As a student of nursing, it is important not only that you understand the role research plays in developing nursing's theoretical body of knowledge, but also that you become a sophisticated consumer of research that has the potential to influence your practice. Research is discussed more throughout this chapter and in Chapter 9.

Reasoning

Reasoning, which is derived from the Latin word *ratio*, is the cognitive process that allows us to think, identify relationships, and form judgments about information. Reasoning also provides us with the basis and justification for our actions. For example, as a nursing student, if you enter a patient's room and see his hand at his throat and realize that he cannot speak, is cyanotic, and has a breakfast tray in front of him, you would connect all of these pieces of information and make a judgment that the patient is choking. This judgment would be based on your knowledge of theory related to airway obstruction, which would also guide your decision to call for help and perform the Heimlich maneuver to try to clear his airway. It is reasoning that allows you to determine the nature and significance of knowledge gained from theory and research and then use this knowledge appropriately in your practice to answer questions, solve problems, explore phenomena, and generate new theory. Reasoning is, in part, a function of intellectual ability, but it is also a skill that can be intentionally and continually developed over time. The more you learn about theory and research, the more they become intentional factors in your reasoning. Being able to operationalize, or use what you know effectively and efficiently, is extremely important in nursing. Just as important is the ability to recognize what you do not know and seek out that information. Reasoning is discussed in more detail in Chapter 4.

The Language of Theory, Research, and Reasoning

According to Reynolds (1971), knowledge provides us with a method of organizing or classifying information (a typology). Theory, research, reasoning, and even knowledge itself share the same basic typology or classification system of words and meanings. Words within this typology include phenomenon, idea, concept, proposition, variable, hypothesis, assumption, research, fact, principle, and law. These terms are also collectively referred to as the building blocks of theory, research, and reasoning. In the following pages, you will study each of these words and their various meanings, and see how they are connected to one another to form theory and research and provide the basis for effective reasoning.

Phenomena

The most fundamental building block is a **phenomenon** (plural, phenomena), which is derived from the Greek word *phainomen*, which means to appear or be revealed (McKean, 2005). Today, phenomena are observable connections or relationships between objects, events, people, or ideas. For example, observations that plants grow better in sunlight, lightning occurs during a storm, an infected wound is red and swollen, and hospitalized children eat better when their mothers are present are all considered phenomena because they each have two or more objects, events, people, or ideas that are in relationship with one another.

Another source of researchable ideas are noumena. Noumena are similar to phenomena in that there is an awareness of a connection or relationship between objects, events, people, or ideas, but the connection or relationship is more of a perception than an observation. This type of connection or relationship is intangible and cannot always be clearly identified in the form of facts; however, it may be perceived as being just as real. Examples of noumena include intuition that guides behavior, the importance faith plays in health, and the effect of personal beliefs on decision making. The study of tangible phenomena is far more common and easier to grasp than the abstractness of noumena; however, study of noumena is very valuable, especially in the field of human services. Human beings are a holistic, pandimensional combination of mind, body, and spirit and encompass both phenomena and noumena; however, for the purpose of this book, the word phenomena will be used.

Ideas, Concepts, and Constructs

Once phenomena are identified, ideas can be generated about them. The term **idea** is derived from the Greek word *idein*, which means to see a pattern or relationship (McKean, 2005). Ideas are the product of organized thought about the origin, nature, boundaries, and significance of a phenomenon. For example, if you observed that plants in your garden receiving direct sunlight were bigger than plants located in the shade, you could generate the idea that the amount of sun a plant receives influences its growth. Ideas generated by nurses when providing care are often the source of researchable questions and theory development. For example, in the mid-18th century, Florence Nightingale, the mother of modern nursing, had an idea that environmental factors such as fresh air, warmth, light, nutrition, and cleanliness contributed to a patient's ability to recover from illness and injury. Her idea proved to be right and her work surrounding this idea provided the basis of one of nursing's first textbooks, *Notes on Nursing: What It Is and Is Not* (1859, 1992). "*Notes* contains timeless wisdom still appropriate for today's professional nurses"

(Chinn & Kramer, 2008, p. 31). Andrist, Nicholas, and Wolf, in their book *A History of Nursing Ideas* (2006), explored the historical development of some of the more significant nursing ideas and their impact on nursing knowledge development from Nightingale's time to the 21st century.

Ideas consist of two or more concepts. The word concept is derived from the Latin word *concipere*, which means to conceive or form a mental image (McKean, 2005). **Concepts** are the words or phrases that identify, define, and establish structure and boundaries for ideas generated about a particular phenomenon. In other words, concepts name and frame phenomena. Concepts included in the previous example would include sunlight, time, and plant growth. From the nursing perspective, some of the concepts used by Nightingale included fresh air, warmth, light, nutrition, cleanliness, and recovery from illness and injury. Without clearly identified concepts, structured theory that helps us answer questions, solve problems, explore phenomena, and generate new theory could not exist.

Concepts may be naturally occurring or they may be "constructed" by a theorist, researcher, or practicing nurse to assist in answering a question, solving a problem, or exploring a particular phenomenon. Concepts that are created for a specific purpose and have measurable specificity are referred to as **constructs.** For example, the naturally occurring concepts of sunlight and time may be developed into constructs by defining them as the amount of direct sun that reaches an outdoor plant for 8 hours every day for 30 days in May. With regard to Nightingale's concepts, fresh air could be constructed to mean open windows and doors to allow for ventilation; nutrition for the very ill could be constructed to mean "beef-tea, of arrowroot and wine, of egg flip, every hour"; and cleanliness for patients could be constructed to mean daily ". . . sponging, washing, and cleansing of the skin . . ." (Nightingale, 1859/1992, p. 36).

Variables

The identification of concepts and constructs is essential to the identification of the next building block, variables. The word variable is derived from the Latin word *variae*, which means to vary (McKean, 2005). Concepts and constructs that have the ability to vary in their characteristics are called **variables.** In theory and research, variables may be used in several ways. They may be considered internal in that they are actually part of a specific relationship being examined. For example, in the relationship among sunlight, time, and plant growth, all of the concepts have the potential to vary. The amount of sunlight could be low on cloudy days but high on clear days. The amount of chlorophyll in each plant may be different, and the clock used to determine the time may be slow or fast. With regard to Nightingale's concepts, fresh air, warmth, light, nutrition, and cleanliness all have the potential to vary in degree, as does the patient's ability to recover from illness and injury. Therefore, the concepts involved in these relationships are called variables.

Variables may also be external to the relationship being examined but still have the ability to exert varying degrees of influence. For example, external variables that could influence plant growth include the amount of rain it receives and whether the plant has any disease-carrying insects on it; however, rain and disease-carrying insects are not part of the original variables in the relationship being examined, so they are considered external. It is important to note that external variables may also be referred to as confounding variables, especially in research.

Defining Variables

Definitions of variables can either be conceptual or operational. **Conceptual definitions** are broad and define a particular concept while usually retaining the root meaning or definition of the word(s) involved. For example, the conceptual definition of sunlight may simply be the light that emanates from the sun. However, for an **operational definition,** you would need to put this conceptual definition into a very specific and measurable form. For example, the operational definition of sunlight may be the amount of light emanating from the sun between 9 AM and 5 PM during the first 30 consecutive days in May. Using one of Nightingale's constructs, the conceptual definition of nutrition could have been simply the "taking of food" and the operational definition for nutrition, at least for the very ill, could have been a spoonfull of beef-tea every fifteen minutes until the patient can tolerate solid food (Nightingale, 1859, 1992, p. 36).

Independent and Dependent Variables. Variables that are in relationship are also considered to be either independent or dependent. **Independent variables** influence or cause something to happen to another variable. The variable that has been influenced then becomes a **dependent variable.** For example, sunlight and time are the independent variables that cause the dependent variable of plant growth to occur. With regard to Nightingale's theory, fresh air, warmth, light, nutrition, and cleanliness are independent variables that influence the recovery from illness to occur (dependent variable). A key step in analyzing relationships in theory, research, and reasoning is the identification of independent and dependent variables in any situation.

While it is important to understand what variables are and how independent and dependent variables differ, fundamentally, they are still concepts, so both of these terms are used within this text.

Propositions, Axioms, and Theorems

The word proposition is derived from the Latin word *proponere*, which means to put forward (McKean, 2005). Today, a **proposition** is a statement that has been put forward to describe the directional relationship between two or more variables. For example, the statement "increasing the amount of time a plant is in direct sunlight increases plant growth" is a proposition because it identifies the directional relationship sunlight and time have on plant growth. With regard to Nightingale's variables, "fresh air, warmth, light, nutrition, and cleanliness assists in the recovery from illness" is a proposition because it identifies the directional relationship fresh air, warmth, light, nutrition, and cleanliness have on the recovery from illness and injury.

Propositions also demonstrate which variables are independent and which are dependent. For example, time and sunlight are independent variables and plant growth is the dependent variable; fresh air, warmth, light, nutrition, and cleanliness are independent variables and recovery from illness or injury is the dependent variable.

Two words that may be used in association with or in lieu of proposition are axiom and theorem. An **axiom** is a proposition that is asserted to be true, and a **theorem** is a proposition that has been deduced from an axiom and is either true or needs to be proven as true. For example, if you assert the proposition that plant growth is dependent on sunlight (an axiom), you could therefore deduce that for the plant to live, it must have sunlight (a theorem). In the same light, if recovery from illness is dependent upon fresh air, warmth, light, nutrition, and cleanliness (an axiom), you could deduce that for the patient to live, he or she must have fresh air, warmth, light, nutrition, and cleanliness (a theorem).

The terms axiom and theorem are simply words that help you identify where and how propositions develop in relation to one another. While it is important for you to be aware of these terms, proposition is the single term that will be used in this text.

Assumptions

The term assumption is derived from the Latin word *sumere*, which means to accept as true (McKean, 2005). Today, **assumptions** are concepts or variables and propositions that are accepted as true. These assumed truths influence or have the potential to influence the concepts, variables, and/or propositions being examined.

Theorists and researchers may identify assumptions they are making about their work. For example, when looking at the proposition about sunlight, time, and plant growth, you would assume that the amount of light provided by the sun is constant, that the amount of chlorophyll in each plant is relatively consistent, and that the clock keeps accurate time. With regard to Nightingale, you would assume that windows and doors could be opened to let in fresh air and light. You could also assume that beef-tea and other forms of food were available and that there was fresh water, soap, and towels for bathing. However, assumptions are not always evident; they may be embedded within concepts, variables, and propositions and go unrecognized. Unrecognized assumptions may be problematic if they influence the proposition unexpectedly. For example, if some of the plants in your experiment were diseased and you assumed they were healthy, the degree of plant growth could be influenced regardless of sun exposure. If Nightingale assumed that the food she was giving to patients was safe and it was not, then the therapeutic relationship between food and recovery would be influenced.

It is important to be intentional about identifying assumptions whenever possible, whether in formulating theories, in conducting research, or reasoning during actual nursing practice, because of their potential to influence and possibly change variables and propositions in significant ways.

Hypotheses

Propositions provide the basis for the formation of hypotheses. The term hypotheses is derived from the Greek word *hypothesis*, which means foundation (McKean, 2005). **Hypotheses** are formal, foundational statements describing an anticipated and measurable relationship between two or more variables. Hypotheses form the basis of quantitative research. As with propositions, these expected relationships are usually directional or causal in nature. For example, you may assert that providing direct sunlight to outdoor plants with chlorophyll for 8 hours every day for the first 30 days in May is associated with a 50% increase in plant growth over original size when compared to similar plants that received 4 hours of sunlight daily during the same period. Proving or disproving cause is a function of quantitative research. You could also hypothesize that injured patients who receive the Food and Drug Administration's daily recommended amounts of proteins, complex carbohydrates, and fats will be hospitalized for fewer days than those who do not.

Research

Earlier in this chapter, you were introduced to how the word research is used to describe a process of scientific inquiry, an outcome of scientific inquiry, and a course that teaches how to conduct scientific inquiry. Now it is time to look at research as a building block of theory. Once an epistemologically significant hypothesis is formed, it needs to be investigated through research. Depending on the nature of the hypothesis, the research may either assist in generating new, speculative theory or in validating and refining existing theory. Research is the dividing line between speculative and established theory because speculative theory that has consistently proven to be valid and reliable through research becomes established theory. Epistemologically significant research is essential to the development of evidence that supports nursing practice.

There are two major types of research, quantitative and qualitative. Research that follows scientific, empirically based research methods involving hypothesis testing and statistical analysis is referred to as **quantitative** research and is the more historically prominent method. For example, a recent study by Gies, Buchman, Robinson, and Smolen (2008) used an empirically based, quantitative design to determine the effectiveness of a nurse-directed smoking cessation program for hospitalized patients who wanted to quit smoking. The second type of research, which is referred to as qualitative or phenomenological, began to emerge more prominently in the mid-20th century. **Qualitative** research focuses on analyzing phenomena (or, more accurately, noumena) as they exist and occur naturally. This methodology has historically been used in the study of human and animal behavior. For example, Jane Goodall, noted behavioral scientist and author, studied chimpanzees in the Gombe National Park in Africa beginning in 1960. Goodall lived among and studied the chimpanzees for decades, observing their behavior and society and drawing parallels to human behavior and society. These observations have proven to be extremely valuable to sociologists and anthropologists globally; however, when Goodall first started publishing her work, it was highly criticized by academicians of the day because it did not follow traditional scientific and empirical research methods. This fact later proved to be beneficial because it prevented empirical bias from influencing the day-to-day observations and conclusions about the natural experiences of these chimpanzees (Goodall, 2000).

It was also during this same period that researchers realized that many nursing phenomena could not be explored or explained through traditional empirical methods. For example, it would be almost impossible to empirically explore the impact of feelings, perceptions, emotions, faith, experiences, and intuition on health and wellness; however, many nursing phenomena involve these, or similar, qualitative concepts. In a recent qualitative study, Standing and Anthony (2008) explored how acute care nurses perceive the meaning of the word delegation and how those perceptions influenced their day-to-day practice.

In some instances, nursing phenomena have both quantitative and qualitative concepts, which requires research designs that combine methodologies. The use of combined methodologies in research is often referred to as **triangulation** research. The term triangulation evolved from the Latin word *triangulum*, which means triangle (McKean, 2005). The term has historically been used in navigation and surveying to determine location and distance when two triangulation points are known and the third is not. An example of triangulated research is the 2008 study by Gillespie, Wallis, and Chaboyer that explored the impact of the culture of the operating room work environment (a qualitative concept) on the ability to retain new nurses in that setting (a quantitative concept).

The dialogue and, at times, tension between quantitative and qualitative researchers regarding the benefits and drawbacks of the different methodologies continue (Gilbert, 2006); however, ultimately nurses must rely on all three types of research to better understand human beings and their health. Ultimately, the profession may, over time, see the emergence of new research methodologies that more easily allow for the integration of quantitative and qualitative concepts.

Facts, Principles, and Laws

The term fact is derived from the Latin word *factio*, which means reality or truth (McKean, 2005). Research findings consistently proven true through replication over time become **facts.** For example, if the research concerning sunlight, time, and plant growth is repeated or replicated many times, and each time the plants that received more direct sunlight had more growth, then your findings would become fact. Over time, this fact would become part of a principle. The term principle is derived from the Latin word *principium*, which means foundation (McKean, 2005). Today, **principle** is defined as a truth that is foundational to other truths. For example, the fact that plants receiving more sunlight experience greater growth helps to establish the principle that plant growth is proportional to the amount of sunlight it receives. Eventually, this principle may become part of a law. The term law is derived from an Old English term that means laid down or firmly fixed (McKean, 2005). Today a **law** is considered to be a truth that guides thinking and behavior. For example, the scientific principle of plant growth being proportional to the amount of sunlight may result in a botanical law that guides horticulturists in developing larger plants.

Facts, principles, and laws are derived from theory and are considered usable knowledge that supports decisions you make every day. For example, as a nursing student, you understand the fact that a blood pressure reading represents the pressure exerted against the walls of arteries during systole (ventricular contraction) and diastole (the heart at rest). This fact supports the principle that blood volume flows from an area of high pressure (left ventricle and arteries) to an area of low pressure (capillaries, veins, right heart). This principle supports Ohm's law, which indicates that blood flow is produced by the size and pressure differences between two ends of a vessel and the degree of resistance encountered along the inside of the vessel (Guyton & Hall, 2005). Understanding this allows you to make informed decisions when assisting the patient who is making lifestyle changes and taking vasoactive drugs to control hypertension.

The 21st century ushered in a new era for nursing with the emergence of nursing's first discipline-specific laws. Nursing laws have the potential to focus the discipline on a global scale and establish nursing's international agenda for decades to come. Refer to page 25 for the reprint of an article (Webber, 2008) that highlights this historic time.

The emergence of nursing laws represents an exciting time for the discipline. These laws will for the first time give clear direction for nursing education and service on a global scale. There will be additional information on both the Law of Self-Care and the Law of Culture Care in Chapter 7, where specific nursing theory is discussed in greater detail.

Putting It All Together

Why is it important in nursing to understand the building blocks of theory, the nature of their relationships with one another, and their ultimate importance to nursing and global society? It is important because they provide structure for your thinking and behavior, which in turn provides internal consistency and reliability for what you do as a practicing nurse. The purpose of knowledge development in nursing is shaped by its practice orientation, and developing knowledge that underlies practice is one of the highest priorities in creating an appropriate future for nursing (Meleis, 2007; Schlotfeldt, 1999).

Knowledge development is based on observation of phenomena; phenomena generate ideas; ideas are defined by concepts and variables; relationships among concepts and variables lead to the formation of propositions; and propositions generate hypotheses, which form the basis of speculative theory. Hypotheses are tested and retested through research; research findings consistently proven true over time become facts, principles, and laws, which form established theory; and established theory forms the basis of knowledge and stimulates the formation of new theory. Table 2.1 demonstrates how these building blocks build upon one another and how they and their interrelationships apply to nursing and relates to Nursing Story 2.1.

When first learning about theory, it may be easier to think about how the building blocks relate to each other in a sequential or straight-line manner. With this approach, you start with the observation of a phenomenon and formation of an idea and then progressively work up through the remaining building blocks until the final destination of theory is reached. It is perfectly acceptable to be introduced to the basic components of theory in this linear manner; however, the relationships among building blocks are not always linear or unidirectional. In fact, there is potential for pandirectional movement of all the building blocks during the use of theory and in theory development, which makes the interrelationships among the building blocks quite dynamic. For example, you could identify a hypothesis and in the process generate another idea; you could be conducting research and observe an unexpected phenomenon; or you could identify an assumption that makes a proposition you were formulating irrelevant. Within the constraints of this two-dimensional page, Figure 2.2 demonstrates this dynamic and pandirectional relationship.

NURSING STORY 2.1

Building Blocks in Practice

Sarah Walker is a 22-year-old, senior-level nursing student who is participating in a month long clinical experience on the pediatric ward of a large urban hospital. One of Ms. Walker's responsibilities is to record food and fluid intake for each of the children under her care. By the third week, Ms. Walker observes the phenomenon that children under her care consistently eat better at mealtime if their mothers are present. Ms. Walker realizes that if this observation is true, it could have a significant effect on how the pediatric unit approaches meeting nutritional needs of children.

Ms. Walker has to develop a research question, or hypothesis, for the nursing research class she is taking. She decides to use her observations about the relationship between children eating and the presence of their mothers to demonstrate the various theoretical building blocks and to form the research question for her class. This application is demonstrated in Table 2.1.

Table 2.1 Comparison of Meanings

Word	Root[a]	Common Meaning[c]	Theory-Based Meanings[d]	Example (based on story)
Phenomenon Observed →	Greek *phainomen*: a thing appearing	Something to be explained; an occurrence	Observable connections or relationships between objects events, or ideas	Ms. Walker observes that *hospitalized children eat better when their mothers are present at mealtime.*
Idea Generated →	Greek *idein*: to see	A thought with a plan	Organized intellectual thought about the origin, nature, boundaries, and significance of phenomena	Ms. Walker forms the idea that *mothers influence the eating habits of hospitalized children.*
Concepts/Constructs/ Internal Variables Identified →	Latin *concipere*: to conceive Latin *variae*: to vary	Components of organized thought	Words or phrases that identify, define structure, and establish boundaries for ideas generated by phenomena	Ms. Walker identifies two concepts: *(1) mother's presence and (2) the eating habits of hospitalized children.*
Proposition Formed →	Latin *proponere*: to put forth	To put forth a relationship between concepts	Identifies the direction and nature of the relationship between concepts: which is the dependent variable (DV) and which is the independent variable (IV)[b]	Ms. Walker identifies the following relationship between the concepts: *mother's presence (IV) increases how much hospitalized children eat (DV).*
External (confounding) *Variables Identified* →	Latin *variae*: to vary	Variables outside the proposition	Variables that can change and have the potential to influence relationships	Examples of variables that may influence how much a child eats include *(1) the quality and type of the food, (2) the mother's interest in assisting, and (3) the time the meal arrives.*
Assumption(s) Identified →	Latin *sumere*: to take	Accepting as true	Assumed truths that influence or have the potential to influence other concepts or propositions	When formulating the hypothesis, Ms. Walker assumes: *(1) the children are capable of eating; (2) the children are hungry; and (3) the mothers want their children to eat better.*
Research Question/ Hypothesis Formulated →	Greek *hypothesis*: to place under	An educated guess	A formal statement describing an anticipated and measurable relationship(s) between concepts	Ms. Walker hypothesizes that *increasing mothers' participation during mealtime will increase the amount that hospitalized children eat.*

	Origin[a]	Common definition[c]	Theoretical meaning[d]	
Research Conducted and Replicated →	Old French *recerchier*: seek for, search	To study in depth	Diligent and systematic inquiry or investigation	*Ms. Walker compares how much hospitalized children eat when their mothers are present and when they are not.*
Fact(s) Revealed →	Latin *factio*: a doing	What actually happened	Observations consistently proved true over time	*Ms. Walker's research identifies the fact that hospitalized children ate more when their mothers were present.*
Principle(s) Evolve →	Latin *principium*: a beginning	What you believe	A truth, built on facts, that is foundational to other truths	*Mothers influence children's eating habits.*
Law(s) Evolve →	Old English *lagu*: a thing laid down	Written (formal) rules of behavior	An absolute truth, built on facts and principles, that guide thought and behavior	*Mothers influence children.*
Established Theory →	Greek *theoria*: speculation	Information that helps explain phenomena	Organized information that is *intended to explain*; may be established or speculative in nature	*Increasing the presence of mothers during mealtime **may** improve how much hospitalized children eat; or, increasing the presence of mothers during mealtime **will** increase how much hospitalized children eat.*
Established Knowledge Leads to the identification of new phenomena, concepts, ideas, propositions (speculative theory)	Old English *cnawan*: to know	To be smart; to have answers	The culmination of the integration of what is known through education and experience	*The presence of the mother can have a positive influence on how much hospitalized children eat.*

[a]The origin and original meaning of the word.

[b]Remember, concepts within a proposition are also identified as independent and dependent variables (variables that are internal to the proposition). Variables outside of the proposition but capable of influencing it are known as external variables.

[c]Common definitions are based on a survey of about 50 high school students and college freshmen.

[d]Theoretical meanings are adapted from *New American Oxford Dictionary* (2001) and *Roget's Thesaurus* (1997); *The World Book Dictionaries*, Volumes I and II (1996); and the authors.

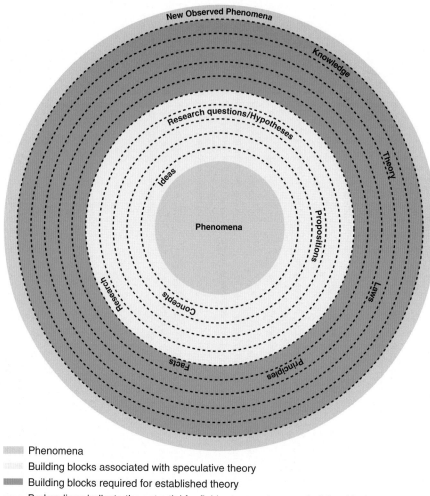

Phenomena
Building blocks associated with speculative theory
Building blocks required for established theory
- - - - Broken lines indicate the potential for fluid movement among building blocks

Figure 2.2 Dynamic relationships in theory.

Summary

This chapter introduced you to words, meanings, relationships, and organizational structure that collectively form the typology or building blocks for theory, knowledge, research, and reasoning (Fig. 2.3). The importance of this typology to nursing's ongoing knowledge development as well as day-to-day practice was highlighted. Also highlighted were some of the landmarks that continue to influence nursing's epistemological development, such as various research methodologies and the emergence of nursing's first discipline-specific laws.

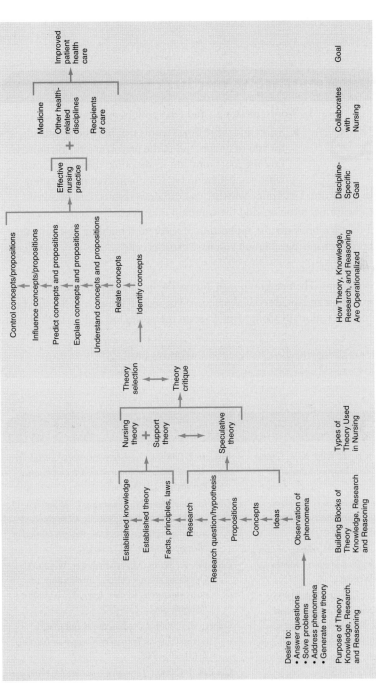

Figure 2.3   As the flowchart depicts, theory, knowledge, research, and reasoning enable you to answer questions, solve problems, explore phenomena, and generate new theory. You begin by making observations about the question, problem, or phenomenon confronting you. You then generate ideas and identify essential concepts and variables associated with your observations. You put these concepts into relationship(s) in the form of propositions and research questions or hypotheses, which are tested through research. Research and its replication lead to the identification of facts, principles, and laws, which form established theory and become part of established knowledge. Speculative theory flows from the generation of ideas and progresses to the development of research questions or hypotheses that are then tested through research. The established theory you select and use in practice helps you identify, relate, understand, explain, predict, influence, and/or control variables and propositions in nursing situations. Nursing joins with other health care professions, such as medicine, physical therapy, and occupational therapy, and families, groups, and communities to improve health care for individual patients and society.

This introduction should provide you with a strong basis for understanding and assimilating later chapters. The content of this chapter is foundational to understanding many subsequent chapters in this book. Do not hesitate to return to this chapter to refresh your vocabulary and understanding as needed.

Learning Activities

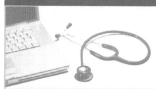

1. Words, meanings, and relationships exercise:

   a. Select and write down words that have been difficult for you to understand in the past. Using the dictionary, find the root word and its meaning, then write down what you believe to be a common everyday meaning associated with that word. Determine whether you can draw connections between the root word, the formal meaning, and the common meaning.

   b. Draw a model that demonstrates the application of theoretical building blocks to an actual clinical problem-solving situation you have experienced.

2. Discourse and exploration

   a. Divide into two groups. The first group is to discuss the impact of the Law of Self-Care on the profession and on individual practice. The second group is to discuss the impact of the Law of Culturally Congruent Care on the profession and on individual practice.

   b. Reconvene as one group and share major implications for each.

References

Andrist, L. C., Nicholas, P. K., & Wolf, K. A. (2006). *A history of nursing ideas.* Boston: Jones and Bartlett Publishers.

Benner, P. (1984). *From novice to expert: Excellence and power in clinical nursing practice.* Menlo Park, CA: Addison-Wesley.

Benner, P., & Wrubel, J. (1989). *The primacy of care: Stress and coping in health and illness.* Menlo Park, CA: Addison-Wesley.

Benner, P., Tanner, C. A., & Chesla, C. A. (1996). *Expertise in nursing practice: Caring, clinical judgment, and ethics.* New York: Springer.

Benner, P. (2000). Links between philosophy, theory, practice, and research. *Canadian Journal of Nursing Research, 32*(2), 7–13.

Chinn, P. L., & Kramer, M. K. (2008). *Integrated theory and knowledge development in nursing* (7th ed.). St. Louis: Mosby.

Fawcett, J. (2004). *Contemporary nursing knowledge: Analysis and evaluation of models and theories.* Philadelphia: F. A. Davis.

Gies, C., Buchman, D., Robinson, J., & Smolen, D. (2008). Effect of an inpatient nurse-directed smoking cessation program. *Western Journal of Nursing Research, 30*(1), 6–19.

Gillespie, B., Wallis, M., & Chaboyer, W. (2008). Operating theater culture: Implications for nurse retention. *Western Journal of Nursing Research, 30*(1), 259–277.

Gilbert, T. (2006). Mixed methods and mixed methodologies. *Journal of Research in Nursing, 11*(3), 205–217.

Goodall, J. (2000). *Through a window: My thirty years with the chimpanzees of Gombe* (Rev. ed.). New York: Mariner Books.

Guyton, A. C., & Hall, J. E. (2005). *Textbook of medical physiology* (11th ed.) Philadelphia: W. B. Saunders Company.

Laerdal. (2008). *Patient simulators.* Retrieved February 8, 2008, from http://www.laerdal.com/document.asp?docid=1022609

Leininger, M. M. (Ed.). (1985). Transcultural care diversity and universality: A theory of nursing. *Nursing and Health Care, 6,* 209–212.

Lewin, K. (1951). *Field theory in social science.* New York: Harper & Row.

Maslow, A. H. (1954). *Motivation and personality.* New York: Harper & Brothers.

McKean, E. (2005). *The new Oxford American dictionary* (2nd ed.). New York: Oxford University Press.

Meleis, A. I. (1997). *Theoretical nursing: Development and progress* (3rd ed.). Philadelphia: Lippincott Williams & Wilkins.

Meleis, A. I. (2007). *Theoretical nursing: Development and progress* (4th ed.). Philadelphia: Lippincott Williams & Wilkins.

Nightingale, F. (1859, 1992). *Notes on nursing: What it is and what it is not* (Commemorative ed.). Philadelphia: J. B. Lippincott. [*Notes on nursing* was published originally by Harrison in London, England, in 1859. The above is an unabridged replication of the first American edition, from D. Appleton and Company in 1860.]

Orem, D. (1971). *Concepts of practice.* New York: McGraw-Hill.

Powers, B. A., & Knapp, T. R. (2006). *Dictionary of nursing theory and research* (3rd ed.). New York: Springer Publishing Company.

Reynolds, P. D. (1971). *A primer in theory construction.* New York: Macmillan.

Schlotfeldt, R. M. (1999). Structuring nursing knowledge: A priority for creating nursing's future. In J. W. Kenny (Ed.). *Philosophical and theoretical perspectives for advanced nursing practice* (2nd ed., pp. 5–9). London: Jones & Bartlett.

Selye, H. (1956). *The stress of life.* New York: McGraw-Hill.

Standing, T. S., & Anthony, M. K. (2008). Delegation: What it means to acute care nurses. *Applied Nursing Research, 21*(1), 8–14.

von Bertalanffy, L. (1968). *General system theory: Foundations, development, applications.* New York: Braziller.

Webber, P. B. (2002). A curriculum framework for nursing. *Journal of Nursing Education, 41*(1), 15–24.

Webber, P. B. (2008). Yes, Virginia, nursing does have laws. *Nursing Science Quarterly, 21*(1), 68–73.

The Emergence of Nursing Laws

(reprint from *Nursing Science Quarterly (NSQ)*, January 2008)

In 1897, when *New York Sun* columnist Francis Pharcellus Church penned the now famous editorial entitled "Yes, Virginia, there is a Santa Claus," he succeeded not only in touching hearts, but also in helping people begin to view tradition differently and to recognize a different truth that moves beyond the obvious (Church, 1897/2007). Looking beyond tradition and the obvious is also characteristic of nursing's century-long journey into scholarship and knowledge development. In seeking to understand and move the profession forward, academics have debated issues such as technical versus professional education prepara-

tion, theory-based practice versus practice-based theory, philosophies versus models versus theories, and empiricism versus phenomenology.

Another phenomenon has evolved that will no doubt stimulate similar discourse. This phenomenon is the possibility of the emergence of nursing laws. These are not the laws of jurisprudence governing nursing practice that are traditionally associated with individual state practice acts, but they are, instead, laws associated with the natural maturation and evolution of selected areas of essential nursing knowledge. While the idea of nursing laws may sound far-fetched or neomodernistic, it is the next logical step in the evolution of nursing knowledge. Unfortunately, recognizing, naming, and framing nursing laws may be as foreign to us now as discipline-specific theory was to practicing nurses in the mid-1900s.

Evolution of the Meaning

To understand the emergence of nursing laws, one must first understand the diverse meanings of the word *law*. Hermeneutically, we know and understand that meanings of words evolve over time according to the nature, needs, and sophistication of society and subsets within society (Johnson & Webber, 2005). The term *law* evolved from the old Norse term *lag* and the old English term *lagu,* both of which mean "to be *laid down* or *firmly affixed"* (Jewel & Abate, 2001). The term quickly became associated with social and cultural rules of behavior as seen in the early Greek and Roman civilizations. During Biblical times the term *law* was used to describe the first five books of the Old Testament. These five books, which were also called the Pentateuch or Torah, established very specific rules governing religious behavior of the early Jews (Life Application Bible, New International Version, 1991). By the time of the Renaissance, which occurred between the 12th and 16th centuries, the definition and use of *laws* had expanded to include social, political, and scientific contexts. Social and political laws focused on expanded rules of human behavior, while scientific laws emerged that established rules associated with the occurrence of phenomena in nature.

By the end of the 16th century, the desire for discovery had prompted the initiation of a scientific revolution. While scientists prior to this revolution used logic and philosophical or Aristotelian analysis to explore natural phenomena, scientists and other authors during the scientific revolution moved toward measurement and numerical analysis (Kuhn, 1970). This approach resulted in the nature, or the perception of the nature, of science becoming *mechanical* and *empirical* (Veltman, n.d.). A byproduct of this empirical focus is that scientists of the time began using mathematical, or empirical, evidence as a criterion for forming scientific laws, an approach that per-

sists today. Scientific discovery focused on quantification through experimentation as the primary method for examining phenomena and forming associated facts, principles, and laws.

Experimentation, by its nature, involves quantification and predictability. These concepts also emerged as essential characteristics of scientific laws and play an essential role in advancing specific areas of knowledge to the status of a law. In 1965, Hempel defined a general law as "a statement of universal conditional form which is capable of being confirmed or disconfirmed by suitable empirical findings" (1965, p. 231). He also indicated that laws serve the purpose of connecting events to patterns, which forms a basis for both prediction and explanation (p. 232). Explanation that supports predictability also supports reliability of the information being used, which is essential in science. The association of empiricism, explanation, predictability, and reliability significantly influenced nursing's journey into scholarship since the profession's foundation is, in part, built on science and our early research foundation was quantitatively based.

Empirical Validation

Concurrent with the development of scientific laws was the emergence of a "mania for measurement" or the at-times frenzied requirement for empirical validation of theory, facts, principles, and laws, which was considered an essential feature of early modern science (Koyré, 1966; Veltman, n.d.). Today, the idea that a law must have empirical evidence supporting 100% predictability is still widely accepted (Hempel, 1965; Hickman, 2002; Polifroni, 1999). According to Hickman (2002, p. 5), scientific laws "predict the results of given experiments 100% of the time. Laws compose the basis of most of the natural sciences. As nursing is a human science, the rigor and objectivity of the laboratory are both impossible and inappropriate to duplicate." The requirement for empirical testing with 100% predictability in defining a law furthered the separation between social and scientific laws, since social laws or rules of social behavior involve more than empirical validation (Kuhn, 1970; Bird, 2004).

By the mid-20th century scientists, theorists, and educators began questioning the adequacy of empirical validation and the accuracy of 100% predictability as the primary criteria for forming scientific laws. In 1959, Scriven, at the annual meeting of the American Association for the Advancement of Science, proffered that laws of science, with few exceptions, are inaccurate and, at best, only approximations of the truth, with a limited range of applicability (Swartz, 2006). This notion was supported by the work of Glanz (1997) and others who demonstrated that Einstein's long-standing laws of physics do not allow 100% predictability, especially when considering the constancy of the speed of light and black holes. Furthermore, Katz and Katz (1995), medical researchers, tell us that while science provides a beautiful picture of the natural world and insight into disease, it can also lead us to error. They argue that our understanding of science is imperfect and that scientific laws are assailable. Katz and Katz base their argument on the fact that modern clinical research trials commonly reveal inconsistencies in scientific laws, and that these inconsistencies represent a reality that disagrees with the previously demanded predictability of science. In conjunction with this observation, Katz and Katz question whether these inconsistencies reflect the imperfections in our ability to interpret the law or the illusory nature of laws themselves (Katz & Katz, 1995).

Of particular importance to the changing nature of scientific laws are the major premises behind Chaos and Complexity Theories, which assert the existence of infinitesimal known and unknown variables, with known and unknown levels of interaction and significance in almost all phenomena, which makes 100% predictability unlikely, even in the best science (Johnson & Webber, 2005). Do these variables minimize the need to strive for empirical evidence to support laws that provide underpinnings of a particular body of knowledge? Of course not, but it does suggest two things. The first is that laws, even scientific laws, like theory, evolve. The second is that it keeps us mindful that empirical predictability is no longer the sole defining characteristic of a law, which opens the possi-

bility of the emergence of new types of laws or, at minimum, a redefining of the term law.

Logical Adequacy

If empirical evidence and 100% predictability are no longer the defining characteristics of a law, is it possible that laws may emerge from behavior-based disciplines, such as nursing, in which knowledge is supported only in part by empirical science? This is, perhaps, one of the most significant questions nursing scholars need to ask in this century. If the answer is "yes," then it represents an epistemological landmark that may result in a paradigm shift for the discipline. Thomas Kuhn, author of *The Structure of Scientific Revolutions* (1970), states that all epistemological crises begin with a blurring paradigm, followed by the consequent loosening of rules, and the eventual emergence of a new paradigm, along with vigorous discourse over its acceptance. Kuhn's view is supported by Bird (2004), who indicated that revolutionary new paradigms are derived from the failure of existing paradigms to resolve certain questions. Nursing has selected areas of knowledge where the traditional descriptors of facts, principles, scientific laws, theories, and philosophies do not adequately describe the occurring phenomena.

So how do we evaluate these areas to determine if they are significant enough to become nursing's first discipline-specific laws? The most likely choice is through determination of logical adequacy. Simply stated, logical adequacy is a method of explaining and validating theory, facts, principles, and laws that may include, but go beyond, empirical testing. Logical adequacy, like empirical predictability, has gone through periods of revolution. In 1965, Hempel indicated that scientific explanation offered through logical adequacy needed to contain at least one law of nature, logical consequences, and be either empirically based or empirically testable. However, Kuhn (1970) and Bird (2004) indicated that science is more than a group of empirical outcomes and that scientists do not make their judgments as a result of consciously or unconsciously following rules, empirical or otherwise. Kuhn further indicated that *values* play an important role in guiding scientists' judgments. Kuhn's interpretation allows for a broader definition of logical adequacy and expands the criteria by which knowledge can be evaluated and put forth as facts, principles, theories, and laws. Collectively, the broader definition of logical adequacy involves, in varying degrees of influence, truth, order, precision, coherence, comprehensiveness, reasonable predictability and reliability, values, consequences, and hermeneutic interpretation and reinterpretation (Bird, 2004; Kuhn, 1970; Polifroni, 1999; Silva, 2004).

Understandably, societal laws, and their subsets, have evolved more frequently through logical adequacy than as a consequence of empirical testing and 100% predictability. Empirical evidence, when available, certainly plays a role in the development of laws guiding the individual and collective behavior of society and its subsets; however, empirical evidence is not as decisive a factor in societal or behavioral law as it is in science. Nursing is an example of a societal subset in which logically adequate laws that guide selected aspects of practice may have begun to emerge.

Redefining Laws

The vast majority of nursing phenomena are a mix of scientific (quantitative) and phenomenological (qualitative) variables; thus, the profession will inherently require integration of both. Does this mean that the profession will never be able to develop nursing laws? No, it does not. However, it does suggest that our traditional definition of law needs to be expanded to encompass the evolution of knowledge associated with these combined phenomena. It further suggests a need to be more representative of the current reality, and to be capable of providing relevant, safe, and effective rules of behavior to guide nursing practice. Im and Chee (2003) indicated that exploration and validation of phenomena containing empirical and qualitative characteristics requires the use of fuzzy logic or reasoning, which respects the benefits of both and which recognizes the gray areas where they merge. In the other words, our paradigms may need blurring, our rules may need loosening, and our discourse may need initiating.

When relating the advancing of selected knowledge to the status of a law, the profession certainly needs to utilize the elements of logical adequacy; however, any rule of behavior significant enough to be advanced to the status of a law and capable of influencing and guiding global nursing practice should also demonstrate:

- Teleologia, a Latin word meaning *end goal* (Jewel & Abate, 2001). In the formation of any law, the goal is to guide behavior toward a goal inherently imbedded in the law itself. Any nursing law must have a clear and concise goal, consistent with the intent of safe and effective nursing care.

- Practical applicability or implementable usefulness. Guidelines and rules that meet the criteria for logical adequacy but do not consistently guide behavior or demonstrate longitudinal achievement of desired outcomes are incapable of being evaluated and, as a result, are not sustainable as laws. Any law with practical application must guide behavior to achieve a desired goal or, at least, indicate what not to do.

- Universality or applicability to all human beings. Global acknowledgment of the desirability and applicability of the goal and premise of a proposed law is necessary to achieve the intent of the law, and ultimately to guide a global nursing practice.

Transitioning Our Thinking

No doubt some of those among us would argue that it is not necessary to elevate selected areas of nursing knowledge to the position of laws or that nursing knowledge is simply not capable of producing laws, at least as we now define them. Perhaps it is our traditional understanding of theory and knowledge development that prevents us from embracing the idea. The word *theory* originated from the Greek word *theoria*, which means to speculate. This speculative origin inherently raises questions regarding validity and reliability of theory. However, like the word *law*, the meaning of *theory* has evolved over time to mean *organized information intended to explain and guide* (McKean, 2001). Organized information begins as speculative theory (concepts, propositions, hypotheses) and, over time, is evaluated in terms of empirical testing and/or logical adequacy for its ability to explain and guide. Theory that is affirmed as a consequence of this process moves to the status of established theory and is used as a valid and reliable tool for answering questions, solving problems, explaining phenomena, and generating new or speculative theory. Established theory and the facts, principles, and laws that emerge from it are taught in every required course in nursing. The evolution of the meaning of theory is apparent when we hear nurses say they understand the "theory" behind a particular phenomenon or skill and when nursing educators say they teach theory-based classes. Nursing educators are using theory in the established, as opposed to the speculative, sense. Articulation of the duality of speculative versus established theory helps students, nurses, and faculty differentiate and operationalize the knowledge typology, which, in turn, allows them see and understand the interrelationships among theory, research, practice, and reasoning (Johnson & Webber, 2005) (refer to Fig. A). Ultimately, this typology facilitates understanding of the progressive intricacies of interaction among the components of knowledge, especially with regard to how and where laws may emerge. Silva (2004), when discussing components of theory, makes the link that is perhaps most significant to this point of view, by indicating that facts, principles, and laws do not constitute theory unless they are interrelated and have relevance to a common problem or issue (p. 5). If a common problem, issue, or other teleological activity is significant enough to force evolution of guiding facts and principles from the-

ory, and if the demands for logical adequacy, practical applicability, and universality have been met, the profession should consider the elevation of that information to the status of law.

Examples of Nursing Laws

While nursing currently has no discipline-specific laws, selected areas of nursing knowledge do meet the revised criteria for formation of laws. Perhaps the most prominent of these areas is self-care. Self-care, as a theoretical concept, first entered mainstream nursing in 1971 with the publication of Dorothea Orem's *Concepts of Practice,* which challenged the health-related wisdom of "doing for" patients and redirected nurses toward the healthier approach of facilitating patients to "care for self" whenever and however possible. Nurses balked at the atypical language and complexity of the theory itself; however, they embraced the logic of self-care as therapeutic. Over time, nurses ceased focusing on "doing for" such as feeding, bathing, and turning patients who could perform these activities themselves and began directing their care toward helping individuals, families, groups, and communities maximize their ability to meet their own self-care demands. An essential assumption in self-care is that, when necessary, nursing will fulfill necessary care requirements of individuals until such time as the individual and/or other care providers, such as family members, can assume that responsibility, such as in the case of infants, children, the elderly, and the infirmed. Orem's *Concepts of Practice* is now in its sixth edition and has expanded to include three separate theories. These

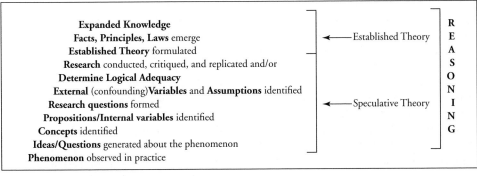

Figure A   Knowledge Typology.

theories have undergone extensive global research that has supported the benefits of self-care. This support also is evidenced by the International Orem Society for Nursing Science and Scholarship (http://www.scdnt.com/ newsl/newsl.html) and by their journal dedicated to publishing self-care research.

The vast majority of nurses, both past and present, do not practice the promotion of self-care as Orem packaged it; they have extrapolated the facts and principles from this theory that were most valuable, specifically those associated with the promotion of the therapeutic benefits of self-care, and repeatedly and successfully integrated them into diverse practice settings. The elevation of the value of self-care beyond the constraints of some of the individual subconcepts and propositions within Orem's original theories made it easier to integrate self-care within nursing practice across the country, different cultures, and the world. Today, nursing's focus on helping people care for themselves is evident from the bedside to the global community and has gained both national and international momentum (Department of Health and Human Services, 1995; Holmes & Gastaldo, 2002; National Health Service, 2006). In 2002, when discussing governmentality and nursing's role in public policy, Holmes and Gastaldo highlighted the role nursing played in bringing the importance of self-care and self-responsibility to the forefront of socially responsible policy. Promotion of self-care is a primary focus in Great Britain's National Health Service and the health care trusts that provide care (National Health Service, 2006). In 2003, Sigma Theta Tau (2003) convened a conference in Sorrento, Italy, to discuss how nurses in southern Europe and the Mediterranean could best contribute to the health of communities in the new millennium. The result, in part, called for encouraging self-care through partnerships between nurses and individuals, families, and communities.

Elevating promotion of self-care to the status of a law would clearly focus the profession on a globally desirable goal, increase practical awareness, and guide students, nurses, and faculty in the delivery of care. It would also positively impact health care effectiveness and costs on a long-term basis. These approaches have the potential to make a significant difference in the health and well-being of global society. Nursing's goal of promoting self-care meets the criteria for logical adequacy, teleologia, practical applicability, and universality, and, as a result, promotion of self-care constitutes one of nursing's first laws. Figure B provides a sample pathway demonstrating the evolution of this law.

THE LAW OF SELF-CARE: Effective nursing care promotes the highest level of self-care possible for individuals, families, groups, communities, and global society.

Another nursing law that may be emerging is that of culturally congruent care. This concept entered mainstream nursing in 1985 with the articulation of Madeleine Leininger's Culture Care Theory. Leininger's theory, which has been expanded several times, brought into focus the profession's need to recognize, value, and consistently integrate the unique needs of the culturally diverse. Unfortunately, like self-care theory, Culture Care Theory was burdened with atypical language and complexity that made it difficult for nurses to utilize in its original form. As with most theory, however, nurses extracted the most valuable facts and principles associated with the theory and imbedded them into their practice, nursing textbooks, classrooms, and clinical experiences. Delivery of culturally congruent care in this era of rapid globalization has emerged as more than just a focus within nursing care. It has become fundamental to nursing behavior in the 21st century and beyond (Murphy, 2006). This change is evidenced by the development of the Transcultural Nursing Society (www.tcen.org), an international organization whose mission is to advance culturally congruent nursing care. Nursing's goal of promoting culturally congruent care meets the criteria for logical adequacy, teleologia, practical applicability, and universality, and, as a result, promotion of culturally congruent care constitutes another law of nursing. Figure C provides a sample pathway demonstrating how this law evolved.

Expanded Knowledge: Promotion of the maximum level of self-care possible is desirable and a goal of nursing.

Facts, Principles, and Laws Emerge:
- **Law:** Effective nursing care promotes the highest level of self-care possible for individuals, families, groups, communities, and global society.
- **Principle:** Nurses meet self-care needs and/or assists individuals, families, groups, and communities in meeting self-care needs.
- **Fact:** Individuals, families, groups, and communities have varying ability to meet self-care needs.

Established Theory is Formed, Developed, and Tested:
- A theory of self-care
- Self-care deficit theory of nursing
- A theory of nursing systems

External/Confounding Variables and Assumptions:
- Self-care is necessary to maintain physical and mental wellbeing
- Human beings want to care for self.

Proposition: Nurses provide care for or assist individuals, families, groups, and communities achieve the maximum level of self-care possible.

Concepts:
- Self-care
- Human beings with self-care needs
- Nurses

Idea: Nurses provide care for those who cannot care for themselves and/or assist those who can until such time as they become independent

Observed phenomenon: Human beings function better and are happier when they can care for themselves; however, human beings vary in their capacity to care for self because of ability, illness, age, and education.

Figure B Pathway to the Law of Self-Care.

Expanded Knowledge: Promotion of culturally congruent care is desirable and therapeutic and a goal of nursing care

Facts, Principles, and Laws Emerge:
- **Law:** Effective nursing care integrates cultural values and beliefs of diverse individuals, families, groups, communities, and global society.
- **Principle:** Diverse cultures have specific values and beliefs that influence health and health care.
- **Fact:** Individuals, families, groups, and communities belong to different cultures and/or subcultures that influence their values and beliefs related to health and well being.

Established Theory is Formed (Developed and Tested)
- Culture Care Diversity and Universality Theory

External/Confounding Variables/Assumptions:
- Level of cultural awareness
- Desire to provide culturally congruent care
- Value of cultural diversity

Proposition: Effective nurses provide culturally congruent care.

Concepts:
- Cultural Uniqueness
- Effective nursing care

Idea: Effective nurses provide culturally congruent care.

Observed Phenomenon: Every individual belongs to a culture and/or subculture that has unique beliefs and values that influence health, well-being and the delivery of nursing care.

Figure C Pathway to the Law of Culturally Congruent Care.

THE LAW OF CULTURALLY CONGRUENT CARE: Effective nursing care integrates cultural values and beliefs of diverse individuals, families, groups, communities, and global society.

Have the concepts of self-care and culturally congruent care matured to the point that they provide rules of behavior that guide all of nursing practice and have global applicability? Have they matured beyond simple facts and principles, and, if so, do they constitute nursing's first laws? If students in schools of nursing or nurses within the profession are not integrating self-care and culturally congruent care into their daily practice, should they be? Should the profession let these and other emerging laws establish the direction for all of nursing practice on a global scale? These questions, over the next few decades, will no doubt stimulate needed and valuable discourse regarding nursing's knowledge development. Epistemologically, from this author's perspective, we need nursing laws to provide clear and unprecedented direction for effective global nursing practice and to crystallize our professional intent in a time of dramatic change. So yes, Virginia, nursing does have laws. If we can recognize them, keep a clear vision regarding how and when they evolve, and then facilitate their development, then the best is yet to come.

References

Bird, A. (2004). Thomas Kuhn. *Stanford encyclopedia of philosophy.* Retrieved October 10, 2006, from http://plato.stanford.edu/entries/thomas-kuhn/

Church, P. (1987/2007). Yes, Virginia, there is a Santa Claus. Retrieved September 22, 2007, from http://www.newseum.org/yesvirginia/

Department of Health and Human Services. (1995). The informed consumer: Self-care, self-help, and selecting health care. Retrieved September 5, 2006, from http://www.health.gov/nhic/Partnerships/1995/inform.htm

Glanz, J. (1997). Visions of black holes. *Science, 275,* 476–478.

Hempel, C. G. (1965). *Aspects of scientific explanation.* New York: Macmillan.

Hickman, J. S. (2002). An introduction to nursing theory. In J. B. George (Ed.), *Nursing theories: The base for professional nursing practice* (5th ed.). Upper Saddle River, NJ: Prentice Hall.

Holmes, D., & Gastaldo, D. (2002). Nursing as a means of governmentality. *Journal of Advanced Nursing, 38* (6), 557–565.

Im, E., & Chee, W. (2003). Fuzzy logic and nursing. *Nursing Philosophy, 4* (1), 53–60.

Jewel, E. J., & Abate, F. (Eds.). (2001). *The new Oxford American dictionary.* New York: Oxford University Press.

Johnson, B., & Webber, P. (2005). *Introduction to theory and reasoning in nursing.* Philadelphia: Lippincott Williams & Wilkins.

Katz, A. M., & Katz, P. B. (1995). Emergence of scientific explanations of nature in ancient Greece: The only scientific discovery? [Electronic version]. *Circulation, 92,* 637–645. Retrieved July 31, 2006, from http://circ.ahajournals.org/cgi/content/full/92/3/637

Koyré, A. (1978) *Galileo studies.* (J. Mepham trans.). Atlantic Highlands, NJ: Humanities Press (original work published in 1939).

Kuhn, T. (1970). *The structure of scientific revolutions.* Chicago: University of Chicago Press.

Leininger, M. M. (1985). Transcultural care diversity and universality: A theory for nursing. *Nursing & Health Care, 6,* 209–212.

Life Application Bible: New International Version. (1991). Wheaton, IL: Tyndale House Publisher, Inc., and Grand Rapids, MI: Zondervan Publishing House.

Murphy, S. (2006). Mapping the literature of transcultural nursing. *Journal of the Medical Library Association, 94* (2), E143–E151.

National Health Service. (2006). *Self-care.* Retrieved July 31, from http://www.dh.gov.uk/PolicyAndGuidance/OrganisationPolicy/SelfCare/fs/en

Orem, D. (1971, 2001). *Nursing: Concepts and practice.* New York: McGraw-Hill.

Polifroni, E. C. (1999). Explanation in science. In E. C. Polifironi & M. Welch (Eds.), *Perspectives on philosophy of science: A historical and contemporary anthology* (pp. 149). Philadelphia: Lippincott.

Sigma Theta Tau International. (2003). Preferred future for nursing professionals. Retrieved September 5, 2006, from www.nursingsociety.org/programs/Arista_SouthernEurope.doc

Silva, M. C. (2004). Philosophy, science, theory: Interrelationships and implications for nursing research. In P. G. Reed, N. C. Shearer, & L. H. Nicoll (Eds.), *Perspective on nursing theory* (4th ed., pp. 3–9). Philadelphia: Lippincott Williams & Wilkins.

Swartz, N. (2006). Laws of nature. *The internet encyclopedia of philosophy.* Retrieved August 20, 2006, from http://www.iep.utm.edu/l/lawofnat.htm

Veltman, K. H. (n.d.). The emergence of scientific literature and quantification 1520–1560. Retrieved July 17, 2006, from www.sumscorp.com/articles/art14.htm

Operationalizing Relationships

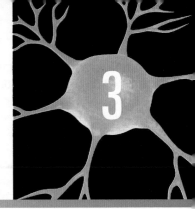

3

Intent: This chapter explores different types of theory; the relationships among theory, knowledge, research, and reasoning; and how they are operationalized in clinical practice.

Key Words/Concepts

cause	influence	predicting
controlling	identify	relating
effect	knowing	significance
established theory	logical adequacy	speculative theory
explain	operationalize	understanding

Introduction

Now that you have learned the language and meanings associated with the building blocks of theory, knowledge, research, and reasoning, it is time to take a closer look at how these building blocks reflect different types of theory. In addition, this chapter explores how these building blocks play an essential role in operationalizing theory in practice.

Types of Theory

Theoretical building blocks provide meaning and structure for the use and development of theory. In addition, they also allow for a natural separation between two basic types of theory: established theory and speculative theory.

Established Theory

Established theory represents the collective culmination of facts, principles, and laws that nurses use when making effective clinical decisions. Established theory provides valid, reliable, and predictable information that has been derived from replicated research and/or determination of its **logical adequacy** over time.

You select and interpret the meaning of established theory based on your knowledge, skills, values, meanings, and experiences, and use this interpreted meaning when answering questions, solving problems, exploring phenomena, and generating new theory. For example, as a first-year nursing student, you learn the facts, principles, and laws of chemistry. As a second-year student, the meaning and significance of these facts, principles, and laws begin to expand as you apply them to the study of pharmacology. By the time you are a third- or fourth-year student and are administering potentially lethal intravenous medications, the meaning and significance of the facts, principles, and laws of chemistry as applied to nursing have expanded dramatically. If you become a nurse practitioner, then you will prescribe these potentially lethal drugs and will participate in clinical research trials to test the effectiveness and safety of new drugs, both of which require a knowledge of chemistry. It is the continued effective application of established theory in practice that provides ongoing evidence of its validity, reliability, and predictability. Nursing Story 3.1 demonstrates how established theory and expanded meanings can be used in a nursing situation.

Speculative Theory

Speculative theory is that which has yet to be adequately tested and where its logical adequacy has yet to be determined. When looking at speculative theory, remember that the root word of

---

NURSING STORY 3.1

Using Established Theory in Practice

Cindy Walters is the registered nurse for a large middle school. At lunchtime, Ms. Walters consistently observes that many adolescents skip lunch or select "junk" food to eat instead of foods with more nutritional value. She decides that this phenomenon presents a significant health risk to students and wants to educate them and their parents about the problem. Ms. Walters identifies established theory that is relevant to the problem, such as the nutritional value of healthy and nonhealthy foods and the long-term negative health effects of consuming insufficient calories or consistently eating foods with low nutritional value. She integrates this established theory with established theory associated with teaching adolescents and adults and then designs posters, printed information, and special classes in an attempt to influence eating patterns of students and educate their parents. In addition, she evaluates the effectiveness of her efforts. Because Ms. Walters is using established theory, she can also predict short- and long-term health consequences for students electing not to change their eating behaviors, such as weight gain or weight loss, poor attention span, weakness, and decreased school performance.

theory is *theoria*, which means to speculate (McKean, 2005). This meaning was expanded over time to include organized and established information, which gives us a dualistic, yet highly functional, way of looking at the meaning of theory.

Building blocks associated with speculative theory are the same as for established theory—up to a point. Speculative theory consists of concepts/variables, propositions, assumptions, and, hopefully at some point, a researchable question or hypothesis. However, what is missing in speculative theory is the validity, reliability, and predictability associated with replicated research and logical adequacy over time. After these criteria have been met, then speculative theory evolves into established theory. Nursing Story 3.2 demonstrates how speculative theory may influence a nursing situation.

Speculative theory is a creative and valuable tool in advancing nursing knowledge because it allows for the exploration of new phenomena. In fact, many original nursing theories were developed through this speculative process. However, use of speculative theory is risky because of its unpredictable nature. As a result, students and inexperienced staff nurses should not independently integrate speculative theory into their practice because it may influence their ability to practice safely and reliably within established practice standards.

Speculative theory is sometimes applied in practice during the conduction of clinical research. Usually, this type of research is guided by masters or doctorally prepared nurses who can successfully and safely guide its application, measure its outcomes, and limit potential risks to the patients and staff involved.

Obviously, there is a significant relationship between established and speculative theory. Indeed, in some cases, the two are so intertwined that it becomes difficult to separate them. However, your skill in identifying, integrating, and using established and speculative theory will increase with education, experience, and guided practice.

NURSING STORY 3.2

The Influence of Speculative Theory in Practice

Cindy Walters, RN, a baccalaureate-prepared school nurse, observes the phenomenon that there were fewer occurrences of anorexia in adolescent girls who participated in team sports at school when compared with other school activities. Ms. Walters forms a speculative proposition that if adolescent girls could participate in team sports on a regular basis, the number developing anorexia would diminish. Before using this proposition to guide her work with anorexic adolescents, Ms. Walters would need to search existing literature to determine whether there is sufficient research on the effect of team sports on the development of anorexia in adolescent girls. Findings in the literature would then need to be analyzed regarding implications for her practice. If there is little or no research support in the literature, Ms. Walters would need to refer the proposition to individuals qualified to help her conduct research on human subjects. Any findings from this research would then need to be scrutinized, analyzed, and replicated before being accepted as valid and reliable theory that Ms. Walters could safely integrate into her practice.

Nursing Theory's Speculative Roots

Between 1950 and the early 1980s, nursing theorists produced many speculative theories that were widely published in both nursing books and journals. This was an important time for nursing because, except for Florence Nightingale's work 100 years earlier, there had been little nursing knowledge development.

These theories were rapidly integrated into nursing education and practice. In some cases, entire health care delivery systems and nursing education curricula were designed around a single nursing theory. By the late 1980s, nursing had gathered sufficient research evidence to realize that using theories in this manner was ineffective and that a single theory, regardless of how good it was, was not adequate to house all of nursing education and practice. As a result, nursing education and practice began to move away from single-theory frameworks. Fortunately, these theories were not discarded, but were studied, tested, and placed within nursing knowledge as useful tools for answering questions, solving problems, exploring phenomena, and generating new theory. Nursing, as a profession, learned that to limit thinking to the boundaries of a single theory is to limit the ability to reason effectively in nursing practice.

Over time, many of these early theories developed a sufficient research base and/or demonstrated sufficient logical adequacy to support their continued use; however, some theories developed little or no support for their continued use. As a result, nursing's landscape became "littered" with theories that were of little epistemological value because they could not provide sufficient validity, reliability, and predictability in practice. While most nurse scholars and scientists of the time could readily differentiate between speculative and established theory, most nursing students, most practicing nurses, and many nursing educators could not. Many became confused and began to question the value of nursing theory itself.

Part of the cause for this was that many early theorists, in an attempt to differentiate their theories, used atypical words and meanings to define concepts and propositions within their theories. The use of atypical words and meanings that had little obvious connection with the existing language used in nursing practice resulted in complaints from nursing educators and practicing nurses alike. They complained that reading nursing theory was like trying to read a foreign language. For example, Orem's theory of self-care (Orem, 1971) used words such as "requisites" and "agency" to describe patients' self-care needs and their ability to provide self-care. Parse's 1981 theory of human becoming used "rhythmicity" to describe human patterning and the term "transcendence" to describe one's hopes and dreams. Decades later, it is easy to see how use of such atypical language obstructed the original intent and value of the theory and contributed to the formation of a gap between theory and practice. Most current-day theorists and researchers learned from this misstep and have made the use of common language a priority.

Nursing theory that contains multiple language obstacles and lacks clarity in practical applicability, regardless of how creatively it is designed, may be doomed to "sit on the shelf" until knowledge and language develop to the point that it is easily understood and applied. By then, however, it may be obsolete.

Nursing learned three valuable lessons from the era of early nursing theorists. These lessons include:

1. Remember the purpose of theory and try not to make it do something it is not intended to do.
2. Ensure that the intent and language of future nursing theory are explicitly clear and meaningful to those who need to use it.
3. Recognize that a theory's value may lie more in what it has to offer to the future than what it has to offer the present.

It is also important to note that many of the most important concepts and propositions from these early nursing theories survived without the atypical language; for example, today nurses commonly speak to a patient's ability to meet his or her own self-care needs without using the terms "requisite" or "agency."

Named Versus Unnamed Theory

As you read about different types of theory, you may notice that sometimes theory is grouped according to discipline and special interests, such as biological theory, feminist theory, family theory, conflict theory, role theory, and leadership theory. You may also notice that some theories have the names of the theorist who developed them in the title, such as Albert Einstein's theory of relativity, Hans Selye's stress adaptation theory (1956), Ludwig von Bertalanffy's general and open system theories (1968), and Dorothea Orem's theory of self-care (1971). Theory grouped by discipline subsumes named theory and is generally a culmination of theory that guides that particular discipline. Individual theories that have the theorists' names attached are ones that, generally speaking, have had a significant impact on a particular discipline, multiple disciplines, or even society as a whole. In some instances, using the theorist's name is simply a pattern used within a particular discipline, which is the case in nursing. Named theories frequently started out as speculative theory and through research and determination of logical adequacy they may have been shown to have significant epistemological value. Sometimes individual theorists and their work have had such a significant impact and developed such a following that the theory has grown into a discipline of its own. For example, Freud's (1938) theories about human behavior have influenced sociological thought for generations; von Bertalanffy's general and open system theories (1968) have had such a tremendous impact on global society that there is now an International Society for Systems Science; and Orem's theory of self-care (1971) has had such an impact on nursing that facilitating patients' ability to care for themselves is now a nursing law.

Historically, most of nursing's theories have been named theories. This most likely occurred because many of the theories were developed in the mid-20th century when nursing was trying to establish itself in academia and naming theories was a trend of the period. Today most nursing theory is generated through research and logical adequacy and is not named. However, whether a theory is named or not, it is important to remember that a true test of any theory's value lies in its ongoing ability to help answer questions, solve problems, explore phenomena, and generate new theory.

Stimulating New Theory

Applying theory, knowledge, research, and reasoning ultimately stimulates new questions, poses new problems, and makes evident new phenomena, thereby providing a stimulus for the development of new theory. Even established knowledge is not static but dynamic, which means that it is constantly evolving. Knowledge evolves over time as new theory develops and allows for new interpretation of previously accepted facts, principles, and laws. This does not mean that previously proven, long-standing theories are not theories, nor that laws derived from them are not laws. It simply means that over time, new research generates new ideas or exposes new variables, propositions, and assumptions, which raises questions about existing theories.

Lessons Learned From Albert Einstein

Albert Einstein's theory of relativity was initially penned in 1905 when Einstein was 26 years old. The theory asserted new meanings associated with time, space, mass, motion, and gravity and built on earlier established theory developed by Sir Isaac Newton. Over time, Einstein's work gave the discipline of physics a mechanism of answering previously unanswerable questions associated with energy and light, the origin of the solar system, and quantum relationships between space and time. For years, the scientific community accepted and used these theories; however, in the late 1980s one aspect of his theoretical work was called into question by scientists who thought that it failed to answer questions associated with the constancy of light and black holes (Bethell, 1990; Cowen, 1997; Glanz, 1997). Today, scientists are still questioning the assailability of Einstein's theories (Fernie, 2005; University of Missouri-Columbia, 2007; Huler, 2008). These questions were generated, in part, by scientific knowledge, techniques, and technology that were not available during Einstein's time. Hence, ongoing analysis and integration of new knowledge over an 80-year period have resulted in re-evaluation of Einstein's theory and the stimulation of new questions and ideas that, through ongoing research, may provide a foundation for new and better theory.

You could reasonably ask that since a component of Einstein's original theory has been called into question, was it really a theory? The answer is yes. Einstein's theory was and is a theory because it has demonstrated consistent validity, reliability, and predictability over time; however, his theory will continue to evolve as knowledge and technology evolve. Another important point to remember is that it was the application of Einstein's theory that originally stimulated the idea that something was missing, which demonstrates that theory is the catalyst for the formation of new theory. Even Einstein said that the theory of relativity is nothing but another step in the centuries-old evolution of science, one that preserves the relationships discovered in the past, deepening their insights and adding new ones (Calaprice, 2000). The eventual obsolescence of theory or parts of theory should not be a deterrent to theory development and testing primarily because these processes are essential for the ongoing development of new and improved theory and ultimately new knowledge. This continuum is essential for sound and responsible knowledge development.

In nursing and other health-related disciplines, it is necessary to have the flexibility to draw on a diverse theory base to be effective in today's complex health care delivery systems. It is equally important, however, to ensure a relevant and diverse theory base for the future, primarily because tomorrow's answers may lie in the speculative theories of today or in the revision of yesterday's established theory.

Operationalizing Theory, Knowledge, Research, and Reasoning

To **operationalize** something means to use it or make it ready for use (McKean, 2005). To operationalize theory, knowledge, research, and reasoning in nursing means that you select and analyze information in the form of variables, propositions, and assumptions to determine their applicability to a particular clinical situation. In Chapter 2, you learned how building blocks are used to construct theory, knowledge, research, and reasoning. These same building blocks can be used to deconstruct theory, knowledge, research, and reasoning when necessary in particular situations. Deconstructing means that you isolate and examine variables, propositions, and assumptions within a particular situation, such as a patient care situation, in an attempt to answer questions or solve problems. Conclusions identified by the theory will help draw conclusions about the clinical situation and guide subsequent actions in a valid, reliable, and predictable manner. Reynolds (1971) indicated that using theory and knowledge in this manner enabled the user to (1) explain past events, (2) predict future events, (3) develop a sense of understanding

> ## Box 3.1   Operationalizing Theory, Knowledge, Research, and Reasoning
>
> **Control** one or more concepts within relationships to bring about desired outcomes ⎤
> **Influence** others to change one or more concepts/variables within a proposition to bring about desired outcomes ⎦ Performance
>
> **Predict** significance of reoccurrence of the same or similar propositions ⎤
> **Explain** significance of propositions to others
> **Understand** significance of propositions, external variables, and assumptions ⎟ Reasoning
> **Relate** concepts/variables within phenomena and form propositions
> **Identify** concepts (internal and external variables and assumptions) related to phenomena ⎦
>
> Observe phenomena in nursing practice ⎤ Observing

about the events, and (4) develop some element of control of the variables and propositions making up the events. For example, if you were caring for an elderly patient with congestive heart failure, you would draw information from biological and pathophysiological theory concerning congestive heart failure and physiological changes in the elderly. Using this established theory, you would then be able to draw parallels to the clinical situation and use the information to make clinical decisions. You would also use the same process when selecting nursing theory to guide your choice of nursing interventions that are applicable to the situation.

For the purpose of this book, we have modified and expanded Reynolds' original work into more clearly articulated and progressive steps that demonstrate how theory, knowledge, research, and reasoning are operationalized in nursing practice. These steps are demonstrated in Box 3.1 and are explained in more detail in the following sections.

Identifying and Relating Concepts

As a nursing student, you learn to answer questions, solve problems, explore phenomena, and **identify** new theory by identifying essential variables within clinical situations and making a determination about how they **relate** to one another. This process of identifying relevant variables and putting them into a directional relationship is referred to as naming and framing a proposition. When trying to name and frame propositions, it is important that you identify not only the variables involved in the proposition, but also any external or confounding variables and assumptions that may have significance to the situation. For example, consider the following: You are caring for a patient with congestive heart failure who is complaining of feeling weak. His assessment findings were unremarkable; however, in reviewing his chart, you realize that his serum potassium level is low and that he has been receiving the loop diuretic Lasix. You remember from pharmacological theory that loop diuretics cause excessive loss of fluid and electrolytes at the site of the loop of Henle in the renal tubules. This can contribute to the development of hypokalemia, which can contribute to feelings of weakness. You may have also assumed that he was on a potassium supplement, which is customary for patients receiving a loop diuretic. However, your review of his medications reveals that no potassium supplement has been ordered. In

> ## Box 3.2 A Closer Look at the Cause-and-Effect Nature of Propositions
>
> When using theory to answer questions, solve problems, and explore phenomena, propositions can usually be identified among relevant concepts or variables. Most propositions have a cause-and-effect nature, meaning that one concept causes something to happen to another concept. Cause is defined as that which produces an outcome or result. The causal nature of a relationship is usually identified within a proposition. For example, if you use sun exposure and skin cancer as concepts, then you can form a proposition that identifies cause and effect by saying that prolonged, unprotected sun exposure can cause skin cancer. Hence, the proposition identifies a causal relationship between concepts.
>
> Obviously, when looking at the causal nature of propositions, it is important to determine what is the *effect* and what is *causing* it. Generally speaking, questions that need asking, problems that need solving, and phenomena that need exploring are generated by the significance of the effect something has on us. For example, you may want to know why your ankle hurts after you step in a hole, or you may want to know why you got lost while traveling. Although the questions may be generated by the significance of the effect on us, the answer lies in identifying the cause of that particular effect. For example, the question of why your ankle hurts when you step in a hole is answered by your knowledge that stepping in a hole twists muscles, ligaments, and tendons, which can result in pain. The question of why you got lost while traveling may be answered by the knowledge that you took the wrong exit. Twisting muscles, ligaments, and tendons when you stepped into a hole *caused* your ankle to hurt, and taking the wrong exit *caused* you to get lost. Knowing these causes provides you with basic answers. However, knowing the cause is not the same as understanding the cause, and it is understanding the cause that provides us with the ability to reason.

coming to this realization, you have named variables and framed a possible proposition in this situation, which is that the patient's hypokalemia and resulting weakness may be the result of the use of a loop diuretic and the omission of a potassium supplement.

The thinking you do as you rule in and rule out variables, form propositions, and examine assumptions constitutes the foundation of basic clinical reasoning. Reasoning in clinical situations frequently involves determining **cause** and **effect** as illustrated in Box 3.2.

Understanding Relationships Among Concepts

Once you have named and framed the propositions in a clinical situation, it is important that you begin to develop an appreciation of their significance to the health and well-being of the patient. To accomplish this, you need to be able to differentiate between knowing and understanding.

Knowing Versus Understanding

What does it mean when you say you "know" something? Is there a difference between knowing and understanding? Absolutely! Knowing and understanding are not synonyms. In conversational English, these two words are sometimes used interchangeably, but there are some important differences, especially when it comes to reasoning. **Knowing** simply means to *be aware of* (McKean, 2005). You can be aware of something without having too much information about it. On the other hand, **understanding** means to *comprehend or grasp the significance of* (McKean, 2005). From these two definitions, you can determine that knowing and understanding are not synonyms but do have a distinct hierarchal relationship. You can have knowledge of, or know, something without understanding it, but you cannot understand it without first knowing or having knowledge about it. An example of this is that many people know what a computer is and how to use it, but few understand how a computer works. With regard to the building blocks of theory, understanding, in any particular situation, means that you comprehend or grasp the importance of the variables, the propositions they form, and any related assumptions. Based on this comprehension you assign importance when reasoning and making clinical decisions. Understanding then results in your being able to answer the "who," "what," "what if," "when," "where," and "why" questions often associated with clinical situations.

The Significance of Significance

Significance is defined as meaning or importance (McKean, 2005). As indicated above, to understand means that you comprehend the importance of variables, propositions, assumptions, and their complex relationships in a particular situation and have made a determination about their significance to you and others. For example, if scientists were to discover a cure for cancer, it would have great significance to all of us. However, if astronomers were to discover another star, it would be profoundly significant to other astronomers, but only mildly interesting to those in the general population.

The degree of significance you assign to information changes as you learn and experience new things. For example, beginning nursing students know how to count a pulse. However, they may not understand the significance of variations in the characteristics of that pulse, such as those associated with atrial versus ventricular arrhythmias, heart blocks, peripheral artery disease, and hemodynamic instability, until they have learned relevant theory and had related clinical experiences. They may also know what an oximeter is, how to put the sensor on the patient's finger, and how to take an oxygen saturation reading. However, they may not have an appreciation of the limitations of the oximeter until they understand the significance of the oximeter reading in relation to the patient's arterial blood gasses, the oxygen dissociation curve, and the patient's clinical picture.

What makes the process of determining significance so important for nursing is that the significance assigned to information in clinical situations dictates what nursing actions should and should not be taken on behalf of patients. Consequently, these actions will influence patients' health and well-being. For example, consider the patient with congestive heart failure and hypokalemia that was discussed previously. Most likely you would assign a great deal of significance to the fact that the patient is taking a loop diuretic but is not taking a potassium supplement at the same time. Because this information is important to the patient's health, it is important to you and warrants specific nursing actions. Therefore, determining significance of information in the form of variables, propositions, and assumptions is essential to safe and effective nursing practice.

Explaining and Predicting Propositions

Once you understand the significance of information (variables, propositions, assumptions), then you need to be able to **explain** it. Explaining is an upper-level skill that involves interpreting information and its significance to others. This may sound like a simple process, but it is not. While you need to understand before you can explain something, not everyone who understands has the skills necessary to interpret the information so others understand. For example, have you ever been in a classroom where it was obvious the teacher understood the information but was not explaining it in such a way that you understood as well? Have you ever had a clinical instructor ask you to explain something that is going on with your patient and you simply could not put the words and rationale together, even though you knew what the teacher was asking? Consider what happens when nurses have to explain diagnoses, surgeries, medications, and treatments to patients or lead discharge planning and education in such a way that patients understand well enough to make informed decisions about caring for themselves. Developing skill in explaining involves making language and intellectual connections with another person and requires that you use your personal and professional knowledge, skills, values, meanings, and experiences to connect meaningfully with someone else who has different knowledge, skills, values, meanings, and experiences. For example, you may have to explain to the patient with congestive heart failure and hypokalemia why it is necessary that he take a potassium supplement and/or eat foods that are a rich source of potassium every day. In addition, he will need to know how often to take the medication, which foods are high in potassium, what portions should be used, and how often they must be eaten. The patient will also need to understand the consequences should he choose not to do this. You may also have to factor in confounding variables such as the patient has a fifth-grade education, is on a fixed income with Medicaid, and is not responsible for buying and preparing his own food. A second example is that as a nursing student, you understand the significance of overexposure of the sun and probably use sunscreen on a regular basis. However, you may have to explain the significance of this to a beach-going, suntan-loving patient who just had a melanoma removed. This patient would need to know and understand how overexposure to the ultraviolet rays of the sun adversely influences the melanocytes in the epidermal layer of the skin, resulting in the development of this type of cancer. You will also need to explain that it is particularly hazardous to continue excessive sun exposure because of the tendency of melanoma to reoccur and its high mortality rate. In addition, you may have to interpret what you understand about the relationship between sun exposure, skin, and the chronicity of melanoma to someone who loves tanning and indicates that she has no intention of stopping.

A skill that goes hand in hand with explaining is predicting. **Predicting** is explaining what may happen in the future based on existing variables, propositions, and assumptions. The only true difference between explaining and predicting is the element of time. Explaining is based in the past and present, whereas predicting is based in the future. The intent of both, however, is to establish meaning and significance and set the stage for action. Nurses use their understanding about a particular situation and their language skills and intellect to explain important information to patients, and they can use these same abilities to predict related future events. For example, you could predict that if the patient with congestive heart failure who is taking Lasix and is hypokalemic does not take a potassium supplement or increase his dietary intake of potassium-rich foods, then the hypokalemia will worsen, which could worsen the weakness and lead to dangerous cardiac arrhythmias. You could also predict that a postoperative patient who does not get out of bed and begin walking around could be predisposed to developing a deep vein thrombophlebitis, which could lead to the development of pulmonary emboli. Can you imagine what would happen if a nurse practitioner were to prescribe or a nurse were to administer a medicine for which the therapeutic and adverse effects could not be identified, understood, explained, and predicted? Once you can predict what can happen, you will be in a position to try and influence or control one or more of the variables involved in an attempt to change the situation and bring about a desirable outcome.

Influencing and Controlling Concepts

Just as understanding assists you in being able to explain and predict, being able to explain and predict assists you in influencing or controlling situations when necessary for safe and effective patient care. **Influencing** is simply an attempt to alter a situation indirectly by persuading someone to alter or change one or more concepts or variables in a situation to bring about a desirable outcome. For example, as a nurse you know what can happen to the patient with congestive heart failure who is on Lasix if he does not take a daily potassium supplement or eat potassium-rich foods. You could attempt to influence the situation by reminding the physician that the patient needs a potassium supplement, and you could ask the dietary department to add a banana to the patient's tray every day. You could also influence the patient directly by explaining to him and his wife the need to take a daily potassium supplement and eat potassium-rich food, and the consequences should he decide not to. You could also let the patient know which potassium-rich foods are covered by food stamps and that less expensive, generic forms of potassium are available. With regard to the patient with melanoma, to influence her and improve her health outcomes, you advise her to use sunscreen with a minimum SPF of 45 every day, wear protective clothing that has been treated with SPF, and significantly limit her exposure to the sun and artificial tanning beds in an attempt to decrease exposure to ultraviolet light and ultimately decrease her chance of developing more malignant lesions.

If attempting to influence a situation is not successful in achieving the desired health outcome, then in selected situations, you may have to try to control the situation instead of simply influencing it. Remember, when influencing a situation, you are most likely attempting to work through someone else, so your actions are indirect; however, when you are attempting to control a situation, you are taking direct action. It is very important to point out that **controlling** is not a matter of trying to dominate or do what is unreasonable or unwanted, but simply a matter of directly altering or changing one or more variables within a situation to bring about a desirable outcome. For example, if you walked in on a patient who was choking, you would attempt to control the situation by performing the Heimlich maneuver and calling for assistance. If a patient was unconscious and could not take care of meeting his daily needs, then you control the situation by meeting his daily needs until such time that he could resume caring for himself.

Controlling is not indicated in every situation. For example, consider the patients with hypokalemia and melanoma who were discussed previously. Ultimately, it is up to each of them to elect to follow your advice or not. They are fully capable of making that decision and are responsible for doing so. While moving to control outcomes in selected situations may bring about mutually desirable outcomes, you must remember that, except for selected emergencies, the decision to allow you, a nurse practitioner, physician, or other health care provider, to influence or control a situation lies with the patient if he or she is coherent and responsible, and with the family if he or she is not. There is a fine line between influencing and controlling nursing situations, and you must be careful not to cross the line and impinge on the patient's rights. Ultimately, it is the patient's decision. Your responsibility lies in ensuring that the patient or family has sufficient information concerning the significance of the situation to make decisions. Box 3.3 is an example of how nurses operationalize theory, knowledge, research, and reasoning.

As indicated in Box 3.1 and Figure 3.1, the complexity associated with operationalizing theory, research, and reasoning parallels the complexity of nursing judgments. Nursing Story 3.3 demonstrates this complexity.

It is important to note that everyone has different levels of expertise in a variety of areas. For example, an expert nurse would easily be able to influence or control common nursing situations in his or her field of expertise; however, that nurse may be at the novice level of identifying variables and propositional relationships when working in an area that is outside his or her expertise, such as the experienced labor and delivery nurse who is sent to work in the intensive care unit one day because of short staffing.

Box 3.3   Operationalizing Theory, Knowledge, Research, and Reasoning in Nursing Actions

The following example combines the actions of identifying, relating, understanding, explaining, predicting, influencing, and controlling into one nursing situation.

As a home health nurse, you are asked to care for an elderly, occasionally confused male patient who lives alone and has been discharged home from the hospital following an episode of self-induced, atenolol-based bradycardia. As his home health nurse, you would do the following:

Identify the variables involved and indicate whether you think they are internal, external, or confounding, or assumptions:

- Elderly male patient
- Desire to live independently
- Episodic confusion
- Atenolol-induced bradycardia (potentially lethal)
- Incorrect dosing of medication
- Physical safety
- Psychological well-being

Relate these variables in the form of a proposition:

- Inappropriate dosing of atenolol is contributing to bradycardia and confusion, which in turn leads to physical safety issues, such as syncope, falls, and possible death.
- This patient is trying to live independently, but may have significant safety issues.
- This patient may be taking additional atenolol when confused.

Understand the significance of the situation:

- Atenolol is a beta-receptor blocker that suppresses the rate of electrical impulses entering the sinoatrial node in the electrical pathway of the heart, resulting in bradycardia. Bradycardia leads to decreased cardiac output and lowered systemic blood pressure, which may also result in decreased cerebral perfusion resulting in dizziness, syncope, falls, trauma, and even death.
- The patient does not understand how atenolol works.
- The patient may not realize that he is taking extra doses of atenolol because of the confusion.
- The patient desires independence and autonomy.

Explain the situation in words the patient understands and emphasizing what has meaning and value to him:

- He may be getting confused at times and forget that he has taken his atenolol.
- There are significant consequences of taking too many atenolol tablets.
- To maintain health and independence, some changes need to occur in how he takes his medicine.

Predict what will happen in future if one or more concepts in this relationship are not changed:

- If he continues to take too much atenolol, the bradycardia will recur and dizziness, syncope, trauma, or even death may occur.
- He may have to have additional help in taking his medication.
- He may lose his ability to live independently if a solution to the situation cannot be found.

Influence the situation:

- Provide the patient with a written explanation of what you have explained to him, and post it where he can readily see it for future reference.
- Provide the patient with a medication box that is marked for each day of the week and has only one atenolol pill per day in it. Visit him each week and refill his medication box from his supply bottle. Count the number of pills that he has in his supply bottle and record the amount.
- Teach the patient to take his own pulse or use a small handheld device that will measure his pulse for him and to notify you if his pulse goes too low or if he is getting dizzy.
- Monitor the patient weekly. If, when monitoring the patient's progress, you realize that his pulse is below 60 and/or the supply bottle of atenolol is missing more tablets than it should, you may have to move to the next step.

Control the situation:

- Notify the physician and family of the dangerous situation.
- Remove the supply bottle from the home and have family members check his pulse and administer medications daily.
- Discuss the situation with the patient and family. Have a family member remove the drug from the home and take the responsibility of checking the patient's pulse each day and administering the correct dose of atenolol.
- Continue to check the patient and monitor for adverse drug reactions and confusion.

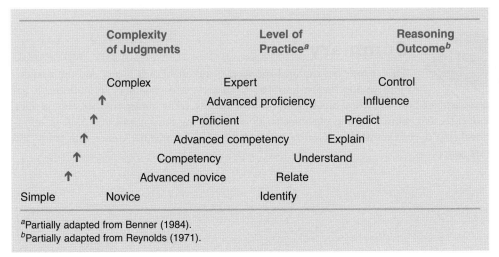

Complexity of Judgments	Level of Practice[a]	Reasoning Outcome[b]
Complex	Expert	Control
↑	Advanced proficiency	Influence
↑	Proficient	Predict
↑	Advanced competency	Explain
↑	Competency	Understand
↑	Advanced novice	Relate
Simple	Novice	Identify

[a]Partially adapted from Benner (1984).
[b]Partially adapted from Reynolds (1971).

Figure 3.1 Correlations among reasoning, judgments, and competency.

NURSING STORY 3.3

Operationalizing Theory

Michael Williams is a 24-year-old nursing student who assesses an elderly male patient and **identifies** that he has dry skin and poor skin turgor. Because of his knowledge from the biological sciences and nursing, Mr. Williams understands that dry skin and poor skin turgor may be **related** to aging, dehydration, and/or thyroid dysfunction. Mr. Williams notes that, according to the chart, the patient is 70 years old, has normal thyroid and cardiac function, and has had less than 2000 mL of fluid in 4 days. He now reasonably eliminates thyroid dysfunction as a contributing external variable, but determines that the patient's age and the amount of fluid he is taking in may be internal variables contributing to the dry skin and poor skin turgor. As a nurse, Mr. Williams **understands** that the only variable he can influence is the amount of fluid the patient is taking in, so he **explains** to the patient that the dry skin and poor skin turgor he is experiencing are most likely related to the fact that he (the patient) is not drinking enough liquids and that they will need to work together to increase the amount he is drinking. Mr. Williams also **predicts** that increasing the patient's fluid intake will help resolve the dry skin and poor skin turgor. He can **influence** the amount of liquids the patient drinks by frequently offering him a variety of fluids and encouraging him to drink, keeping a full glass of water at the bedside, and encouraging him to eat foods that have sodium. If this does not help resolve the dehydration, then Mr. Williams and the provider may have to **control** the situation by starting intravenous fluids.

Summary

This chapter has explored speculative and established theory and the relationships among theory, knowledge, research, and reasoning. In addition, it has demonstrated how theoretical building blocks help identify, relate, understand, explain, predict, influence, and control nursing phenomena, thus influencing nursing practice. Skill in operationalizing theory, knowledge, research, and reasoning in this manner comes with study and experience.

Learning Activities

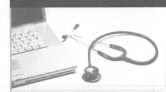

1. Using a simulated clinical situation where there is a patient problem that needs to be resolved:

   - Identify the variables in involved.

   - Relate the variables to each other in the form of a proposition (looking for cause and effect).

   - Determine if you understand the significance of the propositions you formed.

   - Explain the significance of the propositions to your peers.

   - Predict what may happen if action is not taken.

   - Influence the patient, peers, or staff to change one or more variables to improve the situation.

   - Identify how you might control a situation where effective influence is not possible.

2. Under the guidance of a clinical faculty member, repeat the above using an actual clinical situation.

References

Bethell, T. (1990, November 5). A challenge to Einstein. *National Review*, 69–70.

Calaprice, A. (2000). *The expanded quotable Einstein.* Princeton: Princeton University Press.

Cowen, R. (1997, November 15). Einstein's general relativity: It's a drag. *Science News, 152*(20), 308.

Fernie, J. D. (2005). Judging Einstein. *American Scientist, 93*(5), 404.

Freud, S. (1938). *The basic writings of Sigmund Freud* (A. A. Brill trans.). New York: Modern Library.

Glanz, J. (1997, January 24). Visions of black holes. *Science, 275,* 476–478.

Huler, S. (2008). Ripple effect. *Duke Magazine, 94*(1). Retrieved March 14, 2008, from http://www.dukemagazine.duke.edu/dukemag/issues/010208/ripple3.html

McKean, E. (Ed.). (2005). *The new Oxford American dictionary* (5th ed.). New York: Oxford University Press.

Orem, D. (1971). *Concepts of practice.* New York: McGraw-Hill.

Parse, R. R. (1981). *Man-living-health: A theory for nursing.* New York: Wiley.

Reynolds, D. P. (1971). *A primer in theory construction.* New York: Macmillan.

Selye, H. (1956). *The stress of life.* New York: McGraw-Hill.

University of Missouri-Columbia. (2007, October 4). Physicist defends Einstein's theory and 'speed of gravity' measurement. *Science Daily.*

von Bertalanffy, L. (1968). *General system theory: Foundations, development, applications.* New York: Braziller.

Theory and Reasoning

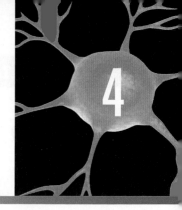

4

Intent: Theory, knowledge, and research are applied in clinical situations through reasoning; however, reasoning is dependent on more than just cognitive awareness of theory, knowledge, and research. This chapter identifies components and processes associated with reasoning, discusses factors that influence reasoning, and demonstrates how they are used in nursing practice.

Key Words/Concepts		
abductive reasoning	deductive reasoning	reasoning
Aristotle	experience	skill
care/caring	emancipatory knowing	Socrates
caring intent	inductive reasoning	Socratic method
cognitive	knowledge	symbols
competence	meanings	values
critical thinking	Plato	

Introduction

Chapter 3 demonstrates how the building blocks of phenomena, concepts, variables, propositions, assumptions, etc., play an essential role in operationalizing theory and research, which is essential to being able to answer questions, solve problems, explore phenomena, and generate new theory in nursing. However, how are theory and research actually applied? The answer is by thinking, but not just any type of thinking. According to Alfaro-LeFevre (2004), thinking refers

Identify	and	Relate	Understand	Act
Concept 1	+	Concept 2 (3,4, . . .) =	Significance of →	Explain
(Actual, potential, perceived)		(Actual, potential, perceived)	Actual	Predict
			Potential	Influence
			Perceived	Control
			Relationships	
			Among	
			Concepts	

Figure 4.1 Deliberate, purposeful thinking.

to any type of mental activity and can be as mindless as daydreaming. The desired level of think-ing in nursing is far from mindless daydreaming. It is an intentional, goal-directed, multistep process that involves (1) making observations about phenomena in clinical situations, (2) identi-fying relationships between and among concepts/variables, (3) understanding the significance of those relationships to the health and well-being of the patient, (4) using that understanding to explain the significance of the situation and possible outcomes to the patient and others, and (5) influencing or controlling one or more concepts or variables in an attempt to bring about a desired outcome (refer to Fig. 4.1). This advanced level of thinking is referred to as reasoning and requires skill to do effectively. Effective reasoning in nursing is influenced by personal and pro-fessional knowledge, skills, values, meanings, and experiences. It is also influenced by your abil-ity to integrate all of these with the knowledge, skills, values, meanings, and experiences of patients, families, peers, and other health care providers.

The ability to reason intentionally and purposefully can be cultivated and developed over time with appropriate teaching and learning methods and through your receptivity to under-standing and expanding how you reason. Perhaps the most significant factor in improving your ability to reason is your own determination and willingness to evolve and change.

There are many textbooks that offer different opinions and models on how to critically think and reason (Alfaro-LeFevre, 2004; Diestler, 2001; Halpern & Riggio, 2003; Jackson, Ignatavi-cius, & Case, 2006; Martinez de Castillo, 2003; Pesut & Herman, 1999; Webber, 2008b), and while they all give us valuable and different perspectives of critical thinking and reasoning, few use the language and meanings that are foundational to theory, research, and reasoning to demonstrate how to develop this skill. The omission of this essential language from these and other nursing textbooks, from learning resources, and by faculty in the classroom results in the loss of integration of the language of theory, research, and reasoning into student and nurse rea-soning, and ultimately in nursing practice. This, in turn, perpetuates an ongoing theory–practice gap and the marginalization of research utilization and conduction in practice. This is not to say that nurses, especially expert nurses, do not use theory; they do, but not within the framework of its language and usually not in a form traditionally recognized as theory or research. For example, an expert nurse will provide ample scientific rationale for a decision to adjust an intravenous vasoactive drug in response to significant blood pressure changes in a patient; however, he or she will usually not recognize or frame that rationale as explaining, predicting, influencing, or controlling dependent, independent, and confounding variables and assumptions associated with biological, hemodynamic, and nursing theory in order to bring about a desirable outcome. In addition, because the language is not an inherent part of how nurses think, they may or may not recognize an atypical response to the vasoactive medication as a phenomenon worth investigating through research. Nurses are also more likely to deconstruct their reasoning into problems and solutions as opposed to phenomena, concepts, independent and dependent variables, confounding variables, propositions, assumptions, and so forth. As a result, they may struggle with understanding and utilizing research or theoretical information that uses this language.

This chapter is an attempt to help you, the next generation of nurses, develop competency in the language of theory, research, and reasoning and forever bridge the theory–research–reasoning–practice gaps.

What We Learned From Socrates

Emphasis on an intentional and purposeful approach to reasoning can be traced back to the ancient Greek philosophers and teachers. The most prominent of these were **Socrates,** his student **Plato,** and Plato's student **Aristotle.** While exploring the philosophical aspects of the human experience, Socrates had his followers discuss abstract topics, such as religion, knowledge, virtue, justice, and wisdom. Socrates wanted to teach his students to replace their vague, unsupported thoughts, opinions, and judgments about these topics with clear and accurate ideas that were supported by a foundation in truth and reality. To accomplish this, he initiated, and his followers continued, a method of purposeful inquiry called the **Socratic method.** The Socratic method involves helping students and others explore their thoughts and opinions about a particular phenomenon and related concepts, propositions, and assumptions by asking "who," "what," "when," "where," and "why" types of questions. He asked students to "define," "describe," "clarify," "relate," "explain," and "justify" their thoughts and opinions in an attempt to reach a truth that was free of bias. Lastly, in an effort to expand students' ability the think beyond the obvious, he would ask them "what if"- and "imagine"-type questions related to the phenomena, concepts, propositions, and assumptions being examined. These intellectual exercises encouraged students to look beyond the basics to multidimensional meanings, causes, effects, and implications (Polifroni & Welch, 1999). Socrates knew that the identification, clarification, and understanding of the origin, nature, context, direction, and boundaries of one's thoughts and opinions would increase the truthfulness, reliability and validity of, and accountability for one's thoughts and opinions. Reasoning in this manner can loosely be related to the use of the concept of "power" in mathematics. Power is the product obtained when a number is multiplied by itself a certain number of times (McKean, 2005). For example, 2 to the 4th power = 16 and 3 to the 5th power = 243. If basic reasoning about a particular phenomenon constitutes reasoning at the 2nd power, then Socrates, Plato, and Aristotle asked their students to think and reason at the 3rd, 4th, 5th, and 6th power and beyond. Remember this concept when your faculty are asking you to think and reason above an introductory level.

Intentional and purposeful inquiry today is not very different. Just as Socrates, Plato, and Aristotle used purposeful inquiry to explore the phenomena of their day, you and your faculty use purposeful inquiry to explore nursing phenomena. For example, if you had a patient who had undergone abdominal surgery and was experiencing pain, you would use purposeful inquiry to explore the origin and nature of the patient's pain and its possible causes and effects. Box 4.1 demonstrates how intentional and purposeful inquiry helps you reason effectively.

Box 4.1   Example of Reasoning Through Inquiry

Observed phenomena

A postoperative patient you are caring for is experiencing pain and is hypoventilating.

WHAT are the concepts involved?

1. Postoperative abdominal surgery patient

2. Pain

3. Hypoventilation

4. Nurse

WHAT is the nature of each of the concepts?

1. Patient

   - 56-year-old male of average weight and height and in relatively good health

   - 24 hours after surgery

   - States that it hurts too much for him to take the 10 deep ventilations every waking hour as directed by the nurse

2. Pain

• Location?	Chest
• Intensity?	Pain scale 7 on a scale of 1 to 10
• Quality?	Sharp and burning
• Onset and duration?	Postoperative and constant
• What makes it better?	Pain medication helps some
• What makes it worse?	Deep breathing
• Effects of the pain?	Shallow breathing

3. Hypoventilation

   - Moving less tidal volume of air (either by rate or volume) during inspiration and expiration than is considered normal for weight and height, which may predispose patient to atelectasis, hypostatic pneumonia, and other serious postoperative complications

4. Nurse

   - Baccalaureate prepared

   - 15 years of surgical nursing experience

   - Has had surgery in the past

(continued)

Box 4.1   Example of Reasoning Through Inquiry *(continued)*

WHAT are possible conceptual relationships?

1. Postoperative patient and pain
2. Postoperative patient and hypoventilation
3. Postoperative patient and nurse
4. Pain and hypoventilation
5. Pain and nurse
6. Nurse and hypoventilation
7. Postoperative patient, pain, and hypoventilation
8. Postoperative patient, pain, hypoventilation, and nurse

WHAT are possible propositions?

1. Surgery causes pain at the patient's incision site and surrounding area.
2. Deep breathing causes pain at the incision site.
3. Postoperative patients may not breathe deeply because of pain.
4. Postoperative patients may hypoventilate if they do not breathe deeply enough postoperatively and develop pneumonia.
5. Nurse understands causes of pain, hypoventilation, and the need for intervention.
6. Nurse can make changes to improve pain relief and thus improve deep breathing.
7. Postoperative patient and nurse work together to resolve hypoventilation.

WHY do these propositions exist (rationale)?

1. Postoperative patients have pain because of the manipulation and disruption of nerves and muscles during surgery.
2. Normal or deep ventilation may cause nerve stimulation and muscle movement in the area of the postoperative suture line.
3. Postoperative patients may avoid movement of the muscles in the surgical area in an attempt to avoid pain.
4. Postoperative patients who do not deep breathe regularly postoperatively may hypoventilate, which could predispose them to other ventilatory complications.
5. Nurses are educated regarding postoperative care of the patient with chest surgery, pain management, and ventilatory management.
6. Nurses have personal experiences that sometimes help them understand patient situations better.

HOW do you know this is true?

1. Biological theory
2. Behavioral theory
3. Nursing theory
4. Observation
5. Experience

Critical Thinking and Reasoning: What Are They, How Are they Different, and Why Are They Important?

In the past three decades, a great deal of attention has been given to teaching nursing students to think effectively and independently (Alfaro-LeFevre, 2004; Bandman & Bandman, 1988; Brookfield, 1990, 1995; Diestler, 2001; Jackson, Ignatavicius, & Case, 2006; Paul, 1985; Penn, 2008; Pesut & Herman, 1999; Rubenfeld & Scheffer, 1995; Shafir, 1995; Webber, 2008b). Nursing has used and continues to use terms and phrases such as clinical decision making, nursing process, problem solving, critical analysis, judgment, evaluation, reflection, and critical thinking (just to name a few) interchangeably with reasoning. In many cases, they use some of these terms interchangeably to define each other. The use of these words and phrases as synonyms has blurred our understanding about what constitutes correct thinking in nursing (Benner, Tanner, & Chesla, 1996).

Since the movement of nursing education from hospitals into universities and the associated movement toward scholarliness through conducting and using nursing research and theory to guide practice, thinking in nursing has had a strong scientific and quantitative slant. This is primarily because most early research used quantitative methodologies, which has shaped our understanding and oriented us toward a scientific rigidity or narrowness that sees critical thinking as a resolution of problems with clearly defined ends (Benner et al., 1996; Meleis, 2007; Webber, 2008b). Today, **critical thinking** is defined as utilizing scientific facts, principles, and laws to identify, relate, understand, influence, and control actual and potential concepts and propositions.

The limiting of critical thinking to the traditionally scientific or quantitative level is not a problem as long as there is equal emphasis on the next level of thinking that integrates phenomenological (qualitative) and experiential aspects of theory, research, and practice at increasingly complex levels. Thinking with this level of inclusion constitutes **reasoning** and is the desired level of intellectual work in nursing. While critical thinking is a term often used synonymously with or in lieu of reasoning, it is actually more of a foundational component of reasoning than a synonym, primarily for the same reason that knowing is different from understanding. Just as one can know without understanding, one can think critically without recognizing all of the other important aspects of what one is thinking about and without translating one's thinking into effective nursing practice.

For example, consider the following true story.

A senior-level student, who had been taught the complexity of scientific relationships among hypoventilation, $PaCO_2$, HCO_3, base excess, and hypoxic drive in a patient with chronic obstructive airway disease (COAD), had significant difficulty translating that information and its implications when attempting to intercede effectively while caring for a 72-year-old female COAD patient who had just undergone a laparoscopic cholecystectomy. In the postanesthesia recovery unit the patient was found to:

- *Be tachypneic and hypoventilating*
- *Have a $PaCO_2$ of 80 mmHg*
- *Have a significantly distended abdomen as a result of her abdomen being filled with air during the laparoscopic cholecystectomy*
- *Be on 6 liters of oxygen (a contraindication in the presence of COAD)*

- *Be agitated and somewhat confused*
- *Be lying in a ball at the foot of the stretcher, which was in high semi-Fowler's position*

The patient was also adamantly refusing the anesthesiologist's insistence on intubation, claiming that "no one was listening" to the fact that she had been intubated before and did not want to be intubated again. The student/staff watched as the expert nurse came in, quickly assessed the situation, and immediately did the following:

- *Turned the oxygen down to 2 liters*
- *Sat the patient upright at a 90-degree angle on the side of the bed (which allowed the patient to again move her diaphragm effectively)*
- *Gave the patient a bedside stand to rest her arms on and support her upper body*
- *Began aggressively working with her to breathe through pursed lips, and "blow out" excess CO_2 with each exhalation*
- *Requested that the patient's pulmonologist be called stat because he better understood the nature of what was happening and had more of a willingness to try alternatives to intubation*

In less than 30 minutes, the patient's $PaCO_2$ was back down to her normal level of 58 (remember COAD patients often have a PaO_2 of 60 and a $PaCO_2$ of 60 normally, because of chronic hypoxia), her confusion had cleared, intubation had been avoided, and she was being moved to the pulmonary floor—not the intensive care unit. The expert nurse kept the student and other staff by her side as she interceded on behalf of the patient, explaining what she was doing and why with each step.

What was the difference between the student, less experienced staff, and expert nurse in this situation? It was the expert nurse's ability to understand the significance of the basic scientific, phenomenonological, and experiential variables involved, and to intercede appropriately. She recognized that this older, chronically ill patient could not move her diaphragm because of the air put in her abdomen during the surgery and because she was lying in a balled-up position. Both of these factors resulted in her not being able to breathe effectively, which in turn resulted in retained CO_2 (worsening hypercapnia) and mild confusion. In addition, she recognized that the patient was receiving too much oxygen, considering she had COAD, and was losing her hypoxic impetus to breathe. The expert nurse also learned that the patient's refusal to be intubated was related to a previous hospital experience that had resulted in a prolonged intubation, severe sleep deprivation, multiple nosocomial infections, and a prolonged and expensive hospital stay. The expert nurse respected the patient's right to self-determination and instituted other options to try to improve the patient's pulmonary status, short of intubation.

Was the anesthesiologist wrong in insisting on intubation? Not completely, considering the patient's precarious arterial blood gas situation; however, what this physician and the surrounding nursing staff did not do was (1) consider the patient's diagnosis of COAD and realize that this was an issue of severe hypoventilation, (2) factor into their thinking the possibility that the air in her abdomen and the position on the stretcher they had allowed her to slide into would prevent her from being able to move her diaphragm and ventilate effectively, and (3) realize that having her on that much oxygen would further suppress her hypoxic drive to breathe. Perhaps most importantly, they did not even attempt to try any interventions short of intubation, despite the patient's adamant refusal.

In summary, the expert nurse demonstrated understanding of the complexity of the nature and significance of actual, potential, and perceived variables, propositions, and assumptions surrounding a situation that had both qualitative and quantitative characteristics. The nurse also demonstrated advanced reasoning skill in explaining, predicting, influencing, and controlling multiple independent variables within the situation to bring about a desired outcome.

While in an ideal world there would be one term that adequately describes the level of reasoning that is desired in nursing practice, the profession is not at the point where it can do that. Too many questions still need to be answered, our collective thinking needs to evolve further, and we must come to some consensus on the term and possibly even conceptual and operational definitions of the desired level of reasoning expected in nursing. As a result, the debate about what constitutes effective reasoning will go on. However, as you prepare to enter the profession, remember that to be truly effective in influencing patient care, you must realize that reasoning is multidimensional and complex and consistently work toward developing this skill.

Developing Reasoning Skills

Reasoning skills may be developed slowly or quickly, depending on the extent of your education, experience, ability, and determination. Beginning reasoning may be slow and awkward, but the more you practice, the better and faster you will become. For example, consider the neuron, which is the electrical transmission cell of the brain that makes all human functioning, including reasoning, possible. All neurons have axons and connect with each other by way of synapses. Electrical impulses that have to travel the axon are slow. As the body matures, the axons of the peripheral nervous system become covered with a supportive and protective covering called myelin. Myelin increases the speed at which electrical impulses travel across neurons so drastically that they appear to be jumping from synapse to synapse. Neurons of newborn infants are immature, so their movement is slow, awkward, nondeliberate, and uncoordinated. As the infant matures and axons become surrounded with myelin, their movement becomes faster, more deliberate, and coordinated. Infants learn to progressively roll over, sit, crawl, stand, walk, and run largely because of this physiological process. Development of reasoning skill follows a similar process. As a student, your thinking initially may be slow and awkward, but as you learn and develop, your thinking becomes faster, more intentional, and purposeful. If you observe expert nurses as they work, you will see that their reasoning moves rapidly, efficiently (jumping from synapse to synapse), and almost effortlessly. Benner et al. (1996) describe this type of reasoning as "nonconscious and nonanalytical aspects of judgment" (p. 2).

As you become immersed in the knowledge, skills, values, meanings, and experiences associated with nursing and progressively develop your ability to reason effectively, you will begin to move from a novice to a competent, even expert practitioner.

The Significance of Pattern Identification

Knowledge, especially discipline-specific knowledge, such as that held by nursing, has patterns of information that are unique and meaningful to the profession and help to establish its disciplinary boundaries (Carper, 1999). Identifying patterns and how they are used during reasoning in clinical situations is extremely important.

Patterning of patient information can be accomplished by trending patient data over time. For example, you can trend a patient's data by assessing baseline information, such as vital signs, 24-hour intake and output, pain level, response to medications, symptoms, and laboratory reports, and then continue to collect similar data over time. Each time additional data are collected, you compare them against previously collected data and monitor for pattern changes and trends. It is important to be able to draw conclusions or explain pattern changes and trends because of the potential impact that information has on patient care. Once you are proficient in explaining trended data, you will be able to make predictions about future changes in those data and, if needed, move to influence or control one or more independent variables to bring about a desired outcome. Consider the following data regarding a male patient who had abdominal surgery 24 hours ago for an intestinal obstruction. He refuses to use the incentive spirometer or take deep breaths and is reluctant to ambulate because of the pain, despite receiving pain medication on a regular basis. He has a 30-pack-year smoking history and has frequent episodes of bronchitis.

Data	Baseline on Admission	Before Surgery	12 Hours Post-operative	24 Hours Post-operative	36 Hours Post-operative	What Is the Trended Pattern?
Blood pressure	140/90	142/88	130/80	120/ 80	116/76	↓
Heart rate	90	88	96	102	108	↑
Ventilatory rate/ Depth	26 Normal	24 Normal	28 Shallow	30 Shallow	32 Shallow	↑ ↓
Temperature	98.6	98.6	99	99	99	Normal to ↑
Hematocrit	52			50	50	Normal
Oxygen saturation (SO$_2$)	92	94	90	88	84	↓
Cough	Occasional	Occasional	Dry	Productive	Productive	Occasional to productive
Immobility	Mobile	Mobile	Reluctant to move	Reluctant to move	Reluctant to move	Mostly immobile
Pain (Pain medication is a synthetic narcotic given IM)	Mild, localized abdominal 2/10	Mild, localized abdominal 2/10	Sharp, general abdominal 9/10 Medication increased	Sharp, general abdominal 9/10 Medication changed	Sharp, general abdominal and distention 8/10	↑ In nature and location

- What conclusions can you draw from these data?
- What are the actual, potential, and perceived relationships among the different types of data?
- What is the significance of the trended data and these relationships to the patient?
- What are the possible consequences if the trend continues?
- How might you influence or control these trends?

Ineffective pain management → ↑ Pain level → ↓ Ability to take a deep
breath → ↑ Hypoventilation → ↑ Complications of hypoventilation
↑

Postoperative patient →
↓

Effective pain management → ↓ Pain level → ↑ Ability to take a deep
breath → ↓ Hypoventilation → ↓ Complications of hypoventilation

Figure 4.2 Reasoning in a picture.

More than likely, in the absence of bleeding and other postoperative complications, these data are the result of a combination of concepts, such as the lack of effective pain control, which makes him reluctant to move, cough, and deep breathe; the fact that he has undergone anesthesia; and his history of smoking and chronic bronchitis. This combination would also lead you to believe that his pain is most likely the reason he is hypoventilating, which is creating a mild drop in oxygen saturation (SO_2) and driving his ventilatory rate up (tachypnea) and his SO_2 level down (hypoxemia). The decreased SO_2 level is causing his heart to work harder, thus increasing the heart rate. The increased heart rate is resulting in decreased cardiac output over time, which decreases the blood pressure. Once all of these variables are put into propositions and their significance is determined, then you can explain and predict what may happen if these trends continue. You can then develop strategies to influence or control one or more of the variables in an attempt to improve the patient's outcomes. For example, in this case, keeping the physician informed of these trends, working with the physician to change the pain medication to something more effective, and administering it intravenously through a patient-controlled administration (PCA) device may significantly reduce the pain and improve the patient's ability to deep breathe and ambulate, as demonstrated in Figure 4.2.

As you can see, the identification of patterns through trending of data can play a significant role in the selection and effectiveness of nursing and medical interventions and ultimately in the patient's health and well-being.

Types of Reasoning

People approach reasoning using several different methods. Three of the most common methods are deductive, inductive, and abductive. Although distinctively different, these methods may be used in combination with each other, which is called dialectical reasoning. Note that this list of methods is not inclusive, nor do authorities always agree on the similarities and differences among them; however, they remain the basis for most reasoning.

Deductive Reasoning

The root word of deductive is deduce, which stems from the Latin word *deducere,* meaning to lead down (McKean, 2005). With **deductive reasoning,** you start with broad established facts, principles, laws, or theories that are known and generally accepted as true and use them to address narrower yet related phenomena, concepts/variables, and propositions. In other words, you use established knowledge to "lead" you to smaller, more specific conclusions. These conclusions may be in the form of an answer, solution, or explanation (Fig. 4.3).

With deductive reasoning, your answers, solutions, and explanations are assumed to be true because the facts, principles, laws, or theory used to explain them are assumed to be true. For

Theory →
Laws →
Principles →   Deductive reasoning →   Explanation of phenomena
Facts →

Figure 4.3 Deductive reasoning.

example, you know and understand that all female mammals secrete milk to feed their young. As a result, you can deduce that female dogs are mammals; therefore, female dogs secrete milk to feed their young. Notice that the reasoning used in this example moves from general to specific. As a nursing example, consider the patient discussed previously who had abdominal surgery. This patient was experiencing pain that worsened with movement and deep breathing and was hypoventilating. When reasoning deductively about this situation, you could formulate the following propositions:

- Pain is contributing to the patient's hypoventilation and reluctance to move (immobility).
- Hypoventilation in postoperative patients may lead to decreased PaO_2 and SO_2, atelectasis, and hypostatic pneumonia.
- Immobility in postoperative patients may lead to the development of venous stasis and possibly deep vein thrombophlebitis, leading to pulmonary emboli; therefore, it is important that the patient ambulate.
- Resolving the pain will help increase ventilation and the likelihood that the patient will ambulate more.

Nursing students use deductive reasoning primarily while in school and while beginning their practices. Because deductive reasoning is generally based on established theory and knowledge, it is one of the safest tools you can use when beginning to make clinical decisions.

Inductive Reasoning

Inductive reasoning is the opposite of deductive reasoning. The root word for inductive is induce, which stems from the Latin word *inducere,* which means to lead to or bring about (McKean, 2005). With **inductive reasoning,** you begin with smaller, narrower concepts/variables and formulate new propositions that may lead to the development of new facts, principles, and laws, and, ultimately, new theory (Fig. 4.4). An example of inductive reasoning is statistical polling, which is conducted during political elections to determine what people think about the various candidates and their platforms, comments, and activities. The pollsters then use these data to project who will win the election in each state and nationally and by what margin. As a nursing example, consider the nurse who has to teach a newly diagnosed type 2 diabetic, who is an illiterate, non–English-speaking, uninsured migrant worker who moves seasonally, what diabetes is and how to test his blood glucose every day, administer the correct dose of insulin, and arrange for routine diabetic follow-up care. All the patient education materials on hand are in print form and are written in English, so the nurse will have to take the concepts/variables she has and inductively build a new, creative, and portable bilingual audio and visual teaching program

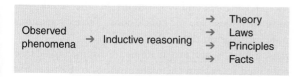

Observed phenomena → Inductive reasoning → Theory
→ Laws
→ Principles
→ Facts

Figure 4.4 Inductive reasoning.

that this patient can use to care for himself. Over time, the program, if effective, may be used with other similar patients and in other health care systems, including free medical clinics for migrant workers. Eventually, this new, creative design may be tested and retested through research and proven to be effective. It then may contribute to the development of facts, principles, and laws used to treat type 2 diabetics who cannot read, who cannot speak English, and who have no consistent health care follow-up.

Essentially, inductive reasoning lends itself to possibilities and probabilities through the discovery of new concepts and propositions, and, ultimately, new theory. When there is no known or identifiable relationship between phenomena and existing facts, laws, principles, or theories, scholars may need to inductively speculate about potential propositions, which, when tested through research over time, may provide the basis for new facts, laws, principles, and theories.

While inductive reasoning may imply some conclusions, there is a degree of uncertainty in those conclusions because of the speculative nature of the reasoning involved. However, inductive reasoning facilitates the use of speculation, creativity, and imagination as reasoning tools. This approach is also important to consider in light of the complexity and speculative origins of some nursing theory.

Abductive Reasoning

The use of the term abductive in relation to reasoning in nursing is relatively new when compared with the deductive and inductive approaches. The root word of abductive is abduct, which is derived from the Latin word *abductus,* which means to lead away (McKean, 2005). When applied to reasoning, it means making a conceptual leap or making an educated guess about concepts and their relationships based on observations, experience, beliefs, and patterns (Polifroni & Welch, 1999). When applied to nursing, **abductive reasoning** means the formation of potential propositions based on personal and nursing knowledge, skills, values, meanings, and experience and not on empirically based evidence or facts. These potential propositions, however, may or may not have links to established or speculative theory. Many scholars (Belenky, Clinchy, Goldberger, & Tarule, 1986; Benner, 1984; Benner et al., 1996; Benner & Wrubel, 1989; Bevis & Watson, 1989; Carper, 1999; Dreyfus, 1980; Dreyfus & Dreyfus, 1980; Gilligan, 1982; Kenny, 1999; Meleis, 2007; Reed & Shearer, 2009; Silva, 1999; Watson, 1999) have indicated that experiential knowing and nonobservable phenomena are as much a part of nursing as empirical facts; however, they are not as easily understood, tested, or integrated into common nursing judgments. For example, consider nursing theorist Jean Watson's abductive assertion that the "... word 'nursing' should be slashed out ..." because it is no longer adequate (Watson, 1999, p. xxii). Why change nursing's name? According to Watson, the term nursing "... is too embedded with the so-called modern nursing practices, procedures, language, and stereotypes which encode and restrict" the profession from becoming what it must become (Watson, 1999, p. xxii). Nursing needs to convey that it has "served the master, masculine archetype script in education and practice ..." long enough and that the profession has moved past stereotypical, "industrial, masculine, archetypal, patriarchal, medical, and institutional thinking" (1999, p. xxii). In 1999, Watson's statements were abductive assertions; in 2008 their truth may be becoming more apparent.

Watson and others who make these types of abductive assertions do so because their culminating knowledge, skills, values, meanings, and experiences allow them to see and speculate about what could be. Abductionists, commonly considered visionaries, facilitate the identification and investigation of previously unidentified or marginally identified human and nursing phenomena that strict deductive and inductive methods could not accomplish.

Factors Influencing Reasoning in Nursing

Nursing scholars have tried for decades to define nursing. Florence Nightingale, who is considered the mother of modern nursing, first attempted to define nursing in 1859 in her text *Notes on Nursing: What It Is and What It Is Not* (1859/1992). Since then, numerous nursing scholars (Bevis, 1997; Newman, 1986; Newman, Sime, & Corcoran-Perry, 1991; Henderson, 1966; Meleis, 2007, Webber, 2002a) and organizations, such as the American Nurses Association (2003), have continued to try to capture the essence of nursing into one global definition or group of characteristics. However, none has been universally accepted. Is there some consensus among these writers and their definitions about the intent and scope of nursing? The answer is no. Nursing appears to be larger and more dynamic than any one author and definition can adequately reflect. However, "there is a constancy of response that speaks to the 'what is' of nursing and nursing science and not to the 'what is' of another profession" (Silva, 1999, p. 222). It is this constancy that helps define the uniqueness of nursing and establishes the parameters of reasoning in nursing. For the purposes of this book, nursing is defined as the desire, intent, and obligation to apply relevant knowledge, skills, values, meanings, and experiences for, with, or on behalf of those requiring or requesting assistance in achieving and maintaining their desired state of health and well-being (Webber, 2002a).

Knowledge

While it may be an example of tautological duplication to have knowledge as a factor that influences the application of theory, knowledge, research, and reasoning, the fact remains that you have to have some knowledge before you can apply knowledge even at an elementary level. In particular, you have to have at least some fundamental information about nursing to be able to identify basic concepts or variables that are relevant in clinical situations. As you read, study, take more classes, and actually practice nursing your level of knowledge grows, and the more it grows, the more concepts and variables you will be able to identify and relate in clinical situations. For example, as a beginning student, you most likely took a class in microbiology. When you took the nursing fundamentals class, you applied what you learned in microbiology when studying the difference between aseptic and sterile technique. The further you advance in nursing, the more your knowledge about microbiology will grow and the more you will be able to apply what you know to nursing situations, such as changing sterile dressings on a burn victim or administering antibiotics to a patient who is in septic shock. In nursing you apply the knowledge you have, and your level of knowledge should be constantly growing and developing. Even after graduation, you will be expected to study and keep abreast of new theory and research being developed and how it impacts practice.

Skills

It is commonly assumed that the word skill means how well you are able to do something and implies action versus thought. However, the word skill originated from the Old Norse term *skill*, which means demonstration of knowledge, and the Old English term *scele*, which means discernment (McKean, 2005). Therefore, by their very meanings, skill and knowledge are intricately connected. Nowhere is this more important than in health care. Knowledge is operationalized through skill, and skill must be rooted in knowledge.

Nursing skills are deliberate acts or activities in the cognitive and psychomotor domains that are selected, performed, and evaluated for, with, or on behalf of those for whom we care (Bevis, 1997). The application of skills requires reasoning that reflects nursing knowledge,

values, meanings, and experiences. Nursing skills have historically been viewed as simply technical acts, such as handwashing, injections, and isolation techniques. Today, nursing skills have
both a cognitive and technical dimension and are dependent on effective reasoning. Nursing
skills include the traditional psychomotor activities, as well as other diverse activities, such as the
effective application of theory and knowledge in meeting diverse patient care needs; utilization of
research findings in practice; communication with other health care professionals, patients, and
families; management of patient care; and financial stewardship. Selection, implementation, and
evaluation of nursing skills depend on the intentional and progressive integration of relevant
nursing knowledge, values, meanings, and experience.

Competence

A concept often associated with skill is that of **competence** or competency. In nursing, competency is defined as the ability to think and act effectively and safely. Competency is not synonymous with experience and is not limited to the performance of psychomotor skills. Competency
in nursing requires the ongoing development of knowledge, skills, values, meaning, and experiences and the ability to apply these when identifying, relating, understanding, explaining, predicting, influencing, and controlling nursing phenomena.

It is assumed that when nurses pass the National Council for Licensure Examination–RN
(NCLEX-RN), they are competent to practice nursing at a level sufficient to protect the safety of the
public. However, minimum competency in patient safety is not equal to the competency level demonstrated by experts in nursing practice. Expert nurses are competent in their ability to influence and
control nursing phenomena, and safety is a fundamental assumption within their practice. In the classic texts *From Novice to Expert* (1984) and *Expertise in Nursing Practice* (1996), Benner et al. describe
stages through which student nurses pass as they graduate and move toward expert practice. These
stages include novice, advanced beginner, competent, proficient, and expert. As nurses progress
through each stage, they deepen their knowledge, skills, values, meanings, and experiences related to
nursing, which in turn progressively influences their clinical reasoning and decision making.

When considering Benner's stages of competency in relation to a nurse's ability to identify, relate,
understand, explain, predict, influence, and control, it becomes apparent that there is a relationship.
To further clarify this relationship, this text has added two additional stages to Benner's model. These
two stages are advanced competence and advanced proficiency. They are intended to demonstrate the
transition periods between competent and expert. In addition, changing Benner's stage of advanced
beginner to advanced novice reflects the difference in the meanings of the two words. To begin (or to
be a beginner) means to start, commence, or take the first step; novice refers to lack of experience
(McKean, 2005), and it is experience that is represented in the transition between the stages. As you
continually gain more knowledge, skills, values, meanings, and experiences and your ability to apply
these in the clinical setting improves, you begin the progression through the stages toward expert practice. Although not articulated in typical theoretical language, Benner's work has been and continues to
demonstrate logical adequacy in facilitating nursing's ability to answer questions, solve problems, and
explore phenomena associated with the development of expertise in clinical practice, which gives it
theoretical validity and reliability. Ultimately, the quality, accuracy, and effectiveness of nurses vary
depending on their level of education, experience, and individual ability to progress (Benner, 1984;
Benner et al., 1996; Flanagan, Baldwin, & Clarke, 2000; Webber, 2002b, 2008b).

Values

Values are enduring beliefs, attributes, or ideals that establish moral and ethical boundaries of
what is right and wrong in thought, judgment, character, attitude, and behavior. They form a

foundation for correct thinking and decision making throughout your life. Values develop over time and reflect individual, family, social, cultural, and religious influences, as well as personal choice. Values provide a sense of individuality, in that you choose personal values, and a sense of community with those who share the same or similar values. Values that are shared collectively by individuals within a particular profession reflect what that profession considers to be good, right, and important (Chinn & Kramer, 2008; Chitty, 2005). Nursing values are operationalized in the context of professional principles, standards, codes, policies, and procedures that guide nursing decisions and actions. Values identified as essential within nursing include altruism, or concern for others; honesty; integrity; ethics; aesthetics or freedom to exercise personal choice; dignity; justice; and truth (American Nurses Association, 2001; Chitty, 2005, Webber, 2002b). These values guide the behavior of nurses and directly influence reasoning in every nursing situation. Collectively these values have not only helped form nurses' professional identity, but also they continue to play a significant role in the public's perception and respect for nurses.

Chinn and Kramer (2008) explored another concept that has potential as a nursing value. This concept is **emancipatory knowing,** which they define as the capacity to identify injustices and to analyze why injustices go unnoticed and/or unaddressed, including injustices toward women, nurses, and nursing collectively. They further assert that emancipatory knowing in nursing requires the identification of "social and structural changes that are required to right social and institutional wrongs" (p. 78). While, historically, nurses have played an important role in addressing social injustices for their patients, in this instance, Chinn and Kramer have identified nurses and nursing as the recipients of institutional, social, and political injustices, especially in the areas of oppressive policies and practices, practice limitations, reimbursement, and roles in health care. They also assert that nurses are aware of these fundamentally unfair and unjust institutional, societal, and political policies and practices, ". . . but rather than pursuing a critical, emancipatory approach" to changing them, we "accommodate" them, foregoing any long-term solutions (2008, p. 80).

Certainly, there is validity in what Chinn and Kramer (2008) assert; however, one could also assert that it is not "knowing" but "understanding" that is the real issue. Remember, understanding is more complex than knowing, and understanding and explaining the real nature and significance of unjust institutional, societal, and political policies and practices, and why they are perpetuated, is essential if we ever hope to be able to influence and control the injustices. Chinn and Kramer (p. 80) also describe nurses as "recipients" of these injustices, which implies a "victim" or a "power and powerless" perception. Even the term emancipatory implies the perception of subserviency. Is it the self-perception of nursing powerlessness that perpetuates these injustices? Are these injustices part of our own making? Most likely, they are. This view is not intended to blame the victim; it is to point out that these injustices have been going on for so long that one has to ask not how we are accommodating them, but how and why we have tolerated, enabled, and empowered them for so long. Is it because the profession is mostly women and women in our society are still largely viewed as less capable than men when it comes to leadership and establishing health care policies and practices? Or is it that we do not see ourselves as capable of doing these things? Most likely it is the latter, because if women and nurses, individually and collectively, viewed themselves as powerful, then the majority of society would as well since women are the majority.

Nursing education must shoulder some of the responsibility for educating a workforce that enables and empowers injustices—not just institutional, societal, and political injustices, but the more basic injustices of men to women, physician to nurse, employer to employee, and women to women, as well. Nursing curricula often speak to educating leaders, and many schools educate midlevel leaders for the practice settings; however, few educate leaders capable of banding together to change institutions, society, and national political environments. How many under-graduate and graduate students ever articulate the goal of sitting at boardroom tables establishing health care practice, policies and procedures, reimbursement levels, and expanding roles of nurses? Not many. Nurses are the largest group of health care providers in the world, yet we persistently fail to recognize and utilize this power. Until nursing education recognizes the need to neomodernistically redesign nursing education and retool nursing faculty to educate sufficient numbers of nurses who view themselves as powerful, equal, and active participates at every boardroom table where health care policy and practices are decided, we will remain in the same position as young Oliver Twist when his prolonged and persistent hunger drove him to say to his oppressors, "Please sir, I want some more."

Perhaps the need for emancipatory knowing to become part of nursing's value set could be overcome if we learn to value ourselves, our power, and our potential.

Care and Caring

Traditional definitions of **care** and **caring** include descriptive words and phrases, such as to have concern for, to value, to protect, to have responsibility for, and to help. All of these words and phrases can be used to describe characteristic feelings and behaviors commonly associated with nursing and other human services professions. However, presenting caring as vague feelings and actions serves neither professionals nor patients (Scotto, 2003). Caring must be operationalized through intentional and purposeful behaviors. Nurses have a caring intent in that their thoughts and behaviors center on valuing and helping others through the application of their knowledge, skill, values, meanings, and experience. Having a **caring intent** influences nursing practice because it attaches expanded meaning and significance to everything nurses do. The intent to care guides all decision making in nursing.

Because care and caring characteristics are frequently associated with nursing, the profession has devoted a significant amount of time to exploring them. For decades it has been debated what care and caring in nursing are and are not (Leininger, 1991; Benner & Wrubel, 1989; Benner et al., 1996; Bevis & Watson, 1989; Bevis, 1997; Watson, 1979, 1985, 1994, 1999; Webber, 2002a). Just as with the definition of nursing, however, the profession has been unable to establish consensus. Perhaps this is because nursing is trying to make caring in nursing something that it is not. Nursing does not have a monopoly on care or caring. Many human beings, families, societies, and other health professions demonstrate characteristics associated with care and caring. So what is it that makes care and caring in nursing unique? It is that they exist and are demonstrated within the context of the application of nursing knowledge, skills, values, meanings, and experiences. This is the constancy that speaks to the "what is" of caring in nursing and not to the "what is" of caring in other professions. This constancy forms an essential assumption upon which a significant amount of nursing theory is based: the assumption that nurses have concern for the well-being of their patients, value them as human beings and individuals, and have knowledge and skills that can help them achieve their health-related goals and accept responsibility for their care. Caring is what motivates the practice of nursing to want to understand, explain, influence, and control phenomena in nursing practice.

Meanings

As you learned in Chapter 2, **meanings** define the context, purpose, and intent of language, the study of which is called hermeneutics. Through hermeneutics, different organizations, cultures, professions, and so on, select, adapt, and organize verbal and nonverbal words, acronyms, abbreviations, and symbols into a subset within existing language. These subsets represent what is believed and valued within a particular profession, and are derived from epistemologically significant information, patterns of use, and traditions within each profession. Nursing, medicine, and law are examples of professions that have their own subset language. These professions also, at times, use the same words, but with different meanings. For example, what does it mean when nurses say they give "holistic" care or when they describe themselves as "professional" nurses? How does this differ from physicians who describe themselves as professionals who provide holistic care? When nurses talk about the practice implications of a new drug, how is it different in meaning from physicians who will be looking at the practice implications of the same drug?

Most health-related professions, such as nursing, medicine, physical therapy, etc., also share words, abbreviations, symbols, prefixes, and suffixes associated with common medical terminology. Most likely, you have taken a medical terminology course or have studied medical terminology within an existing course. Nursing language, often in association with medical terminology, is characteristically used in nursing texts, journals, and day-to-day conversations among nurses. This language includes acronyms, which are words formed from the first letter(s) of words within phrases, titles, etc. (McKean, 2005). For example, most people are aware of the word radar, but few people know that this word is actually an acronym for the phrase "radio, detection, and ranging." Most people are also aware of the term laser, which is simply an acronym of "light amplification by simulated emission of radiation." Common nursing acronyms include T, P, R, BP, which represent temperature, pulse, respirations, and blood pressure. Collectively, T, P, R, BP is represented by another acronym, referred to as VS, or vital signs. Examples of other acronyms nurses use include BRP, which means bathroom privileges; T, C, DB, which means to turn, cough, and deep breathe a patient every 2 hours to prevent hypostatic pneumonia; and FF, which means to force fluids. Acronyms play an important role in nursing language, both in terms of clarity and efficiency; however, as with all shortcuts, it is important for safety reasons that you use only those acronyms accepted by the profession.

Many professions also use **symbols** to represent unique meanings within their language. For example, physicians use the caduceus as a symbol for healing. The caduceus is a staff or wand with two serpents intertwined around it. The caduceus was believed to have been carried by Hermes, the messenger god in Greek mythology. In the 7th century, it became known as a symbol of healing, a meaning that continues today (McKean, 2005). Lawyers use the symbol of Lady Justice, or Justitia, the Roman Goddess of Justice, to personify the moral and ethical underpinnings of the legal system. Since the Renaissance, Justitia has been represented by a blindfolded, bare-breasted female balancing a sword in one hand and scales in the other. This symbol is commonly found in courthouses and courtrooms (McKean, 2005).

Nursing symbols are not quite as clear and appear to be evolving. The mother of modern nursing, Florence Nightingale, gave us one of the earliest nursing symbols, a lamp. While caring for soldiers during the Crimean War, Nightingale would make rounds to her patients at night carrying an oil lamp. She became known as the "Lady with a Lamp" (Dossey, 1999, p. 184). Consequently, the lamp came to represent the consistent and vigilant care and compassion demonstrated by nurses. In the early 20th century the lamp took a back seat to white uniforms, nursing caps, capes, and school pins; however, by the 1970s nurses were letting go of some of these latter-day symbols, in part because of infectious disease control issues and also because of the feminist movement. As women took off their bras, nurses took off their white uniforms, caps, capes, and, in some cases, school pins. Unfortunately, today many in the profession has replaced professional white uniforms with unironed, multicolored scrubs with cartoon characters on them. Nursing caps with hair pulled neatly up and back have been replaced with long flowing hair that seems to be more about making a fashion statement than helping control infectious diseases. Obviously, these are nursing image and safety issues the profession is trying to address.

The majority of schools of nursing still have pins representing their undergraduate programs; however, most practicing nurses no longer wear them. It is questionable as to whether the pin is more of a symbol of unity with a particular school than a symbol of nursing. The most common symbols of nursing today appear to be stethoscopes and syringes, which may or may not be professionally desirable. Noted nursing visionary and leader, the late Dr. Em Olivia Bevis, once lamented that she was concerned that nursing had relinquished most of the meaningful symbols that helped form our professional, and respected, identity (personal communication, May 10, 1997). It may be time for us to consider moving Nightingale's lamp and its rich meaning to modern nursing into a more prominent position as nursing's primary symbol, especially since its meaning is foundational to the role of the profession. It certainly would represent us better than wrinkled, comical scrubs and unrestrained hair falling into sterile fields.

Personal and professional experiences also influence meanings that you assign to every clinical situation. For example, a nurse with 15 years of postoperative nursing experience who has a personal history of postoperative thrombophlebitis and resulting pulmonary emboli will apply different meanings and significance to the postoperative patient complaining of leg pain than would a new graduate with minimal surgical nursing experience and no history of postoperative thrombophlebitis and pulmonary emboli.

Learning the meanings and nuances of nursing's unique language and symbols is essential to delivering safe, effective, and ethical care and is foundational to developing a professional identity (Milton, 2005). Every day that you practice and gain experience changes the meanings and significance you assign within clinical situations, which is an essential part of meaning making in nursing. As you continue your nursing education and begin to practice, make a point of identifying words, abbreviations, acronyms, symbols, and actions that have unique meaning to you as a nurse and watch how these meanings and their significance evolve over time.

Experience

Experience commonly refers to longevity or length of time in a position. However, meanings associated with experience and experiential learning in clinical situations are much more complex and valuable than this definition represents. Nursing **experience** refers to the unique and active process of defining, refining, and evolving personal and professional knowledge, skills, values, and meanings used in clinical reasoning as a result of actively engaging in nursing situations over time. Change, not passage of time, is the defining characteristic of experience (Benner et al., 1996). Experience is laden with richness, false starts, challenges, successes, and failures, and it is how you cope with the responses to these experiences that is crucial to experiential learning (Benner et al., 1996; Benner, 2001).

As a student, you generally have an experiential void in practice, for which you compensate by gathering and relying on established theory and knowledge and by maintaining a certain degree of scientific rigidity in your reasoning. As you move toward competency, you develop more confidence and begin to acknowledge and integrate experiential knowing and understanding into your practice; however, your clinical decisions are still guided primarily by scientific evidence. Expert nurses usually have sufficient confidence in their knowledge and understanding that they easily integrate experience and intuition into effective reasoning.

Although nursing education has made great strides in developing creative teaching and learning strategies that support the development of advanced reasoning ability (Myers & Jones, 1993; Diekelman & Scheckel, 2003; Jackson et al., 2006), experience, as defined by change and not time, is the one thing that nursing faculty cannot provide for you. You must do this yourself. Each clinical encounter, good and bad, has the potential to teach you something new about patient responses or nursing care if you are paying attention. Expert nursing practice requires ongoing development of clinical knowledge through experiential learning, and for experiential learning to occur, it is essential that you involve your body, mind, and spirit in the process. Faculty can plan the clinical and classroom experiences and schedule the time, but it is ultimately up to you to become actively and intellectually engaged in the experience, ultimately improving your reasoning ability through your own experiential learning.

The Role of Nursing Process in Reasoning

Reasoning in nursing is multidimensional and involves several processes. One of the oldest of these is called the nursing process (Hall, 1955) and has been used for decades as a means of introducing nursing students to basic problem solving and thinking in nursing. Today, nursing process is considered a functional process model that calls for the nurse to accomplish the following:

1. Perform an assessment of the patient.
2. Identify specific problems based on the assessment.
3. Identify patient and nursing goals related to the identified problems.
4. Select specific nursing interventions and scientific rationale to address the identified problems and meet the identified goals.
5. Evaluate the effectiveness of the interventions in resolving the problems and meeting the goals.

Nursing process has been used effectively in schools of nursing to introduce students to basic problem-oriented thinking through the identification of basic concepts and propositions. The process facilitates exploration of interrelationships between assessment findings and problems, problems and nursing interventions, and nursing interventions and resolution of identified problems. If nothing more, nursing process focuses the student on the identification of relationships and cause and effect in many nursing situations. However, nursing process is not without its limitations. Although it facilitates basic problem-oriented thinking, not all nursing practice is problem oriented. Nursing process also tends to direct nursing decision making toward resolution of problems and clearly defined ends, which is not an accurate reflection of nursing practice (Benner et al., 1996; Meleis, 2007). In addition, nursing process does not support multidimensional reasoning and the nonanalytical and nonconscious aspects of thinking that are frequently demonstrated in expert nursing practice. According to Benner et al. (1996), expert nurses attune to subtle changes in the clinical situation, attend to salient information, and understand and respond to patient issues or concerns, often without conscious deliberation and with the knowledge that there may not be clearly identified ends. What this means is that while nursing process serves a purpose at the introductory level of nursing education, students and practicing nurses quickly move past it as their reasoning ability develops.

Nursing diagnosis, a component of nursing process that was added in the 1970s, categorizes common problems encountered by nurses according to very prescribed language. It has come under serious question over the past two to three decades because of its rigidity and esoteric language. With regard to facilitating the development of critical thinking—it simply doesn't. The rigid and prescriptive nature of nursing diagnosis restricts you to lower-level thinking, which is inconsistent with facilitating upper-level reasoning capability (Benner et al., 1996; Webber, 2001, 2002a, 2004, 2008b). Meleis (2007, p. 531) contends that the concept of nursing diagnoses ". . . did not emerge from a coherent philosophical approach or from a theoretically defined domain . . . ." She further contends that nursing diagnosis does not and cannot represent the thinking and actions of the "majority of nurses who have been caring for clients and communities for years, and whose level of expertise ranges from novice to the expert." Benner et al. previously demonstrated in a 1996 landmark study that practicing nurses simply do not use nursing diagnosis to help frame any aspect of their practice. For nursing education to be clinically relevant, it must emphasize concepts and theory considered epistemologically significant and relevant to improving nursing practice and facilitate the development of advanced reasoning skills, and it is simply not evident that nursing diagnosis does this. While the language of nursing diagnosis is, for now, embedded in our textbooks and in the computerized documentation systems of health care agencies, it has not proven sufficiently meaningful or valuable enough for practicing nurses to use. The fact remains that nurses do what they are forced to do with nursing diagnosis in computerized documentation systems and then they proceed to practice without it.

With the growing trend of evidence-based practice, it is likely that the nursing diagnosis aspect of the nursing process will be phased out. The remaining framework of nursing process will again be limited to use as an introductory problem-solving process, and nursing education will move toward teaching learning activities that accurately reflect the conscious and nonconscious, analytical, advanced reasoning needed to be effective in today's nursing practice.

Putting It All Together

Purposeful and effective reasoning in nursing is a complex and multifaceted process that takes time to develop. Nursing Story 4.1 demonstrates reasoning in a clinical situation, and Figure 4.5

Theoretical Foundation	Level of Practice	Level of Reasoning	Complexity of Judgments	Reasoning Outcome[b]
Scientific/ phenomenological	Expert	Clinical reasoning	Complex	Control
↑	Advanced proficiency	↑	↑	Influence
↑	Proficient	↑	↑	Predict
Scientific preferred	Advanced competency	Critical thinking	↑	Explain
↑	Competent	↑	↑	Understand
Scientific rigidity	Advanced novice	Linear thinking	↑	Relate
Theory introduction	Novice	Information gathering	↑ Simple	Identify

[a]Partially adapted from Benner (1984).
[b]Partially adapted from Reynolds (1971).

Figure 4.5 Correlations among reasoning, judgments, and competency.

NURSING STORY 4.1

Using Reasoning Processes in Nursing Practice

The Patient's Story

Peggy Garland is a 20-year-old nursing student assigned to assist Shirley Evans, an elderly left hemispheric stroke patient, with eating breakfast. While eating, Mrs. Evans chokes and starts to have difficulty breathing. Ms. Howard calls for a registered nurse and attempts to have Mrs. Evans cough, but she is unable to clear the food from her throat. Ms. Garland remembers that the Heimlich maneuver is used to clear airways, but is unable to get Mrs. Evans repositioned in the bed to perform the procedure. At this point, an experienced registered nurse, Ann Griffin, comes in, assesses the situation, and immediately suctions the patient's airway with a plastic tonsil suction. After the obstruction is cleared, Ms. Griffin assesses Mrs. Evans' vital signs, listens to her breath sounds, and determines that she is stable. Ms. Griffin and Ms. Garland reposition Mrs. Evans in bed and clear the food tray away. When they return to the nurses' station, Ms. Griffin makes a note to talk with Mrs. Evans' physician about a follow-up chest x-ray to ensure that Mrs. Evans did not aspirate food particles when she choked and to discuss further diagnostic evaluation of her ability to swallow effectively. Ms. Griffin then explains to Ms. Garland that Mrs. Evans' left hemispheric stroke has left her with weakened facial muscles on the right side and ineffective cough and gag reflexes. She continues to explain that patients with this kind of deficit need to be fed on the unaffected side of their mouth, using small portions of semisolid or ground food. Ms. Griffin also explains that Ms. Garland could change the thickness of liquids by adding varying amounts of a commercially prepared gelatin, which enables Mrs. Evans to swallow more easily. Ms. Griffin also predicts that a similar situation may happen again and decides to post an alert sign over Mrs. Evans' bed and to have a patient-care conference for students and ancillary personnel on feeding techniques for patients with impaired swallowing. In addition, Ms. Griffin tells Ms. Garland that when Mrs. Evans' lunch tray comes up, they will feed her together so she can help Ms. Garland practice safe feeding techniques.

Reasoning Processes

The student was able to *identify* and *relate* the concepts of a swallowing deficit, food, choking, and airway obstruction, but she had a lack of *understanding* of the degree of

(continued)

Using Reasoning Processes in Nursing Practice (Continued)

their interrelatedness, their significance, and, while she attempted to intervene, her choice of interventions was ineffective for the given situation. The experienced nurse, however, was able to come in, quickly assess and understand what was happening and move to *influence* and *control* the outcomes by suctioning the patient to clear her airway and assessing the patient for possible complications. The experienced nurse was also able to *explain* to the student why the event happened and *predict* that the patient may have aspirated despite the clear breath sounds, thus determining the need for a chest x-ray and further diagnostic evaluation of the patient's swallowing. She also predicted that a similar situation may happen again and instituted additional education measures to influence and control future situations by working with the student and other staff to increase their awareness and skills needed to feed patients with a swallowing deficit.

demonstrates the progressive relationships among theory, experience, reasoning, and outcomes. As you read the story, try to identify the reasoning processes being used. You will see that there are correlations among theoretical foundation, clinical experience, levels of reasoning, and complexity of variables, judgments, and outcomes. Study the figure and make a determination about where you are in your professional development.

Summary

This chapter provides introductory information with regard to the differences between critical thinking and reasoning; some of the different types of reasoning; and factors that influence advanced reasoning in nursing. In addition, it demonstrates how all of these are used in a progressive and integrated fashion in nursing practice.

Learning Activities

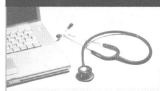

1. Select an interesting issue being debated in one of your nursing classes, apply the Socratic method of investigation through inquiry during the discussion, and then apply how the discussion was different from previous discussions on the topic.

2. Determine how each of the following influenced the discussion in question 1:

Personal	Professional	Others
a. Knowledge	Knowledge	Knowledge
b. Skills	Skills	Skills
c. Values	Values	Values
d. Meanings	Meanings	Meanings
e. Experience	Experience	Experience

3. Using the concepts and propositions associated with question 1, answer the following:

   a. Identify the concepts/variables involved.

   b. Relate the concepts in the form of propositions.

   c. Understand the propositions by describing their significance to you, the class, and nursing.

   d. Explain the significance to others.

   e. Predict what may occur in the future in relationship to the propositions being proposed.

   f. Describe how you would attempt to appropriately influence one or more concepts/variables in an attempt to bring about a desired outcome.

4. Develop a model that demonstrates the above.

References

Alfaro-LeFevre, R. (2004). *Critical thinking and clinical judgment: A practical approach.* St. Louis: Saunders.

American Nurses Association. (2001). *Code of ethics for nurses with interpretive statements.* Washington, DC: Author.

American Nurses Association. (2003). *Nursing's social policy statement* (2nd ed.). Washington, DC: Author.

Bandman, E. L., & Bandman, B. (1988). *Critical thinking in nursing.* Englewood Cliffs, NJ: Prentice-Hall.

Belenky, M. F., Clinchy, B. M., Goldberger, N. R., & Tarule, J. M. (1986). *Women's ways of knowing.* New York: Basic Books.

Benner, P. (1984). *From novice to expert: Excellence and power in clinical nursing practice.* Menlo Park, CA: Addison-Wesley.

Benner, P. (2001). Taking a stand on experiential learning and good practice. *American Journal of Critical Care, 10*(1), 60–62.

Benner, P., Tanner, C. A., & Chesla, C. A. (1996). *Expertise in nursing practice: Caring, clinical judgment, and ethics.* New York: Springer.

Benner, P., & Wrubel, J. (1989). *The primacy of caring: Stress and coping in health and illness.* Menlo Park, CA: Addison-Wesley.

Bevis, E. O. (1997). *Caring, expertise, and fire in the belly.* Unpublished manuscript.

Bevis, E. O., & Watson, J. (1989). *Toward a caring curriculum: A new pedagogy for nursing.* New York: National League for Nursing.

Brookfield, S. D. (1990). *The skillful teacher.* San Francisco: Jossey-Bass.

Brookfield, S. D. (1995). *Becoming a critically reflective teacher.* San Francisco: Jossey-Bass.

Carper, B. A. (1999). Fundamental patterns of knowing in nursing. In J. W. Kenny (Ed.), *Philosophical and theoretical perspectives for advanced nursing practice* (2nd ed., pp. 30–38). London: Jones & Bartlett.

Chinn, P., & Kramer, M. K. (2008). *Integrated theory and knowledge development in nursing* (7th ed.). St. Louis: Mosby.

Chitty, K. K. (2005). *Professional nursing: Concepts & challenges* (4th ed.). St. Louis: Elsevier-Saunders.

Diekelman, N., & Scheckel, M. (2003). Teaching students to apply nursing theories and models: Trying something new. *Journal of Nursing Education, 42*(5), 195–197.

Diestler, S. (2001). *Becoming a critical thinker: A user friendly manual* (3rd ed.). Upper Saddle River, NJ: Prentice Hall.

Dossey, B. (1999). *Florence Nightingale: Mystic, visionary, healer.* Springhouse, PA: Springhouse Corporation.

Dreyfus, H. L. (1980). Holism and hermeneutics. *Review of Metaphysics, 34,* 3–23.

Dreyfus, S. E., & Dreyfus H. L. (1980). *A five-stage model of the mental activities involved in direct skill acquisition.* Unpublished report supported by the Air Force Office of Scientific Research (AFSC), USAF (Contract F49620-79-C-0063). Berkeley, CA: University of California at Berkeley.

Flanagan, J., Baldwin, S., & Clarke, D. (2000). Work-based learning as a means of developing and assessing nursing competence. *Journal of Clinical Nursing, 9*(3), 360–368.

Gilligan, C. (1982). *In a different voice: Psychological theory and women's development.* Cambridge, MA: Harvard University Press.

Hall, L. E. (1955, June). *Quality of nursing care.* Public Health News. Newark, NJ: State Department of Health.

Halpern, D. F., & Riggio, H. R. (2003). *Thinking critically about critical thinking* (4th ed.). Mahwah, NJ: Lawrence Erlbaum.

Henderson, V. (1966). *The nature of nursing.* New York: Macmillan.

Jackson, M., Ignatavicius, D. D., & Case, B. (2006). *Conversation in critical thinking and clinical judgment.* Boston: Jones and Bartlett.

Kenny, J. W. (1999). *Philosophical and theoretical perspectives for advanced nursing practice* (2nd ed.). London: Jones & Bartlett.

Leininger, M. (1991). *Culture care diversity and universality: A theory of nursing.* New York: National League for Nursing.

Martinez de Castillo, S. L. (2003). *Strategies, techniques, & approaches to thinking: Case studies in clinical nursing.* St. Louis: Saunders.

McKean, E. (2005). *The new Oxford American dictionary* (2nd ed.). New York: Oxford University Press.

Meleis, A. (2007). *Theoretical nursing: Development and progress* (4th ed.). Philadelphia: Lippincott Williams & Wilkins.

Milton, C. L. (2005). Symbols and ethics: Integrity and the discipline of nursing. *Nursing Science Quarterly, 18*(3), 211–214. Philadelphia: Lippincott-Raven.

Myers, C., & Jones, T. B. (1993). *Promoting active learning: Strategies for the college classroom.* San Francisco: Jossey-Bass.

Newman, M. (1986). The continuing revolution: A history of nursing science. In N. Chaska (Ed.), *The nursing profession: A time to speak.* New York: McGraw-Hill.

Newman, M., Sime, A. M., & Corcoran-Perry, S. A. (1991). The focus of the discipline of nursing. *Advances in Nursing Science, 14*(1), 1–6.

Nightingale, F. (1859/1992). *Notes on nursing: What it is and what it is not.* (Commemorative ed.). Philadelphia: J. B. Lippincott. [*Notes on nursing* was published originally by Harrison in London, England, in 1859. The above is an unabridged replication of the first American edition, from D. Appleton and Company in 1860.]

Paul, R. W. (1985). The critical thinking movement. *National Forum, LXV*(1), 32.

Penn, B. K. (2008). *Mastering the teaching role: A guide for nurse educators.* Philadelphia: F. A. Davis.

Pesut, D. J., & Herman, J. (1999). *Clinical reasoning: The art and science of critical and creative thinking.* Boston: Delmar.

Polifroni, E. C., & Welch, M. (1999). *Perspectives on philosophy of science in nursing: A historical and contemporary anthology*. Philadelphia: Lippincott Williams & Wilkins.

Reed, P. G., & Shearer, N. B. C. (2009). *Perspectives on nursing theory*. Philadelphia: Wolters Kluwer/Lippincott Williams & Wilkins.

Rubenfeld, M. G., & Scheffer, B. K. (1995). *Critical thinking in nursing: An interactive approach*. Philadelphia: J. B. Lippincott.

Scotto, C. J. (2003). A new view of caring. *Journal of Nursing Education, 42*(7), 289–291.

Shafir, E. (1995). Uncertainty and the difficulty of thinking through disjunctions. In J. Mehler & S. Fanck (Eds.), *Cognition on cognition* (pp. 253–279). Cambridge, MA: MIT Press.

Silva, M. C. (1999). The state of nursing science: Reconceptualizing for the 21st century? *Nursing Science Quarterly, 12*(3), 221–226.

Watson, J. (1979). *Nursing: The philosophy and science of caring*. Boston: Little, Brown. (Second printing, 1985. Boulder, CO: University Press of Colorado.)

Watson, J. (1985). *Nursing: Human science and human care*. Norwalk, CT: Appleton-Century-Crofts. (Second printing, 1988. New York: National League for Nursing.)

Watson, J. (1994). *Applying the art and science of human caring*. New York: National League for Nursing.

Watson, J. (1999). *Postmodern nursing and beyond*. New York: Churchill Livingstone.

Webber, P. B. (2001). Clinical decision-making: Components, processes, and outcomes. In *Teaching clinical decision making in advanced nursing practice* (Monograph, pp. 17–26). Washington, DC: National Organization of Nurse Practitioner Faculties.

Webber, P. B. (2002a). A curriculum framework for nursing. *Journal of Nursing Education, 41*(1), 15–24.

Webber, P. B. (2002b). From novice to expert: Reasoning in theory-based practice. *Enhancing the practice experience*. European Nursing Honor Society, 57–66.

Webber, P. B. (2004). Relationships: The matrix of effectiveness. *Enhancing the practice experience* (2nd Vol.). European Nursing Honor Society.

Webber, P. B. (2008a). Yes, Virginia, nursing does have laws. *Nursing Science Quarterly, 21*(1), 68–73.

Webber, P. B. (2008b). Facilitating critical thinking and effective reasoning. In B. Penn (Ed.), *Mastering the teaching role: A guide for nurse educators* (pp. 361–384). Philadelphia: F. A. Davis.

Wikipedia. (2006). Caduceus. Retrieved May 26, 2008, from http://en.wikipedia.org/wiki/Caduceus

Support Theory

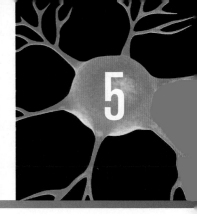

5

Intent: The intent of this chapter is to introduce you to examples of essential theories from the arts, sciences, and humanities that have had, and still have, a significant influence on nursing theory, knowledge, practice, and research.

Key Words/Concepts

adaptation	equifinality	personality
arts	feedback	refreezing
behavior	fields	restraining forces
boundaries	general adaptation syndrome	sciences
change	general system theory	stress
chaos theory	grounded theory	support theory
communication	hierarchy	system
complexity theory	humanities	subsystem
developmental stages	human needs	teleology
discipline-specific theory	interaction	theoretical DNA
driving forces	local adaptation syndrome	unfreezing
entropy	motivation	wholeness
environment	moving	
electronic medical record (EMR)	open system theory	

Introduction

As discussed in earlier chapters, health-related disciplines rely on **discipline-specific theory** to establish boundaries of what is and is not part of their interest and knowledge domain and to provide a rich resource of information to answer questions, solve problems, and explore phenomena associated with improving the health and well-being of the people they serve. However, no one body of discipline-specific theory is completely distinct or isolated from another. This is especially true in nursing. Nursing's body of knowledge contains discipline-specific theory that is enhanced and supported by a wealth of theory from the arts, sciences, humanities, and related disciplines.

A Common Theoretical Base

In health care, discipline-specific theory is intricately connected by a common theoretical foundation based in the **arts, sciences,** and **humanities.** This theoretical foundation is achieved by taking courses in biology, microbiology, immunology, genetics, chemistry, physics, kinesiology, religion, art, music, psychology, growth and development, sociology, nutrition, English, technology, research, and so on. However, different disciplines emphasize some theory more than others based on their particular needs. For example, physical therapy relies more heavily on physics and kinesiology than on microbiology and nutrition, whereas nursing and medicine rely heavily on microbiology and nutrition.

Having a common theoretical base is unifying for all health disciplines in that it provides a basis for understanding when working collaboratively, sharing theory, or conducting interdisciplinary research.

Nursing's Theoretical Roots

The roots of modern nursing began with Florence Nightingale in the mid-1800s with the publication of her classic text, *Notes on Nursing: What It Is and What It Is Not* (Nightingale, 1859/1992). Nightingale's formative years were significantly influenced by her family, as well as the social forces of the time, which were, at minimum, restraining on women (Gill, 2005). During her years of providing care for the sick and injured, especially during the Crimean War, Nightingale made essential observations regarding the relationship between environmental concepts of clean air, clean water, efficient drainage, physical cleanliness, light, warmth, quiet, and nutrition and the mortality of patients under her care. Nightingale was not the first to identify and define these concepts; however, she was the first to identify and describe a significant relationship between these collective concepts and the health and well-being of the sick and injured. In addition, she was the first to organize these concepts into a framework that provided structure for the delivery of nursing care. In other words, Nightingale demonstrated how modern nursing could draw from supporting theory in the arts, sciences, and humanities to help deliver focused and effective nursing care.

Since Nightingale's time, more than 100 years of research, education, and practice have had a dramatic effect on the development, scope, and complexity of nursing theory and supporting theory from the arts, sciences, and humanities. There is a connectedness among these diverse theories that is mutually beneficial and progressive. Just as humans have DNA by which their entire genetic makeup can be identified, most nursing theories have a type of **theoretical DNA** that can be traced back to supporting theory from the arts, sciences, and humanities.

Some authors (Barnum, 1990; Chinn & Kramer, 2008; Fawcett, 2000; Johnson, 1968; Nunnery, 1997) suggest that supporting theory, such as that from the arts, sciences, and humanities, is simply borrowed theory. This implies, however, that nursing can use it whenever it wants and then simply give it back when it is not needed, which is not the case. To assume that nursing theory, practice, and research are isolated from supporting theory and research in the arts, sciences, humanities, and other disciplines is to ignore some of the very roots of nursing's practice and theoretical development. Nursing practice relies heavily on the best theory and research available to help answer questions, solve problems, and explore phenomena in nursing regardless of the discipline from which it comes. Some of these supporting theories are intricately embedded in nursing theory, research, and practice and are as much a part of the established foundation of nursing as is any theory that is considered discipline specific. In fact, most nursing theories are based, in part, on concepts and propositions from supporting theories. However, there is one significant factor that must be considered when using concepts and propositions from **support theory,** and this is how they are operationalized for and used within the context of nursing. Attention must be paid to how these concepts translate across disciplines and the new meanings that evolve once they are integrated into nursing (Chinn & Kramer, 2008; DeKeyser & Medoff-Cooper, 2004; Rodgers & Knafl, 2000;).

Several essential support theories that have contributed and continue to contribute significantly to the development of nursing knowledge and practice are discussed throughout this chapter.

Grand Theories That Support Nursing

Von Bertalanffy's General and Open System Theories

Human beings are a system made up of multiple layers of subsystems, such as cells, organs, and blood. Human beings are also subsystems of families, societies, the human race, the universe, and beyond. Biological systems give you life, and other types of systems influence every minute of your life. In this society, you are surrounded by diverse systems—ecological, family, health care, business, government, computer, transportation, political, university, and so on. What exactly is a system? What is it made up of? How does it work? Are there trillions of separate systems, or is everything from the subatomic parts of an atom to the largest thing in the universe one massive interactive and interdependent system? There are two globally influential theories that help us begin to answer these questions.

General system theory (GST) and **open system theory** (OST) were originally framed in the 1920s by Ludwig von Bertalanffy, a biologist from Vienna. Open system theory, which was generated from GST, was framed in the 1930s and presented to the scientific community at a meeting at the University of Chicago in 1937. However, there was such "bad repute" toward biological theory at the time, because of the human experimentation occurring in Germany prior and during World War II, that GST/OST went unacclaimed and unpublished for decades (von Bertalanffy, 1967, 1968).

By 1947, the war was over and von Bertalanffy felt that there had been enough of a change in the intellectual climate toward biological theory that GST/OST could be safely reintroduced. Once GST/OST was published, it had such a global impact that it started a systems revolution within the scientific community and across all disciplines that is still going on today.

The initial premise of GST was based in the biological sciences and suggested that there was structure, organization, and interdependent function among living things based on systems and subsystems that joined together to form "wholes." The term **system** is operationally defined as connected, interdependent, interacting elements (e.g., components, people) that are hierarchically organized into a single entity for the purpose of maintaining homeostasis and achieving a common goal. A **subsystem** is defined as connected, interdependent, interacting elements that are part of a larger system. Von Bertalanffy (1967) asserted that subcellular components, such as the nucleus, mitochondria, Golgi apparatus, cytoplasm, and so on, are actually separate microscopic systems that joined together to form a larger system called a cell. Cells with similar structure, organization, and function join together and work to form larger, distinct systems called organs (e.g., epithelial cells form skin, smooth muscle cells form the heart, neurons and neuroglia form the nervous system, and so on). These organs then combine and work together to form the even larger system known as the human body. Von Bertalanffy contended that these biological systems and subsystems exist within internal and external environments and work in a specific hierarchical order as a whole to maintain biological homeostasis and achieve the goal of maintaining life. **Wholeness** indicates that although systems and subsystems may be separate in nature, together they constitute a whole that is greater than the sum of the parts. For example, some may view the human body as a compilation of systems or organs; however, to view the human body wholistically (sometimes spelled holistically) is to view it as an integration of body, mind, and spirit.

As GST evolved, von Bertalanffy made additional observations that gave it a new and more global dimension and ultimately formed a new theory. This second theory was OST. Whereas GST focused on the physical aspect of systems, subsystems, and environments, OST focused more on their interactions. **Interaction** is defined as the exchange of energy, information, or matter across systems, subsystems, and environmental boundaries. Von Bertalanffy contended that these interactions were designed to help the whole system, including subsystems and suprasystems, to be self-regulating. He also indicated that these self-regulating interactions were in the form of input, output, and feedback. Input is energy, information, or matter that enters a system from the outside. Output is energy, information, or matter that leaves a system in response to input and either goes to another system or into the environment. **Feedback** is energy, information, or matter that is received by the original sending system from the receiving system or environment in response to input. Because whole systems self-regulate through their interactions, input, and output, feedback leads to changes within the system, subsystem, and environment. For example, in the human body, the endocrine and renal systems help regulate fluid balance. When you become dehydrated, the hypothalamus, which is a subsystem of the endocrine system, senses a change in the osmotic pressure of the serum. It sends a message to the posterior pituitary system to release antidiuretic hormone (ADH), which causes the kidneys to retain sodium and, subsequently, water. When sufficient amounts of sodium and water have been retained by the body, the osmotic pressure within the serum returns to normal. This message is received by the hypothalamus, which in turn tells the posterior pituitary to stop releasing ADH. This is a good example of how interactions help systems, subsystems, and environments to self-regulate.

Environment, defined as the surroundings or conditions in which something exists or operates (McKean, 2005), is an essential concept within OST. Systems and subsystems have both internal and external environments that have the potential to influence and be influenced, just as systems and subsystems have the potential to influence and be influenced by each other. From the biological perspective, everything within the cell membrane is the internal environment, and everything outside the cell membrane is the external environment. Similarly, everything within an organ is part of its internal environment, and everything outside the organ is part of its external environment. In relation to the entire body, internal environment is everything housed within the skin. The external environment is everything outside the body, such as the room a person is in and the characteristics of that room, such as hot or cold, small or large, clean or dirty, and windows or no windows. It could also refer to the characteristics of the earthly environment, such as urban or rural, green as with grass and trees or brown as with desert and cacti, flat or mountainous, rainy or dry, high or low altitude, and polluted or clean. Families, schools, businesses, industries, countries, the earth, the universe, and beyond all have internal and external environments.

Environments can also be nonphysical in nature and include qualitative factors that influence relationships between systems and subsystems, such as values, beliefs, philosophies, behaviors, and attitudes. For example, a nonphysical organizational environment could be described as friendly or unfriendly, caring or uncaring, passive or hostile, rigid or flexible, helpful or not helpful, for profit or not for profit, and professional or unprofessional. Nonphysical environments have the potential to influence and be influenced by systems and subsystems as much as physical environments. Think about your family, school, home, or place of employment and describe their nonphysical environments. See if you can identify each of the systems, subsystems, and environments, as well as what constitutes input, output, and feedback.

With OST, von Bertalanffy needed to be able to differentiate between systems, subsystems, and environments that were interacting, so he used the concept of boundaries. **Boundaries** are traditionally defined as lines, real or imaginary, that separate or enclose. Boundaries sometimes act as stopping points; however, in OST, they are "slowing down" points where input, output, and feedback cross. This type of permeable boundary is similar to that of a semipermeable cell membrane that allows small molecules to pass through but is impermeable to large molecules. An example of this is the blood–brain barrier (BBB). The BBB is not a structure per se but an indication of the permeability of the cells within the brain. These semipermeable cell membranes allow small molecules such as O_2 and CO_2 gases to pass through but are impermeable to large molecules. So the next time you read that a medication does not cross the BBB, you will know that it is the result of the permeability of the cell membranes in relation to the size of the molecules. The concept of semipermeable boundaries could also be applied to an airport security department that closely screens and monitors individuals entering the country for weapons and other undesirable objects, but loosely monitors them as they are leaving. It could also apply to a school of nursing that has admission criteria that applicants must meet prior to being admitted and graduation criteria that they must meet prior to earning a degree.

As previously discussed, von Bertalanffy indicated that a **hierarchy** exists among a system, its subsystems, and its environments that is based on predetermined, directional characteristics (e.g., small to large, high to low, weak to strong, simple to complex, follower to leader, or vice versa). Hierarchy may also be based on organizational functioning. For example, the unit nurse reports to the charge nurse, the charge nurse reports to the supervisor, the supervisor reports to the director of nursing, the director of nursing reports to the chief executive officer, the chief executive officer reports to the board of trustees, and the board of trustees is accountable to the public it serves. Hierarchy is not only important to the structure and function of the systems, subsystems, and environments, but it also frequently sets the path of interaction.

Other essential concepts within OST include teleology, entropy, and equifinality. Yes, the words sound complex, primarily because you may not have been exposed to them previously because they are used mostly in the biological and systems sciences; however, their meanings are simple and apply to nursing as well. **Teleology** is derived from the Latin word *teleologia*, which means end goal (McKean, 2005). When operationally defined for OST, teleology means that the structure, function, and interactions among the systems, subsystems, and their environments are goal directed. For example, the goal of the systems, subsystems, and internal environments of the human body is to support life. In an organization such as the federal government, which is an extremely large system, the goal or intent is to serve the citizens of the United States, and the goal of for-profit corporations is to make money. **Entropy** is derived from the Greek word *entrope*, which means to transform (McKean, 2005). It is operationally defined in OST to mean that systems, their subsystems, and their environments adapt to influences and changing conditions in order to maintain homeostasis. Conditions are constantly changing, and systems, subsystems, and environments are constantly interacting and adapting to these changes in an attempt to maintain homeostasis and achieve their goals. This means that the conditions you start with are not necessarily the conditions you will end with. **Equifinality** is derived from the Latin word *aequi*, which means equal, and *finalis*, which means end (McKean, 2005). It has been operationally defined in OST to indicate that the goal of an open system can be accomplished in more ways than one. In other words, the initial plan does not necessarily dictate how the goal is ultimately achieved, and there are multiple ways to reach the goal.

The following is an example of a nursing situation that represents teleology, entropy, and equifinality.

You have a patient on your unit who developed a decubitus ulcer on his hip after being on the unit for three days. Once the decubitus is discovered, the goal is to get the ulcer to heal. You and the other nurses modified the patient's turning schedule and increased the amount of protein in the patient's diet, among other things, and have made significant progress in getting the ulcer to begin healing; however, the funds available to keep your patient in the hospital have run out, and he has to be discharged. Another way you can keep making progress toward achieving the goal of healing the ulcer is to teach the patient and his family what you were doing, why you were doing it, and how they can do it themselves, as well as how to evaluate progress and potential problems. You could also arrange for the patient and family to have nursing support at home by referring the case to a nursing community case manager. This way, you achieve the goal, but not the way you had originally intended.

Now, go back through this example and identify the systems, subsystems, and environments involved; look at the hierarchy and interactions (input, output, and feedback); identify and describe the environmental influences; and identify examples of teleology, entropy, and equifinality. In doing this, you are integrating all of the concepts of OST in your reasoning. Box 5.1 provides a summary of OST.

GST and OST provided such a revolutionary way of viewing everything in the world that it started a global movement of new thinking. The logical applicability of GST/OST resulted in such rapid acceptance that at the 1954 Annual Meeting of the American Association for the Advancement of Science (AAAS), von Bertalanffy and others proposed the development of a separate society specifically for GST/OST. This society later became known as the Society for General Systems Research, a branch of the AAAS. Ultimately, the society separated from AAAS to form the current International Society for Systems Science (www.isss.org/world/index.php).

Disciplines such as psychology, sociology, business and management, politics, and nursing, to name a few, began to see strong implications for the use of OST. This is demonstrated by the abundance of literature describing the use of OST in various disciplines (Abbey, 1970; Ackoff, 1974; Bourjolly, Hirschman, & Zieber, 2004; de Rosnay, 1979; Duncan, 1994; Dye, 1987; Frey, Sieloff, & Norris, 2002; Gustafasson & Anderson, 2001; Hanney, Gonzalez, & Block, 2008; Katz & Kahn, 1966; King, 1976; Laszlo, 1975; Manning, 1967; Neuman, 1982; Parsons, 1964; Sutherland, 1973; Torsch & Edwards, 1997). Open system theory has now evolved to the point that most of its concepts and propositions are so embedded in so many aspects of our society that they constitute assumptions associated with our daily nonconscious reasoning. In addition, it has

Box 5.1   Summary of von Bertalanffy's Open System Theory

Phenomenon: Systems, subsystems, and environments interact with and influence each other.

Idea: Interactions among systems, subsystems, and their environments are self-regulating and goal directed.

Key Concepts/Internal Variables

- System: connected, interdependent, interacting elements
- Subsystem: a system within a larger system
- Environment: internal and external surroundings of systems and subsystems
- Hierarchy: the ordering or ranking of systems and their subsystems
- Wholeness: systems, subsystems, and environments working as one
- Interaction: the exchange of energy, influence, and matter across a boundary (in the form of input, output, and feedback)
- Teleology: goal-directed interaction
- Entropy: adaptive interaction
- Equifinality: goals accomplished in different ways

Examples of Propositions

1. Systems, subsystems, and their environments form hierarchical wholes that maintain homeostasis and work toward a common goal.
2. Systems, subsystems, and their environments self-regulate based on their interactions.
3. Teleology, entropy, and equifinality are achieved through interactions.

Examples of Assumptions

1. Everyone knows what the goal is.
2. The hierarchical order is actually facilitating the achievement of the goal.
3. The system has the resources for entropy and equifinality if needed.

Examples of External Variables

1. External environments may be influenced by other systems with different goals.
2. Boundaries may be established in such a way as to impede interactions.
3. Input, output, and feedback may be routed to an inappropriate system.

Examples of Facts/Principles/Laws

Fact: Systems, their subsystems, and environments interact.

Principle: Interactions among systems, their subsystems, and environments are self-regulating.

Law: Interactions that influence one aspect of a system have the potential to influence the whole system.

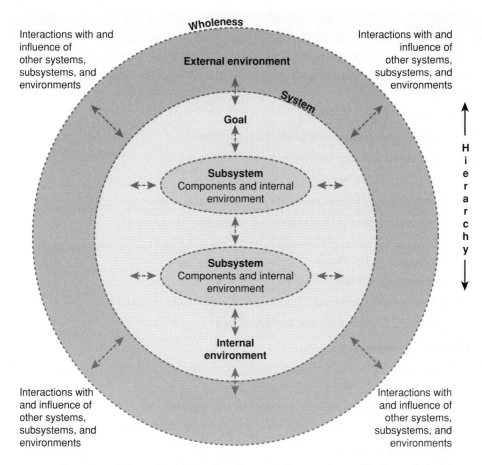

←-➤ = dynamic, multidimensional interaction, demonstrating entropy, equifinality, and teleology.

Figure 5.1 Interaction in open system theory.

stimulated the formation of new system-based theory that now governs most modern thought. Figure 5.1 demonstrates the interaction among the major concepts in OST.

Open System Theory as a Tool for Reasoning

Open system theory is not only a revolutionary theory for analysis, but it is also a dynamic theory for representing the process of reasoning. As you learned in Chapter 4, reasoning is dependent upon the identification of the nature and significance of relationships among concepts. In addition, you have learned that OST emphasizes analysis of the nature and significance of interactions among systems, subsystems, and environments. The common denominator between the two is the analysis of relationships. Both look at the nature and significance of relationships; however, because OST emphasizes multiple levels of relationships, interactions, and influences, it forces you to reason at that pandimensional level as well (Webber, 2008). When attempting to answer a hard question, solve a complex problem, or explore phenomena, it may be helpful to use OST as a framework for your reasoning. Nursing Story 5.1 demonstrates how OST can be applied to reasoning in nursing.

NURSING STORY 5.1

Applying Open System Theory to Reasoning and Decision Making in Nursing

The Patient's Story

Jeff Michaels, RN, is a 34-year-old baccalaureate-prepared staff nurse with 10 years of experience. He works in an open, six-bed pulmonary intensive care unit of a large community-based hospital. While completing his 7:00 am assessment of Sarah Campbell, a 68-year-old white female hospitalized with chronic respiratory failure, he receives a culture report indicating that Mrs. Campbell has a methicillin-resistant *Staphylococcus aureus* (MRSA) infection. He realizes immediately the significance of both the nature of the bacteria that is growing and the fact that Mrs. Campbell has been in an open ward with other patients for several days, which means they also have been exposed. Mr. Michaels immediately places Mrs. Campbell on strict isolation and notifies the following people and departments:

Mrs. Campbell's physician: The physician asks Mr. Michaels to discontinue the methicillin, which is the antibiotic that Mrs. Campbell had been receiving, and to begin administering vancomycin.

The laboratory: Mr. Michaels confirms the MRSA culture and asks the lab to draw a creatinine level before he gives the first dose of vancomycin. This is because Mrs. Campbell also has diminished renal reserve and has been requiring serial creatinine levels to monitor renal function. Mr. Michaels is aware that vancomycin, like methicillin, can be nephrotoxic. He also informs the laboratory that Mrs. Campbell is now on strict isolation and that the technicians will have to use appropriate isolation and universal precautions when drawing blood. Mr. Michaels also lets the laboratory know that Mrs. Campbell was in an open ward and that the other patients may need cultures to screen for MRSA because it is highly communicable, especially in an open unit where there is a lot of interpatient contact.

The nursing supervisor: The nursing supervisor, Jill Courts, will have to make arrangements to transfer Mrs. Campbell out of the open pulmonary unit and into an isolation room. In addition, because she still requires intensive care, Mrs. Courts will have to make arrangements for one-on-one nursing care while Mrs. Campbell is in isolation. Mrs. Courts tells Mr. Michaels that there are no isolation rooms available and that another patient will have to be moved before Mrs. Campbell can be transferred.

(continued)

Applying Open System Theory to Reasoning and Decision Making in Nursing (Continued)

Mrs. Courts also indicates that she has no extra staff available and that a nurse will have to be called in to provide care after Mrs. Campbell moves into the isolation room. It is also possible that Mr. Michaels or another intensive care nurse will be assigned to care for her.

Respiratory care personnel: Mrs. Campbell was hospitalized because of chronic respiratory failure and has been receiving supplemental oxygen and aerosol treatments. The respiratory care department, which is also usually understaffed, will now have to give special consideration to all equipment being used with Mrs. Campbell and follow isolation procedures when providing her treatments.

Epidemiology and infection control services: The epidemiology or infection control department will have to be notified that a patient has acquired MRSA because they are required to keep demographic and statistical information on any nosocomial (hospital-induced) infections, especially those caused by resistant microorganisms. In addition, they may require that a physician specializing in infectious diseases be brought in as a consultant. They are also concerned because the entire hospital has a higher-than-average occurrence of nosocomial MRSA infections.

Environmental services: Environmental services will need to be notified because the unit will have to be thoroughly cleaned after Mrs. Campbell is transferred. In addition, they will need to prepare an isolation room for Mrs. Campbell to move into. Afterward, they will have to follow isolation precautions in cleaning the room.

Dietary services: Dietary services will need to be informed that Mrs. Campbell is on strict isolation and will soon be transferred so that they can make arrangements to provide meals on disposable trays with disposable utensils and deliver them to the appropriate room.

Admissions department: The admissions department will need to be notified when Mrs. Campbell's room changes so that they can change the database in the hospital's computer system and other essential paperwork.

Billing department: The billing department will have to be notified because the charges for the isolation room with one-to-one nursing care are more than the previous room.

(continued)

NURSING STORY 5.1

Applying Open System Theory to Reasoning and Decision Making in Nursing (Continued)

Utilization review: The utilization review department will have to be notified so that they can monitor the evolving diagnosis, the number of patient care days that are needed, and the level of reimbursement from Mrs. Campbell's insurance and Medicare that the hospital can expect to receive.

Family and visitors: Mr. Michaels and other nurses will have to notify the family and visitors of Mrs. Campbell's room change and explain why they have to wear gowns, masks, and gloves when visiting. Although the family and visitors are very concerned and cooperative, Mr. Michaels finds that they frequently forget to put gloves and masks on and to remove them the way he had instructed.

In addition to all of these activities, Mr. Michaels and the other nurses need to follow strict isolation measures while Mrs. Campbell is still in their unit. They must also clean their personal stethoscopes, scissors, and other equipment with an appropriate disinfecting solution and use only equipment that stays at the isolation bedside. Mrs. Campbell is finally transferred to an isolation room at the change of shifts, and Mr. Michaels goes home, where he must wash his uniform and shower to prevent spreading the bacteria to his family.

Applying Open System Theory and Reasoning to the Story

1. What individual and organizational systems, subsystems, and environments can you identify in this story?
2. Identify the multidirectional relationships between the systems, subsystems, and environments and describe the nature and significance of these relationships.
3. Describe the reasoning that Mr. Michaels and others involved with the case are using. How does it influence their decision making?
4. How are Open System Theory and reasoning merging within this story?

Chaos Theory and Complexity Theory

Open system theory has contributed to the development and enhancement of many new theories in such areas as quantum physics, artificial intelligence, cybernetics, and meteorology. In particular, two theories, **chaos theory** and **complexity theory** (which is also known as complex systems theory), are very prominent and need to be introduced. Chaos theory was initially penned by meteorologist Edward Lorenz in 1963. While the term chaos is defined as complete disorder and confusion (McKean, 2005), the term is one, like theory, that has evolved over time to form a type of dichotomy. While the lay person's perception of chaos is that of disorder and

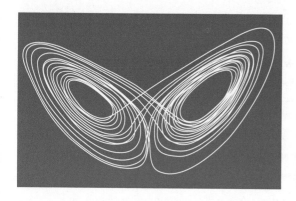

Figure 5.2 The butterfly effect. The Lorenz attractor: Trajectories cycle, apparently at random, around the two lobes.

confusion, the more chaos was studied and researched, the more evident it became that the disorder and confusion was superficial and that at many levels chaos had predictable patterns. Lorenz had been conducting research on making more accurate weather predictions using a set of computerized mathematical equations. The numbers he used in calculating the equations were generally carried out to six decimal places (e.g., 0.506127) and the results printed out in a computer-generated graph. However, one day he calculated the equations using only three decimal places (e.g., 0.506), which was considered an acceptable protocol according to traditional scientific methods. Using this smaller number of decimal places should have provided him with results very similar to those achieved when using six decimal places. However, the results were anything but similar. The mathematical change, which was a miniscule difference of 0.000127, resulted in such a dramatic change in the curves and patterns on the graph that it significantly altered the weather prediction. In fact, the grafted pattern Lorenz identified looked much like a butterfly (Fig. 5.2). Stewart (2002) described the significance of this phenomenon as comparable to a butterfly flapping its wings in Asia and causing a hurricane to form in the Atlantic. Today this phenomenon is commonly known as the butterfly effect. This type of miniscule, yet powerful, source of change is also referred to as behavior that is highly sensitive to slight changes in conditions (McKean, 2005). Systematically speaking, it means that even a miniscule change in the initial conditions can dramatically alter the long-term behavior of a system, its subsystems, and its suprasystems and ultimately influence the ability to achieve desired goals. The ability of chaos theory to demonstrate order and patterning (albeit mathematical) even in the presence of disorder and confusion brings up the likelihood that other phenomena previously thought not to have order or pattern most likely do. For example, consider the human heart that is in ventricular fibrillation (V-fib). The electrocardiogram, at first glance, would show erratic, chaotic electrical waves; however, closer analysis would reveal that even in V-fib there is order and patterning in the electrical activity. Understanding this concept may one day help electrophysiologists prevent V-fib from occurring. One could also consider what happens to the electrical activity of the human brain during chaotic generalized seizures. Scientists have been able to pattern and can now predict these seizures utilizing chaos theory (University of Florida, 1999).

Chaos theory has been significant in helping us understand the potential impact of even the smallest influence or variable on a system, its subsystems, and its environments. Many disciplines, such as economics, medicine, nursing, emergency preparedness, and psychology, are working to understand the applications of chaos theory. Perhaps the most promising aspect of this theory is that if order and pattern can be identified in even the most unlikely phenomenon, then that phenomenon can eventually be recognized and possibly influenced (refer to Fig. 5.2).

Complexity theory, which has elements of OST, chaos theory, and change theory, focuses on complex systems in which subsystems and environments are arranged in structures that exist on many known and unknown levels. It also asserts that these systems are influenced by so many variables and go through so many complex changes that their relationships require multiple levels of explanation (http://www.calresco.org). However, with the emergence of extremely powerful computers, scientists are now able to study not just the large, seemingly more significant variables that influence phenomena, but also the small, seemingly insignificant variables that, previously, would have been ignored. Luckily, Lorenz's work with chaos theory demonstrated what can happen when even the smallest, most seemingly insignificant variables are ignored. Quite simply, complexity theory is changing the way we live. For example, it has already facilitated the mapping of human DNA and the development of artificial intelligence; however, scientists have barely scratched the surface of the theory's potential.

So what do chaos theory and complexity theory mean to you at this point in your education? If you "reduce" the simplest of meanings from both, you can deduce the following: (1) situations are never as simple as they seem—there are always more variables influencing clinical situations than you are aware of and you would be well served to anticipate them and actively look for and think about them when reasoning and making clinical decisions; and (2) the smallest, seemingly insignificant variables can cause dramatic changes, either for the better or for the worse, in almost every situation. Unfortunately, we cannot always predict which it is going to be. Applying this to your practice, you could assume that no patient experience or nursing action is insignificant. It also reinforces the need for you to look for nonobvious patterns in patients, their responses to nursing and medical interventions, and nursing care itself.

The potential impact of chaos and complexity theory on the future of nursing and even global society remains to be seen; however, what we do know is that chaos and complexity theory are to the 21st century what GST and OST were to the 20th century, and their influence is just beginning. "At roughly 40 years of age, complexity theory is still an infant science" (Arora & Barak, 2007).

Selye's Stress Adaptation Theory

Another important support theory for nursing that is rooted in the biological sciences is stress adaptation theory. This theory was first described by Hans Selye (1946), a Canadian physician and scientist known for his research on the various effects of stress on the human body. As a medical student, Selye noticed that many ill patients, regardless of their diagnosis, had a similar pattern of early symptoms, such as loss of energy, loss of appetite, pallor, aches, and pains. Later, as an endocrinologist and researcher, he began studying these early symptoms shared by so many patients and decided to devote his life to investigating this phenomenon, which had been essentially ignored by medicine up to this point. His perseverance led him to believe that this recurring pattern of symptoms was brought on by stress the patients were experiencing. Selye defined **stress** as the body's physiological and psychological response to situations that it considers threatening to its homeostasis or situations that it considers challenging (Selye, 1956, 1978). Examples of physiological threats include the growth of germs associated with an infection and physical trauma. Examples of psychological stress include situations the body may view as challenging, such as sports competitions and work environments where there are high expectations for personal performance. These situations may be real or imagined and may be positive or negative; however, they all result in stress.

Selye (1956, 1978) indicated that when stressed, the body will attempt to adapt its internal environment to maintain homeostasis. **Adaptation** is defined as changes or adjustments made in response to new conditions. Subsumed within Selye's work on stress adaptation are the basic tenets of von Bertalanffy's work, which indicated that systems adapt in order to maintain homeostasis and to achieve a goal. In the biological sense, a body under stress attempts to adapt in such a way that it is able to maintain homeostasis and preserve life. Selye (1956) contended that "Indeed there is perhaps even a certain parallelism between the degree of aliveness and the extent of adaptability in every animal—in every man" (p. 118).

Selye indicated that the body can adapt to stress through a localized response, which he named **local adaptation syndrome** (LAS), or it can have a general response, which he called the **general adaptation syndrome** (GAS). According to Selye (1978), LAS addresses the isolated effects of stress, usually at the point of origin. For example, the redness and swelling at the site of a laceration or infection and the swelling at the site of an insect bite are considered localized responses. General adaptation syndrome addresses the overall systematic effects of stress on the body and is the more serious of the two responses. Local adaptation syndrome and GAS are closely coordinated, and LAS can lead to GAS if it goes unchecked. General adaptation syndrome has three distinct phases: (1) In the alarm phase, the body prepares itself for survival, a time that Cannon (1939) referred to as the fight-or-flight response. During this period, the body's sympathetic or adrenergic nervous system releases stress hormones called catecholamines, specifically norepinephrine and epinephrine, which stimulate the heart rate, raise the blood pressure, and redirect blood flow toward the vital organs, such as the brain and heart. (2) The resistance phase is when the body recognizes the continued threat and "resists" the threat by mobilizing additional physiological responses, such as increasing white blood cells in the presence of infection. (3) The last phase is that of exhaustion, when the cells and organs of the body begin to show deterioration as the body begins to fail in its ability to adapt. Selye contended that failure of the GAS mechanism resulted in the development of "wear-and-tear diseases," such as hypertension and osteoarthritis, which reinforces the assertion that the body's reaction to stress is far more significant than the stressor itself (Selye, 1976).

It is from Selye's work that nursing and medicine learned about the significance of the physiological effects of stress on health. His work also made all health professionals aware that a patient's psychological status directly influences physiological well-being. Today, the acronyms of LAS and GAS are not commonly used, but the thoughts behind them are. For example, the swelling associated with a bee sting or infected insect bite is called a localized response and the whole body effects of chronic stress are called a systemic response. In 1995, the New York Academy of Sciences published what has become the classic comprehensive text on stress, *Stress: Basic Mechanisms and Clinical Implications*, which operationalizes many of the concepts put into motion by Selye (Chrousos et al., 1995). Selye's work, as with von Bertalanffy's work, has evolved to the point that most of his concepts and propositions are so embedded in basic thinking that they constitute assumptions used in everyday reasoning. Box 5.2 provides a summary of Selye's theory.

Since Selye's work began influencing how the world perceived stress and its physical and psychological symptoms, there has been a tremendous amount of research and theory development in related areas, such as stress responses, emotions, relaxation, self-regulation, motivation, coping, psychoneuroimmunology, vulnerability, and resiliency, to name a few. Examples include the type A/type B personality model developed by Friedman and Rosenman (1974). They indicated that personality type influences stress levels as well as the response to stress. Lazarus in 1991 developed a model that integrates emotion into stress and adaptation, called the "cognitive-motivational-relational theory," which asserts that emotions are an integral part of physiological functioning and that stress and coping are a part of emotions. In 2004, Motzer and Hertig

Box 5.2   Summary of Selye's Stress Adaptation Theory

Phenomenon: Patients under stress, regardless of their diagnosis, have a similar pattern of early symptoms.

Idea: Early symptoms are actually a syndrome caused by the body's reaction to stress.

Key Concepts/Internal Variables

- Stress: a syndrome associated with the physiological and psychological responses to situations that the body perceives as threatening
- Adaptation: changes or adjustments made in response to threatening situations in order to maintain homeostasis
- Local adaptation syndrome: isolated effects of stress, usually at the point of origin
- General adaptation syndrome: the body's systematic response to stress, which occurs in three phases:

  Alarm: the first response to a stressor; fight-or-flight response

  Resistance: the period when the body attempts to adapt to the stressor, which may or may not be successful

  Exhaustion: the period when the body's ability to adapt to unrelenting stress is exhausted and begins to fail

Examples of Propositions

1. Stress causes similar physiological and psychological symptoms among individuals.
2. Stress stimulates local or general adaptation as the body tries to maintain homeostasis.
3. Failure of the body to adapt to stress results in exhaustion.

Examples of Assumptions

1. Stress may be good or bad.
2. Prolonged stress is undesirable.
3. Symptoms of stress occur in patterns.

Examples of External Variables

1. Medical treatment can influence some of the effects of the stress (e.g., surgery, antibiotics, antianxiety drugs, exercise).
2. Multiple stressors can exist at the same time.
3. The patient assigns significance to the stress.

Examples of Facts/Principles/Laws

Fact: Prolonged stress leads to physiological and psychological symptoms.

Principle: Physiological and psychological symptoms are proportional to the degree of stress.

Law: Psychological stress adversely influences physiological functioning.

described potential gender differences in the response to physiological and psychological stress. Most recently, the United States Department of Health and Human Services (2008) released a study that built on Selye's work and linked the variability of the stress response to genetics.

Nurses rely heavily on stress-adaptation theory; however, its focus is more on a patient's ability to adapt to stress than on the cellular effects of stress. Nurses use a variety of synonyms to describe a patient's ability to adapt to stress, such as hardiness, resiliency, and vulnerability; however, all of these terms are rooted in stress and the physiological response to it. This is demonstrated by Haase (2004), who proposed a resiliency model demonstrating the process and outcomes associated with quality of life in adolescents with cancer, and by Gillespie, Chaboyer, and Wallis (2008), who determined that resilience against stress is not an inherent characteristic of personality but a process that can be developed at any time during the lifespan based on environment and experience. They also asserted that nursing can use this information to help build resiliency in patients.

The impact of Selye's work has been so significant that the Hans Selye Foundation and the Canadian Institute of Stress (www.stresscanada.org) were formed to help continue this important work. In 1988 the first International Congress on Stress was held in Montreux, Switzerland, and, more recently, in July of 2007, the University of Quebec at Montreal hosted the Hans Selye International Symposium on Stress: Basic Mechanisms and Clinical Implications (www.stress2007. med.ucla.edu/). Events such as these assemble leading authorities on stress from all over the world and provide them with a forum for discussing their research and advances in the field. These events also serve to commemorate the work of Selye and provide a forum for awarding the Hans Selye Award, which is bestowed annually upon a senior scientist who has made significant advances to our understanding of stress. Today, Selye is still the most quoted authority on stress.

Maslow's Theory of Human Motivation and Hierarchy of Basic Human Needs

In 1954, Abraham Maslow, an American psychologist, founded a movement called humanistic psychology, which stressed the importance of studying well-adjusted people, as opposed to emotionally and psychologically disturbed people, who had been the previous focus of psychological research. In doing this, Maslow developed what is now considered to be a grand theory called the theory of human motivation and hierarchy of basic human needs. As part of this theory, Maslow (1943, 1954, 1970) identified a hierarchy of basic **human needs** that he contended is the **motivation** behind **behavior**. These motivational human needs were placed in hierarchical order based on priority, with the greatest priority given to needs required to sustain life, such as air, water, food, safety, and shelter. Subsequent priorities addressed more psychological needs, such as self-esteem, love, and self-fulfillment. Maslow assumed that well-adjusted people meet these needs sequentially and that less well-adjusted people may have needs that overlap (1954, 1970). His work was well received, especially by those in the helping or health-related professions, because it helped to establish priorities of care (Fig. 5.3). See Box 5.3 for a summary of his work.

As with all theory, Maslow's work was highly scrutinized by his peers, and two areas of criticism emerged. The first called into question his methodology, which lacked the scientific and empirical rigidity that most researchers of the time demanded. Maslow was neither random nor diverse in the selection of subjects to be studied, which called the generalizability of his outcomes into question. The second criticism had to do with the progressive nature of the hierarchy. Maslow asserted that human beings had to move up the hierarchy, completely satisfying one need before being able to move to the next, which has also proven not to be accurate. While Maslow attempted to address these concerns (1943, 1954), the criticism has continued. In an analysis of

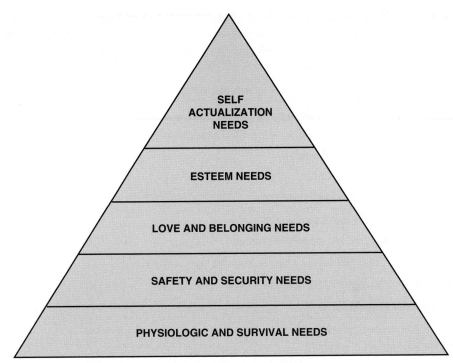

Figure 5.3 Maslow's hierarchy of needs (1954, 1970). (Adapted from www.wikipedia.org/wiki/Maslow's_hierarchy_of_needs. Retrieved April 20, 2008.)

related research, Wahba and Bridgewell (1976) found little evidence for the ranking of needs that Maslow described or even for the existence of a definite hierarchy at all. Despite the criticism, the acceptance of the theory has not been deterred. Maslow's work has enjoyed widespread acceptance despite the lack of empirical evidence to support all aspects of it. There are at least two reasons for this. The first and perhaps most important is the logical adequacy associated with Maslow's basic proposition that needs drive behavior. The second reason is that the nature of Maslow's work is more phenomenological than empirical, which allows for conclusions to be drawn from observation of actual experiences. Maslow, who died in 1970, was very aware of the benefits and limitations of his work and felt that for his theory to reach its own level of self-actu-alization, there needed to be continued research.

Examples of theories stimulated by Maslow's work include Alderfer's (1972) theory of existence, relatedness, and growth, which also focused on needs as the motivation for behavior. Alderfer identified unsatisfied needs as the source of motivation and contended that one could, at times, regress to lower-order needs and that more than one needs could exist at a time. Lawrence and Nohria (2002) built on Maslow's work in presenting a sociobiological theory for business that contends that human beings have four basic needs: acquiring objects and experiences, bonding with others, learning, and defending themselves against harm. Lastly, Lambertus and Yakimchuk (2007) utilized Maslow's hierarchy in examining policing patterns within international contemporary societies. They contend that successful policing patterns are hierarchical and use a need-based approach similar to Maslow's model.

Box 5.3   Summary of Maslow's Theory of Human Motivation and Hierarchy of Basic Human Needs

Phenomenon: Need motivates behavior.

Idea: Needs that motivate behavior are hierarchical in order.

Key Concepts/Internal Variables

- Hierarchy of human needs: those things that humans need to survive and thrive
- Physiological: air, food, water
- Safety: shelter from harm
- Love: affection and acceptance
- Self-esteem: self-worth, positive self-image
- Self-actualization: development of potential
- Motivation: the reason(s) for acting or behaving in a specific way
- Behavior: the way in which one acts

Examples of Propositions

1. Human need motivates behavior.
2. Human needs are ordered according to a survival hierarchy.
3. The majority of needs in one level must be met before moving to the next higher level.

Examples of Assumptions

1. Motivation is hierarchal.
2. Males and females have the same motivation.
3. To be well adjusted, physiological needs must be met first.

Examples of External Variables

1. In the presence of psychological illness, needs may not be recognized.
2. Motivation for one need may outweigh another lower-level need.
3. How well someone is adjusted may depend on how well adjusted those around him or her are.

Examples of Facts/Principles/Laws

Fact: Physiological needs must be met for survival.

Principle: Needs are based on a hierarchy.

Law: Need motivates behavior.

Maslow's work has played a significant role in the development of nursing theory, education, and practice. In the mid-1900s, it was a cornerstone in many nursing curricula. While it plays a smaller role in nursing curricula today, it is still the topic of nursing research (Davis-Sharts, 1986; Leidy, 1994). Maslow's major proposition, that needs motivate behavior, still helps nurses prioritize clinical decision making. For example, nurses make sure that patient's airways are open, that they have adequate food and water, and that their environment is safe. Think about Maslow's hierarchy the next time you are caring for a patient and identify what needs you are helping to meet.

Erikson's Theory of Personality Development

Eric Erikson, a German-born psychoanalyst, identified concepts associated with personality formation that eventually turned into a theory of **personality** development (1963, 1968, 1978). Erikson based many of his ideas on the earlier work of Sigmund Freud, who emphasized the biological and psychological significance of early childhood experiences on later development. In addition to Freud's focus, Erikson included social and cultural experiences as significant to personality development and emphasized that there is continual personality development across the lifespan.

In his theory, Erikson identified eight **developmental stages** that human beings move through. The eight stages are growth categories of infant, toddler, preschool, school, adolescent, young adult, middle adult, and older adult. Each of these categories has a corresponding developmental stage through which an individual progresses, albeit subconsciously, by accomplishing specific tasks associated with each stage. When moving through each stage, the goal is to complete the necessary developmental tasks before moving to the next stage. Erikson felt that if tasks of a particular stage were not accomplished, they would be revisited by the individual during a later stage.

Erikson was just one of several developmental theorists of the time, yet he has had a significant influence on nursing by identifying growth and development stages and emphasizing the importance of achieving growth and development tasks across the lifespan. His work is reflected in the developmental focus of early childhood health assessments and education, as well as in our approach to caring for an ever-growing elderly population. Box 5.4 provides a summary of Erikson's theory.

Contemporaries of Erikson also contributed to the theoretical base of personality development. They included Anna Freud (1974), Sigmund Freud's daughter, who focused on psychoanalysis of children as a tool for helping their parents understand them; Harry Stack Sullivan (1968), who emphasized the importance of children developing a self-concept and awareness of the environmental factors that influence it; Mahler (1975), who studied the evolving independence of an infant; and Lewin (1951), who studied human motivation and change.

Theorists of the late 20th century also built on Erikson's work. Kohlberg (1984) used Erikson's work to develop a theory of moral development that focused on how children learn norms and expectations within their culture and society. Stern (1985), Emde and Buchsbaum (1990), and Rogoff (1990) utilized Erikson's work to explore the impact of the quality of relationship between infant and caregiver, the effects of separation on children and caregivers, and the development of social interactions. On May 13, 1994, following Erikson's death, *The New York Times* stated "His popular recognition reached a peak in the 70's, particularly because of his identification with the development of 'identity crisis,' a term he coined. But his scholarly contributions have assured him of a place of eminence in many disciplines" (NYTimes, 2008, ¶ 7).

Today, there is renewed interest in Erikson's work. For example, in 2007, Burston (2007), in his book *Erik Erikson and the American Psyche: Ego, Ethics, and Evolution*, defended Erikson's work related to basic human nature and the nuclear family and its applicability for contemporary American society against what he considered postmodern attacks.

Communication Theory

If there is one theory that crosses and impacts all disciplines and societies on a minute-by-minute basis, it is communication theory. Communication, as a named discipline, goes back to the days

Box 5.4 Summary of Erikson's Theory of Personality Development

Phenomenon: Human beings have a common pattern of growth and development.

Idea: Patterns of growth and development have distinct levels with specific developmental stages.

Key Concepts/Internal Variables

- Personality development
- Developmental stages

  - Infancy — Trust vs. mistrust
  - Toddler — Autonomy vs. doubt
  - Preschool — Initiative vs. guilt
  - School — Industry vs. inferiority
  - Adolescence — Identity vs. role confusion
  - Young adult — Intimacy vs. isolation
  - Middle adult — Generativity vs. stagnation
  - Older adult — Ego integrity vs. despair

- Progression is based on accomplishing tasks associated with each stage.

Examples of Propositions

1. Humans develop psychologically by progressing through specific developmental stages.
2. Developmental stages correspond with chronological age.
3. The goal of each developmental stage is that the developmental tasks are accomplished prior to moving to the next stage.

Examples of Assumptions

1. Accomplishing developmental tasks in order is necessary for healthy development.
2. If tasks are not accomplished, they will be revisited at future stages.

Examples of External Variables

1. Developmental stage of others, such as parents and siblings.
2. Presence of long-term illness or other chronic stressors.
3. Damage to the neurological system, which can prevent staged development.

Examples of Facts/Principles/Laws

Fact: Human beings progress through specific developmental stages.

Principle: Progression through developmental stages is dependent upon accomplishing developmental tasks.

Law: Developmental stage influences the interactions an individual.

of Socrates, making it the first and most contested of all early sciences and philosophies. Aristotle first attempted to work out a theory of communication in *The Rhetoric*, an ancient Greek treatise, which focused on the art of persuasion (Stanford Encyclopedia of Philosophy, 2002). Since this period, communication has been at the forefront of societal and academic interest, resulting in untold numbers of texts, hundreds of theories, and thousands of academic programs within colleges and universities devoted to different types of communication (public speaking, interpersonal communication, journalism, electronic communication, mass communication, group communication, etc.).

Today, **communication** is defined as exchanging of information (McKean, 2005); however, this definition leaves out an essential concept, which is that communication is often designed to influence. Ruesch, a pioneer in communication theory, asserted that communication consists of any behavior that is used to affect or influence another and that communication may consist of words (written or verbal), gestures, signals, and symbols (Ruesch, 1972). According to Berlo (1960), Ruesch (1972), and Nunnery (1997), key concepts within all types of communication theory include the following:

- An originator, or source of the communication, who establishes the intent of the message
- A sender, who formulates the content and context of the message
- The message itself
- A delivery method
- A receiver, who accepts and interprets the content and context of the message and provides feedback
- Feedback, or a return message to the sender

The sender may be the origin of the communication, or he or she may simply be the vehicle for someone else. However, the sender usually is the one who puts the content of the message into usable form. The sender formulates a message based on his or her knowledge, skills, values, meanings, and experiences (Webber, 2008). The context of the message is the psychological environment in which the message is housed and depends on the attitude of the sender and his or her relationship with the receiver. For example, if someone says "I'm fine" with a smile, you could assume that the meaning of the message is true and the context appropriate. However, if someone says "I'm fine" with a negative tone, a frown, and tightly crossed arms, then the content of the message is in conflict with the context. As you can tell, the content of the message and the context in which it is sent can dramatically influence the meaning and effectiveness of communication. During the process of communicating, receivers become senders when they reply to a received message (feedback), and senders then become receivers. Messages are analyzed and interpreted based on the receiver's knowledge, skill, values, meanings, and experiences, which may or may not be consistent with the sender's. As a result, messages are vulnerable to misinterpretation. In addition, messages may be influenced by external factors during the delivery process, which may also change the message and result in misinterpretation.

In 2007, Owen and Dudley conducted a meta-analysis of communication models and texts in relation to the feedback component of communication. Their study revealed that none of the authors differentiated between informative and reinforcing feedback. Informative feedback enters new information into the message and reinforcing feedback simply supports what has already been said. Both informative and reinforcing feedback result in influencing the listener and, ultimately, communication outcomes. Owen and Dudley (2007) also indicated that while most contemporary authors on communication theory recognize that feedback serves as information and/or reinforcement, this understanding does not get translated into a more useful operational definition of feedback, an issue that may be contributing to communication errors and an overall lack of understanding of the intricacies of the communication process.

Clear, accurate, and timely communication is essential in nursing, medicine, and other health professions. Can you imagine the consequences if (1) the origin of a message concerning a patient's care could not be identified, (2) the sender was in a bad mood, (3) the delivery method was slow, (4) the receiver could not understand the message, and (5) no feedback was given? The next time you are in a clinical situation, observe communication among staff and see if you can identify the essential components of communication and make a determination about the staff's accuracy and effectiveness in communicating with each other. Communication theory is summarized in Box 5.5.

Communication theory has such universal application that multiple disciplines and authors (Berlo, 1960; Leary, 1955; Northhouse & Northhouse, 1992, 2007; Owen & Dudley, 2007; Shannon & Weaver, 1949), including nursing (Arnold, 1995; Balzer-Riley, 1996; Habermas, 1999; Lee, 2007; Mavundla, Poggenpoel, & Gmeiner, 2001; McQuail, 2000; Stuart & Sundeen, 1995), have contributed to the body of knowledge surrounding communication theory. Most literature associated with communication uses the term model in lieu of the term theory. This could be because communication is thought of more as an interactive process that is simply better represented by a model. However, as discussed previously, a model is theory in a picture, and the same components and relationships within a theory (e.g., concepts, propositions, assumptions) can be identified in a model. As a result, models can be just as effective in answering questions, solving problems, and exploring phenomena. They may simply do it in abbreviated form.

Examples of some of the more prominent communication models include the Shannon-Weaver model, which was one of the first models developed and includes the concepts of encoder (sender), message, and decoder (receiver). In addition, Shannon and Weaver introduced a new concept called noise, defined as environmental, psychological, or perceptual interferences that may distort the message (Shannon & Weaver, 1949). The Berlo model, which is also known as the source–message–channel–receiver (SMCR) communication model, indicates that the source of communication depends on the knowledge, culture, and attitude of the sender. The message has structure and is transmitted by sensory pathways (hearing, seeing, touching, smelling, tasting). The receiver then decodes or interprets the message according to his or her own knowledge, culture, and attitude (Berlo, 1960). A model that has specific implications for health professionals is the health communication model, which was developed by Northhouse and Northhouse (1992, 2007). This model builds on previous models; however, its focus is on communication that occurs in health care settings. The model has three basic concepts: relationships, transactions, and contexts. Relationships refer to regular contact among health care professionals, patients, and significant others. All of these individuals have their own knowledge, meanings, culture, and attitude, which influence communication. Transactions include the message as influenced by the relationships and context, which are the settings in which the communication occurs. All three of these concepts have the potential to dramatically influence the effectiveness of communication in health care settings.

In focusing on the dramatic changes in communication theory brought about by the rise of mass media, McQuail (2000) suggests that in our information society, we form a new agenda for the development of new communication theory that includes a focus on social and communication networks, freedom versus containment, interactivity, experience, responsibility, and trust.

The Influence of Computers on Communication Theory

With the onset of the computer age, information technology, and the resulting electronic mail, automated information systems (computers), artificial intelligence systems, and other advances in cybernetics, the way we communicate is changing rapidly. Some of the messages you receive today by phone, computer, or another imaging modality may not come from a person at all, but

Box 5.5   Summary of Communication Theory

Phenomenon: Communication has distinct structure.

Idea: The components of communication are dependent upon one another.

Key Concepts/Internal Variables

- Originator: the source that establishes the intent of the message
- Sender: the one who formulates the content and context of the message
- Message: verbal and nonverbal language, gestures, signals, or symbols that imply specific meaning
- Delivery method: the mechanism by which the message is delivered to the receiver
- Receiver: the one who accepts and interprets the message
- Feedback: a message sent in response to a previous message

Examples of Propositions

1. Messages may move from sender to receiver and back again.
2. Delivery method has the potential to influence the message.
3. Knowledge, skills, values, meanings, and experiences of senders and receivers influence the message.

Examples of Assumptions

1. The message can be understood.
2. The delivery method works for both the sender and receiver.
3. Sender and receiver both want to communicate.

Examples of External Variables

1. Multiple messages may be sent and received at the same time.
2. Messages may be interrupted between sender and receiver.
3. Messages may be misinterpreted.

Examples of Facts/Principles/Laws

Fact: Communication requires both a sender and receiver.

Principle: Direct communication reduces the likelihood of miscommunication.

Law: Communication is vulnerable to misinterpretation and external influences.

rather from a preprogrammed computer that identified you according to your demographic makeup. In the future, you may receive messages by means of virtual reality or an as yet undiscovered imaging or auditory method.

Health care communication is rapidly becoming computer based, with **electronic medical records (EMRs)** providing the fastest-growing mechanism of health care documentation and communication among health care providers, patients, and affiliating organizations (Matheny et al., 2007; McGrath, Arar, & Pugh, 2007). For example, outpatient laboratory orders for a patient being discharged from the hospital may simply be faxed from the patient's hospital room to a laboratory draw station near the patient's home and his prescriptions faxed to his home town pharmacy—all from the computerized EMR used to document his hospital stay. You may have already received a reminder about an upcoming health care appointment via an automated voice messaging system or you may have received results about a recent diagnostic procedure such as a Pap smear, mammogram, or x-ray via e-mail or some other computer-generated system. While this type of communication may save time, energy, and money, we have only begun to see the potential ethical and legal implications of such communication mechanisms and the easy access to confidential records (Curtin, 2005). For example, in the past year, two celebrities have had their medical records illegally accessed and made public by curious health care professionals. Obviously, there are and should be significant consequences for any type of communication that breaches confidentiality; however, the development of appropriate research and theory to support the knowledge, skills, values, meanings, and experiences necessary to protect the public is not keeping up with the speed that communication and information technology is developing.

In the past, nursing school graduates taking the National Council of Licensure Examinations (NCLEX) for registered nurses communicated what they had learned by taking a paper-and-pencil licensing exam; today, they take the exam by computer; and in the not-too-distant future, they will take it by multisensory virtual reality testing, communicating through a multisensory hypothetical reality. This communication revolution has significant implications for nursing theory, research, practice, and education. Therefore, nursing needs to move quickly into research that provides theoretical insight into the significance and impact of these communication changes.

There is no question that electronic communication is here to stay and is desirable in many ways. With instantaneous communication, however, comes instantaneous reactions, which increases efficiency but also takes away the element of controlled restraint and accountability that is associated with person-to-person communication. With today's electronic communication, accountability is at the other end of cyberspace. Nurses who use these methods of instant communication must be aware of the personal and professional pitfalls and work to prevent them. Otherwise, nursing, as well as other disciplines, may be developing a new theory based on the phenomenon of "cyberspace regret."

Lewin's Force Field Analysis Model (Change Theory)

To **change** means to make or become different (McKean, 2005) and may be intentional or haphazard, planned or spontaneous, calm or chaotic, good or bad, or any combination of these characteristics. Many change theories have been developed over the years, including those by Havelock (1971), Rogers and Shoemaker (1971), Rogers (1983), Lippit (1973), and Chin and Benne (1976). However, perhaps the most significant of these theories is Kurt Lewin's force field analysis (or change) theory (1935, 1951). Lewin, a psychologist in the tradition of Erikson and others, studied the motivation and intent behind human behavior. However, he differed from the others in that he not only offered analysis of motivation and associated behavior, but also studied how to improve behavior, especially with regard to bringing about change within systems. His work culminated in the development of a landmark theory of change, which is sometimes referred to as psychological field theory or the force field analysis model. The force field analysis model (FFAM) provides structure for identifying and understanding motivation behind individuals' responses to change and for improving behavior during change. Lewin believed that there were two dynamic and opposing forces, driving and restraining forces, present during any type of change. **Driving forces** move behavior toward a positive state of mind that encourages change. **Restraining forces,** also known as static forces, move behavior toward a negative state of mind that supports maintaining the status quo, thus opposing the change. Driving forces may be the result of external influence on the system (the external environment), or they may be the result of internal influence within the system (internal environment). Remember from the discussion about OST that environment can include beliefs, philosophies, behaviors, and attitudes. Lewin called the environment in which these opposing forces existed and interacted **fields,** hence the name force field analysis. He also indicated that the change process consisted of very specific stages with regard to the behavior of those involved:

- **Unfreezing:** the stage of change where the motivation or need for change becomes apparent. Driving and restraining forces that influence change are identified, and activities are initiated to decrease the restraining forces and increase the driving forces.
- **Moving:** the stage where the details of the change are planned and initiated. This stage involves people who may not have been involved in the decision to make the change and, as a result, may have to be persuaded as to its necessity.
- **Refreezing:** the final stage where changes that have been initiated become integrated, established, and stabilized. Those involved or those influenced by the change become conditioned to it and its consequential effects.

Box 5.6 provides a summary of this model.

Chin and Benne (1976) built on Lewin's work and identified three specific behavioral approaches to planned change. The first approach is called the empirical–rational approach, which is based on the belief that people are rational and that rational people will change if it is in their best interest. The second approach is called normative–re-educative and is based on the assumption that commitment to social and cultural norms motivates people to change. The third, and last, is called the power–coercive approach, which is autocratic in that the power to initiate change is localized with one or more people, and change can be initiated regardless of the social and cultural norms or the ability of people to justify it. Unfortunately, it is the autocratic approach that frequently influences the delivery of patient care as health care systems try to adapt to an environment of scarce financial resources, spiraling costs, and a shortage of nurses. The applicability of FFAM was demonstrated by Schein in 1995 who, as a proponent of Lewin, used it as a model for managing learning (http://www.solonline.org), and by Bozak (2003), who used it in successfully implementing a new nursing information system.

In 2006, Schein not only explored change as a part of learning, but also explored the cultural implication of change. According to Schein, important changes inevitably involve important cultural assumptions and successful change involves the ability to perceive and appreciate the meaning of such assumptions.

"If we want to enrich our understanding of these dynamics further, we also should become cross-cultural learners, to expose ourselves to different cultures and begin to reflect on what it means to try to change cultural assumptions. We may then discover why 'change' is better defined as 'learning,' why cultures change through enlarging and broadening not through destruction of elements, and why the involvement of the learner is so crucial to any kind of planned change or, as we might better conceptualize it—'managed learning'" (Schein, 2006, p. 7).

Never-ending change is a fact of life and, in particular, nursing and health care; therefore, we need to use theories such as Lewin's FFAM to help us learn, change, and improve the provision of nursing care for diverse populations in a constantly and dramatically changing health care environment.

Box 5.6   Summary of Lewin's Force Field Analysis Model

Phenomenon: People respond to change differently.

Idea: Motivation influences an individual's response to change.

Key Concepts/Internal Variables

- Change: to make different
- Motivating forces: factors that influence behavior
- Driving forces: support change
- Restraining forces: resist change
- Field: the environment in which driving and restraining forces are interacting
- Change process: the process of making different
- Unfreezing: the need for change becomes apparent
- Moving: change initiated
- Refreezing: change established

Examples of Propositions

1. Change is influenced by driving and restraining forces.
2. Driving and restraining forces interact within a field.
3. Change is dependent upon unfreezing, moving, and refreezing behaviors.

Examples of Assumptions

1. Change always has opposition.
2. Driving and restraining forces are the only forces influencing change.
3. Moving occurs before refreezing.

Examples of External Variables

1. Motivation may be hidden.
2. Behaviors may be neither driving nor restraining.
3. Change may be ongoing.

Examples of Facts/Principles/Laws

Fact: Response to change is dependent upon motivation.

Principle: Motivation leads to driving or restraining behavior (forces).

Law: For change to occur, driving forces must override restraining forces.

Grounded Theory

A different type of theory that has influenced knowledge development in nursing is **grounded theory.** Grounded theory evolved as the result of an increase in the use of qualitative research methods and is unlike other theories discussed in this chapter in that it is not an organized set of concepts and propositions that support deductive analysis of phenomena. It is a form of qualitative theory that is based on inductive analysis of direct observations of real-time social phenomena. It is included in this chapter because of the tremendous emphasis nursing places on this type of theory. Schreiber and Stern (2001) note that in the last 10 years, grounded theory, or at least what nursing thinks is grounded theory, has become the second most popular method of nursing research.

The idea of grounded theory was originally developed by sociologists Glaser and Strauss (1967). Their goal was to develop new social theory by analyzing and explaining phenomena associated with how people interpret their social structure, processes, and interactions, as well as the language or symbols that they used. Achieving this goal required "real-time" direct observations of the phenomenon as it was occurring; hence, research resulting in grounded theory is based in reality. Glaser and Strauss eventually split and developed different approaches to analyzing data using grounded theory (Walker & Myrick, 2006).

While grounded theory is very popular and has tremendous applicability in nursing because of the social and interpersonal nature of nursing work, it has not been without critics. Dey (1999) indicated that as grounded theory evolved, its authors and other researchers developed differing views about what grounded theory actually was, which has resulted in confusion about its purpose and use as a guiding framework for qualitative research. Schreiber and Stern (2001) caution that nursing's use of grounded theory outreaches its understanding, and they encourage more investigation of exactly what grounded theory is and how it serves as an organizing framework for qualitative research to confirm and ensure its reliability in explaining social and nursing phenomena. Polit and Beck (2008, p. 533) also identified a limitation of qualitative analysis when they stated that grounded theory is guided by "few standardized rules." However, while Burns and Grove (2007) indicate that the quality of the theory being generated through grounded theory is sufficient and that further theory testing is not needed to enhance its usefulness.

As a beginning student of theory, it would be interesting for you to follow the continued development of grounded theory to see if the confusion clears and its reliability and validity are confirmed, especially in light of its current popularity.

Additional Support Theories

There are many more valuable support theories used by nurses and nursing educators. Unfortunately, because of space and time limitations, they cannot all be introduced in this chapter. However, you are strongly encouraged to begin to identify support theories used within your class and clinical activities and to investigate additional theories as you progress through your nursing curriculum. You will find most of them interesting, enjoyable, and, most of all, supportive of your nursing education and practice. Some of these additional theories include advanced systems theory, quantum theory, leadership theory, family theory, conflict resolution theory, teaching–learning theory, cognition theory, organizational theory, and role theory, to name a few. As you progress through your nursing courses, pay attention to new theories that are introduced, and note how they are being integrated into your education and into health care. Ask questions about them, enjoy learning about them, evaluate them, and most importantly, when they consistently and reliably help answer questions, solve problems, and explore nursing phenomena, integrate them into your practice.

The Role of Women in Support Theory Development

Many of the early supporting theories of the time have not been without criticism. Perhaps the most significant criticism was directed toward the research methodology used by Maslow, Freud,

Erikson, Kohlberg, and others, whose research populations were not random or diverse. Specifically, much of theory of the day was developed based on research that used males only, which prompted the logical question as to whether the concepts and propositions identified in these early theories apply to women the same way they do men. Perhaps one of the most classic texts to address the issue of male-oriented research is that of Carol Gilligan. Gilligan was a student of Kohlberg's, the psychologist who developed the theory of moral development. Kohlberg, whose research subjects were male, asserted in his theory that the concept of justice was the primary influence on the development of moral reasoning. Gilligan's complaint, as noted in her popular 1982 text, *In a Different Voice: Psychological Theory and Women's Development,* was not that male-based research leaves women out, but that it is poor psychology to leave out over half of the human race. She proposed an alternative theory to Kohlberg's that asserted that women had their own specific stages of moral development and that caring, as well as justice, plays a role in their moral reasoning. While Gilligan's text was extremely popular, her theory never gained widespread support. However, her work, then and now, demonstrates that research based on one gender is not generalizable to both and that women were and continue to be woefully underrepresented in research guiding the theory and practice of most health professions. Gilligan's work raised awareness of the gender gap in health care and health care research and led to increased scrutiny of previously accepted theories and increased interest in phenomena unique to women. For example, it led to the development of two nationwide research studies, the Nurses' Health Study (NHS) (Speizer, 1976) and the Nurses' Health Study (NHSII) (Willett, 1989). Both studies are longitudinal investigations of risk factors for major chronic diseases in women. The findings of these ongoing studies have resulted in over 700 published articles since 1990 alone and have had a significant impact on improving health care for women (http://www.channing.harvard.edu/nhs). Today, these ongoing studies are a collaborative effort among clinicians, epidemiologists, and statisticians at the Channing Laboratory, which is associated with Harvard Medical School and the Brigham and Women's Hospital; Boston Children's Hospital; Dana Farber Cancer Institute; and Beth Israel Deaconess Medical Center (http://www.channing.harvard.edu/nhs/). As you become sophisticated consumers of research, watch for more findings from these ongoing, history-making studies.

Summary

In the 1950s, schools of nursing were in the process of moving from hospital-based, technical programs to more scholarly, collegiate-based programs. As a result, they were each looking for a framework to guide education and practice. Initially, they tried creating educational frameworks by combining early nursing theory, such as Nightingale's environmental concepts and nursing process, with theories from the arts, sciences, and humanities, such as those of von Bertalanffy, Selye, Maslow, and Erikson. However, these combinations did not adequately reflect what nursing was or did, and as a result, curriculum frameworks built on them did not last. However, these concepts and theories were not abandoned; they were simply put where they belonged, which was as supportive theory within nursing's body of knowledge. They have continued to be scrutinized, replicated, and modified over the years to ensure their continued reliability, validity, and applicability to current times and circumstances. Today, many of the concepts and propositions inherent in these support theories are included in what Benner, Tanner, and Chesla (1996) call nursing's nonconscious clinical judgment. For example, nurses use organizational charts and collaborate with other nurses, units, and organizations every day, but seldom do they say that they are applying von Bertalanffy's OST to do it, nor do they acknowledge Selye when they make assumptions about the effect of stress on a patient's condition. Although these theories may not have been developed by nurses exploring nursing phenomena, they have been integrated and operationalized in nursing in such a way that they now are part of the theoretical DNA that is embedded in nursing's body of knowledge, skills, values, meanings, and experiences. The support theories discussed here, along with other relevant support theories, will continue to be valuable to nursing as long as they continue to contribute to a usable and effective body of knowledge that helps nursing answer questions, solve problems, and explore phenomena. However, nursing and nursing education may need to improve its pedagogy for recognizing and using them (Diekelmann & Scheckel, 2003).

Learning Activities

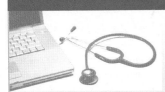

1. Identify theories from the arts, sciences, and humanities courses you have taken and describe how they are influencing your practice.

2. Using open system theory, analyze the origin, pathophysiology, and effects of a common health disorder.

3. Develop a model of your workplace or school using the concepts of open system theory.

4. Analyze how the following theories influenced your most recent clinical experience:

   a. Stress adaptation theory

   b. Theory of human motivation and hierarchy of basic human needs

   c. Theory of personality development

   d. Communication theory

   e. Change theory

References

Abbey, J. C. (1970). General systems theory: A framework for nursing. In J. Smith (Ed.), *Improvement of curricula in schools of nursing through the selection of core concepts of nursing: An interim report.* Boulder, CO: Western Interstate Commission for Higher Education.

Ackoff, R. L. (1974). *Redesigning the future: A systems approach to societal problems.* New York: John Wiley & Sons.

Alderfer, C. (1972). *Existence, relatedness, & growth.* New York: Free Press.

Arnold, E. (1995). Developing therapeutic communication shills in the nurse-client relationship. In E. Arnold & K. U. Boggs (Eds.), *Interpersonal relationship: Professional communication skills for nurses* (2nd ed., pp. 198–232). Philadelphia: W. B. Saunders.

Arora, S., & Barak, B. (2007). Computational complexity: A modern approach. Retrieved April 20, 2008, from http://www.cs.princeton.edu/theory/complexity/introchap.pdf

Balzer-Riley, J. W. (1996). *Communication in nursing* (3rd ed.). St. Louis: Mosby.

Barnum, B. J. S. (1990). *Nursing theory: Analysis, application, evaluation* (3rd ed.). Glenview, IL: Scott, Foresman/Little, Brown.

Benner, P., Tanner, C. A., & Chesla, C. A. (1996). *Expertise in nursing practice: Caring, clinical judgment, and ethics.* New York: Springer.

Berlo, D. K. (1960). *The process of communication: An introduction to theory and practice.* New York: Holt, Rinehart, & Winston.

Bourjolly, J. N., Hirschman, K. B., & Zieber, N. A. (2004). The impact of managed health care in the United States on women with breast cancer and the providers who treat them. *Cancer Nursing, 27*(1), 45–54.

Bozak, M. G. (2003). Using Lewin's force field analysis in implementing a nursing information system. *CIN: Computers, Informatics, Nursing, 21*(2), 80–85.

Burns, N., & Grove, S. K. (2007). *Understanding nursing research: Building an evidenced-based practice.* St. Louis: Saunders.

Burston, D. (2007). *Erik Erikson and the American psyche: Ego, ethics, and evolution.* Lanham, MD, & Toronto: Jason Aronson.

Cannon, W. B. (1939). *The wisdom of the body.* New York: W. W. Norton.

Chin, R., & Benne, K. D. (1976). General strategies for effecting change in human systems. In W. G. Bennis, K. D. Benne, R. Chin, & K. D. Corey (Eds.), *The planning of change* (3rd ed., pp. 22–45). New York: Holt, Rinehart, & Winston.

Chinn, P. L., & Kramer, M. K. (2008). *Integrated theory and knowledge development in nursing* (7th ed.). St. Louis: Mosby.

Chrousos, G. P., McCarty, R., Pacak, K., et al. (1995). Stress: Basic mechanisms and clinical implications. *Annals of the New York Academy of Sciences, 771.*

Curtin, L. (2005). Ethic in informatics: The intersection of nursing, ethics, and information technology. *Nursing Administration Quarterly, 29*(4), 349–352.

Davis-Sharts, J. (1986). An empirical test of Maslow's theory of need hierarchy using hologeistic comparison by statistical sampling. *Advances in Nursing Science, 9*(1), 58–72.

de Rosnay, J. (1979). *The macroscope: A new world scientific system.* New York: Harper & Row.

DeKeyser, F. G., & Medoff-Cooper, B. (2004). A non-theorist's perspective on nursing theory: Issues of the 1990s. In P. G. Reed, N. C. Shearer, & L. H. Nicoll (Eds.), *Perspective on Nursing Theory* (4th ed.). Philadelphia: Lippincott Williams & Wilkins.

Dey, I. (1999). *Grounding grounded theory: Guidelines for qualitative inquiry.* San Deigo: Academic Press.

Diekelmann, N., & Scheckel, M. (2003). Teaching students to apply nursing theories and models: Trying something new. *Journal of Nursing Education, 42*(5), 195–197.

Duncan, K. A. (1994). *Health information and health reform: Understanding the need for a national health information system.* San Francisco: Jossey-Bass.

Dye, T. R. (1987). *Understanding public policy* (7th ed.). Englewood Cliffs, NJ: Prentice-Hall.

Emde, R., & Buchsbaum, H. (1990). "Didn't you hear my mommy?" Autonomy with connectedness in moral self-emergence. In D. Cicchetti & M. Beeghly (Eds.), *The self in transition* (pp. 35–60). Chicago: University of Chicago Press.

Erikson, E. H. (1963). *Childhood and society* (2nd ed.). New York: W. W. Norton.

Erikson, E. H. (1968). *Identity: Youth in crisis.* New York: W. W. Norton.

Erikson, E. H. (1978). *Adulthood.* New York: W. W. Norton.

Fawcett, J. (2000). *Analysis and evaluation of contemporary nursing knowledge: Nursing models and theories.* Philadelphia: F. A. Davis.

Freud, A. (1974). *Normality & pathology in childhood: Assessments of development* (writings of Anna Freud, Vol. 6). Madison, CT: International Universities Press.

Frey, M. A., Sieloff, C. L., & Norris, D. M. (2002). Research issues. King's conceptual system and theory of goal attainment: Past, present, and future. *Nursing Science Quarterly, 15*(2), 107–112.

Friedman, M., & Rosenman, R. H. (1974). *Type A behavior and your heart.* New York: Knopf.

Gill, G. (2005). *Nightingales: The extraordinary upbringing and curious life of Miss Florence Nightingale.* New York: Random House, Inc.

Gillespie, B. M., Chaboyer, W., & Wallis. M. (2008). Development of a theoretically derived model of resilience through concept analysis. *Contemporary Nurse*. Retrieved May 18, 2008, from http://www.contemporarynurse.com /archives/vol/25/issue/1-2/article/2247/ development-of-a-theoretically-derived-model-of

Gilligan, C. (1982). *In a different voice: Psychological theory and women's development.* Cambridge: Harvard University Press.

Glaser, B. G., & Strauss, A. L. (1967). *The discovery of grounded theory: Strategies for qualitative research.* Chicago: Aldine.

Gustafasson, B., & Anderson, L. (2001). The nine-field model for evaluation of theoretical constructs in nursing: Part two: Application of the evaluation model to theory analysis, theory critique, and theory support of the SAUC model. *Theoria Journal of Nursing Theory, 10*(2), 19–38.

Haase, J. (2008). The adolescent resilience model as a guide to interventions. *Journal of Pediatric Oncology, 21*(5), 289–299.

Habermas, J. (1999). Towards a theory of communicative competency. In E. C. Polifroni & M. Welch (Eds.), *Perspectives on philosophy of science in nursing* (pp. 360–370). Philadelphia: Lippincott Williams & Wilkins.

Hanney, S. R., Gonzalez, A., & Block, M. (2008). Why national health research systems matter. *Health Research Policy and Systems, 6*(1). Retrieved May 18, 2008, from http://www. healthpolicysystems.com/search/results.asp? terms=open+system&db=jou10049& searchoperator=and&usq_param1=all &Submitted=Yes

Havelock, R. G. (1971). *Planning for innovation through dissemination and utilization of knowledge.* Ann Arbor: University of Michigan.

Johnson, D. E. (1968). Theory in nursing: Borrowed or unique? *Nursing Research, 17,* 206–209.

Katz, D., & Kahn, R. L. (1966). *The social psychology of organizations.* New York: John Wiley & Sons.

King, I. M. (1976). The health care systems: Nursing intervention sub system. In H. H. Werley, A. Zuzuck, M. N. Zailowski, & A. O. Zagornik (Eds.), *Health research systems: The systems approach* (pp. 51–60). New York: Springer.

King, I. M. (Winter, 1997). King's theory of goal attainment in practice. *Nursing Science Quarterly, 10*(4), 180–185.

Kohlberg, L. (1984). *The philosophy of moral development: Moral stages and the idea of justice.* New York: Harper Collins.

Lambertus, S. L., & Yakimchuk, R. (2007, November). Maslow revisited: Conceptualizing a hierarchy of police approaches. Paper presented at the annual meeting of the American Society of Criminology, Atlanta Marriott Marquis, Atlanta, Georgia. Retrieved May 14, 2008, from http://www.allacademic.com/meta/p200722_ index.html

Laszlo, E. (1975). The meaning and significance of General System Theory. *Behavioral Science, 20,* 9–24.

Lawrence, P. R., & Nohria, N. (2002). *Driven: How human nature shapes our choices.* San Francisco: Jossey Bass.

Lazarus, R. S. (1991). *Emotions and adaptation.* New York: Oxford University Press.

Leary, T. (1955). The theory and measurement of methodology of interpersonal communication. *Psychiatry, 18,* 147–161.

Lee, C. J. (2007). Educational innovations. Academic help seeking: Theory and strategies for nursing faculty. *Journal of Nursing Education, 46*(10, 468–475.

Leidy, N. K. (1994). Operationalizing Maslow's theory: Development and testing of the basic need satisfaction inventory. *Issues in Mental Health Nursing, 15*(3), 277–295.

Lewin, K. (1935). *A dynamic theory of personality.* New York: McGraw-Hill Book Co.

Lewin, K. (1951). *Field theory in social science.* New York: Harper & Row.

Lippit, G. L. (1973). *Visualizing change: Model building and the change process.* La Jolla, CA: University Associates.

Lorenz, E. (1963). Deterministic nonperiodic flow. *Journal of Atmospheric Sciences, 20,* 130–141.

Mahler, M. S. (1975). *The psychological birth of the human infant.* New York: Basic Books.

Manning, H. (1967). *Political realignment: A challenge to thoughtful Canadians.* Toronto: McClelland & Steward.

Maslow, A. H. (1943). A theory of human motivation. *Psychology Review, 50,* 370–396.

Maslow, A. H. (1954). *Motivation and personality.* New York: Harper & Brothers.

Maslow, A. H. (1970). *Motivation and personality* (2nd ed.). New York: Harper & Row.

Matheny, M. E. , Gandhi, T. K., Orav, E. J., et al. (2007). Impact of an automated test results management system on patient's satisfaction about test results communication. *Archives of Intern Medicine, 167*(20), 2233–2239.

Mavundla, T. R., Poggenpoel, M., & Gmeiner, A. (2001). A model of facilitative communication for support of general hospital nurses nursing mentally ill people: Part I: Background, problem statement and research methodology. *Curationis, 24*(1), 7–14.

McGrath, J. M., Arar, N. H., & Pugh, J. A. (2007). The influence of electronic medical record usage on nonverbal communication in the medical interview. *Health Informatics Journal, 13*(2), 105–118.

McKean, E. (2005) *The new Oxford American dictionary* (2nd ed.). New York: Oxford University Press.

McQuail, D. (2000). *McQuail's mass communication theory* (4th ed.). London: Sage Publications.

Motzer, S. A., & Hertig, V. (2004). Stress, stress response and health. *Nursing Clinics of North America, 35*(3), 663–669.

Neuman, B. (1982). *The Neuman systems model: Application to nursing education and practice.* Norwalk, CT: Appleton-Century-Crofts.

Nightingale, F. (1859/1992). *Notes on nursing: What it is and what it is not* (Commemorative ed.). Philadelphia: J. B. Lippincott. [*Notes on nursing* was published originally by Harrison in London, England, in 1859. The above is an unabridged replication of the first American edition, from D. Appleton and Company in 1860.]

Northhouse, P. G., & Northhouse, L. L. (1992). *Health communication strategies for health professionals* (2nd ed.). Norwalk, CT: Appleton & Lange.

Northhouse, P. G. & Northhouse, L. L. (2007). *Health communication strategies for health professionals* (4th ed.). Norwalk, CT: Appleton & Lange.

Nunnery, R. K. (1997). *Advancing your career: Concepts of professional nursing.* Philadelphia: F. A. Davis.

NYTimes. (2008). Erik Erikson, 91, Psychoanalyst Who Reshaped Views of Human Growth, Dies (May 13, 1994). *The New York Times: On the Web*, Books Section. Retrieved May 16, 2008, from http://www.nytimes.com/books/99/08/22/specials/erikson-obit.html

Owen, J. L., & Dudley, J. E. (2007). A content analysis of the treatment of informative and reinforcing feedback in contemporary communication theory textbooks *American Communication Journal, 9*(4). Retrieved May 16, 2007, from ttp://www.acjournal.org/holdings/vol9/winter/articles/treatment.html

Parsons, T. (1964). *Essays in sociological theory.* London: Free Press.

Polit, D. F., & Beck, C. (2008). *Nursing research: Generating and assessing evidence for nursing practice.* Philadelphia: Wolters Kluwer/Lippincott Williams & Wilkins.

Rodgers, B. L., & Knafl, K. A. (2000). *Concept development in nursing: Foundation, techniques, and applications.* Philadelphia: W. B. Saunders.

Rogers, E. M. (1983). *Diffusion of innovations* (3rd ed.). New York: Free Press.

Rogers, E. M., & Shoemaker, F. F. (1971). *Communication of innovations: A cross-cultural approach* (2nd ed.). New York: Free Press.

Rogoff, B. M. (1990). *Apprenticeship in thinking: Cognitive development in social context.* New York: Oxford University Press.

Ruesch, J. (1972). *Disturbed communication: The clinical assessment of normal and pathological communicative behavior.* New York: W. W. Norton.

Schein, E. H. (1995). Kurt Lewin's change theory in the field and in the classroom: Notes toward a model of managed learning. *Reflections: The SoL Journal, 1*(1). Retrieved August 4, 2003, from http://www.sol-ne.org/static/research/workingpapers/10006.html

Schein, E. H. (2006). Kurt Lewin's change theory in the field and in the classroom: Notes toward a model of managed learning. *A2ZPsychology.* Retrieved May 16, 2008, from http://www.a2zpsychology.com/articles/kurt_lewin's_change_theory.htm

Schreiber, R. S., & Stern, P. N. (Eds.). (2001). *Using grounded theory in nursing.* New York: Springer Publishing.

Selye, H. (1946). General adaptation syndrome and diseases of adaptation. *Journal of Clinical Endocrinology, 6,* 117–230.

Selye, H. (1956, 1978). *The stress of life.* New York: McGraw-Hill.

Shannon, C. E., & Weaver, W. (1949). *The mathematical theory of communication.* Urbana, IL: University of Illinois Press.

Speizer, F. (1976). Nurses health study I. Retrieved July 28, 2003, from http://www.channing. Harvard.edu/nhs

Stanford Encyclopedia of Philosophy (2002). Aristotle's Rhetoric. Retrieved November 4, 2008 from www.plato.stanford.edu

Stern, D. N. (1985). *Interpersonal world of the infant: A view from psychoanalysis and development psychology.* New York: Basic Books.

Stewart, I. (2002). *Does God play dice? The mathematics of chaos.* Oxford: Blackwell Publishers.

Stuart, G. W., & Sundeen, S. J. (1995). *Principles and practice of psychiatric nursing* (5th ed.). St. Louis: Mosby.

Sullivan, H. S. (1968). *The interpersonal theory of psychiatry.* New York: W.W. Norton.

Sutherland, J. (1973). *A general systems philosophy for the social and behavioral sciences.* New York: Braziller.

Torsch, V. L., & Edwards, K. A. (1997). World system theory and nursing's decision making position: A qualitative study. *Journal of Theory Construction and Testing, 1*(2), 54–59.

University of Florida. (1999). Chaos' theory empowers VA and University of Florida researchers to predict epileptic seizures. Retrieved April 20, 2008, from http://news.ufl.edu/1999/12/08/epilepti/

U.S. Department of Health and Human Services. (2008). Scientists find genetic factors in stress response variability. *NIH News.* Retrieved May 18, 2008, from http://www.nih.gov/news/health/apr2008/niaaa-02a.htm

von Bertalanffy, L. (1967). *Robots, men and minds: Psychology in the modern world.* New York: Braziller.

von Bertalanffy, L. (1968). *General system theory: Foundations, development, applications.* New York: Braziller.

Wahba, A., & Bridgewell, L. (1976). Maslow reconsidered: A review of research on the need hierarchy theory. *Organizational Behavior and Human Performance, 15,* 212–240.

Walker, D., & Myrick, F. (2006). Grounded theory: An exploration of process and procedure. *Qualitative Health Research, 16*(4), 547–559.

Webber, P. (2008). Facilitating critical thinking and effective reasoning. In B. Penn (Ed.), *Mastering the teaching role: A guide for nursing educators* (pp. 361–384). Philadelphia: F. A. Davis.

Willett, W. (1989). Nurses health study II. Retrieved July 28, 2003, from http://www.channing. Harvard.edu/nhs

Internet Sites

http://www.isss.org

http://www.channing.harvard.edu/nhs

http://www.calresco.org/intro.htm

http://www.stresscanada.org

http://www.sol-ne.org/static/research/workingpapers

Foundations of Nursing Theory

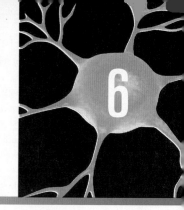

6

Intent: As nursing slowly moved into higher educational institutions, nurse leaders developed graduate education programs, became more research oriented, and developed the base for theory.

Key Words/Concepts		
apprenticeship model	conceptual framework	nurse traineeships
body of knowledge	licensure	

Introduction

You have learned the language and structure of theory; explored relationships between knowledge, theory, and practice; and discovered how to use reasoning in the application of theory and knowledge. You are acquainted with nonnursing theories that support nursing practice and now you are ready to examine the historical background that has led nurses to develop theories.

At the beginning of the 20th century, almost 500 hospitals offered diploma programs in nursing in the United States. Nursing was not taught in colleges or universities as it is today. There were no theoretical foundations, no funds to conduct research studies, no scholarly journals, and no governmental control of the education and practice of nursing. Even in the middle of the 20th century, there were few opportunities for nurses to further their education beyond the hospital-based diploma program.

Nurse leaders in the 1890s faced many challenges in an attempt to regulate the education and practice of nurses. With almost 500 basic nursing programs at the turn of the century, the distance between them and the difficulty of communication and travel hampered nurse leaders from discussing concerns and developing solutions. Nurses began to organize as early as 1893, and the first licensing laws were enacted in three states 10 years later in 1903. The first state to enact a nurse practice act was North Carolina on January 20, 1903, with New York and Virginia to follow later that year (Kalisch & Kalisch, 2004).

Although increasing numbers of states adopted nurse practice legislation, the laws were permissive, not mandatory. Permissive licensure allowed lay and graduate nurses who had not attended or graduated from a school of nursing to practice as long as they did not declare themselves to be licensed (Kalisch & Kalisch, 2004). Mandatory **licensure** in every state did not occur until the 1950s. This was when hospitals owned and ran nursing programs, and physicians taught most of the classes. The emphasis of the program was medical diagnosis, medical treatment, and medical prognosis, rather than nursing care, therapeutic nursing interventions, and nursing science.

This chapter will look at the historical base for nursing theory and examine the direction nursing was taking during the 20th century. States began to define nursing and enact regulations to license nurses. Education slowly moved into the university and graduate programs became available. Private and federal funds became available for basic and advanced education and for research projects, leading to the development of scholarly journals to disseminate the findings of research. As you examine these changes, you will learn how important each step was in the building of a theoretical foundation that enabled nurses to take charge of nursing practice, education, and research.

The Influence of Education on the Growth of Nursing Theory

Basic Nursing Education

The development of basic education for nurses extended over 136 years from the time of the first three Nightingale schools of nursing to today's plethora of doctoral, master's, baccalaureate, and associate degree programs. By 2003, the 2500 hospital diploma programs that existed in 1929 had dwindled to less than 60 (Kalisch & Kalisch, 2004).

In 1873, three 2-year nursing programs opened, the first in May at Bellevue Hospital in New York City, the second in October at New Haven Hospital in Connecticut, and the third in November at Massachusetts General Hospital in Boston. Although other smaller efforts to teach women to be nurses preceded these three, these became known as the first Nightingale programs in the United States. At the time, nursing was considered women's work, so nursing was largely isolated from higher education until well into the 20th century. Students in hospital-based training programs, as they were called, cared for hospitalized patients, most of whom were terminally ill and under the direction of physicians. Students attended lectures generally presented by a physician. Although Florence Nightingale is credited with advising the founders of many schools of nursing in America, there was little resemblance between the early schools and what we currently know and see in universities and colleges across the country (Kalisch & Kalisch, 2004). Every basic nursing program in the United States from 1873 until 1909 was located in a hospital (Roberts, 1963).

The first nursing program located on a university campus was in 1909 at the University of Minnesota, 100 years prior to the third edition of this theory textbook. The University of Minnesota nursing program was offered by the College of Medicine and Surgery and was 3 years in length. However, graduates received a diploma, not a baccalaureate. Within 7 years, 16 colleges and universities had opened programs on university campuses that did award the baccalaureate, although most students completed only the nursing portion of the program (Kalisch & Kalisch, 2004). In the 1920s, both physicians and superintendents of hospital-based nurse training schools insisted that nurses only needed technical skills and manual dexterity, and many expressed concern that nurses were becoming overeducated (Kalisch & Kalisch, 2004). The number of collegiate schools of nursing continued to slowly increase, with only 106, or less than 10%, of the 1148 programs at the midcentury (West & Hawkins, 1955).

Graduate Education

In 1899, Teachers College of Columbia University in New York City offered a 1-year course for graduate nurses, the first such course in the country (Roberts, 1963). The course focused on hospital economics, however, not nursing, which says something about the body of nursing knowledge at the time.

The first master's program in nursing in the United States opened at Teachers College, Columbia University, in the 1920s. During the next 50 years, the number of programs leading to a master's degree in nursing slowly expanded. As late as the mid-1970s, however, there were insufficient numbers of nurses with doctorates and master's degrees to meet the need for faculty in schools of nursing.

In the 1960s, research studies explored the possibility of expanding and extending the nurse's role. In 1965, the term "nurse practitioner" was introduced, demonstrating that nurses could be prepared to provide well-child care and could ultimately serve as a research topic for future changes in the nursing role (Kalisch & Kalisch, 2004). Starting from a 3- to 4-month program in the 1970s, the nurse practitioner movement grew to a popular graduate nursing program, with 20,000 graduates by 1984. As the numbers grew, the length of programs did as well, until many required a program of 54 to 60 credits, more comparable in length to doctoral than to master's programs.

In 1933, Teachers College, Columbia University, established the first doctoral program in nursing in the country, a doctor of education (Matarazzo, 1971). By 1970, there were only five doctoral programs in nursing, including Teachers College. The other programs and the dates they were established were New York University, opening the first PhD program in nursing in 1934; the University of Pittsburgh in 1954; the University of California at San Francisco in 1964; and The Catholic University of America in 1967. Boston University opened a program in 1960, but closed it in 1970 (Kalisch & Kalisch, 2004). The dearth of doctoral programs that emphasized nursing practice, research, theory, and knowledge forced nurses to select disciplines other than nursing, such as education, administration, or one of the sciences. Nurses who completed doctorates generally took positions as college deans or faculty; few were involved in practice or research. In 1969, there were just above 500 nurses in the United States with earned doctoral degrees (American Nurses' Foundation, 1969).

During the 1970s, the nurse faculty members were engaged in feasibility studies, institutional and state approval, and funding efforts to support the need for graduate studies. To support these programs and gain approval from university committees, the faculty was again engrossed in identifying subject matter for master's and doctoral education focusing on the body of nursing knowledge to determine when specific content should be taught.

In 1988, there were 46 doctoral programs, and by 1999, there were 69, with other universities planning and opening programs (Doheny, Cook, & Stopper, 1997; Jones & Lutz, 1999). The distribution of programs improved, and the number increased. In 1999, 35 states offered at least one doctoral program in nursing, with 11 of them offering more than one. Thirty-four, or 49.3%, of the programs were located in 10 states: California, Florida, Georgia, Illinois, New York, Ohio, Pennsylvania, Tennessee, Texas, and Virginia (Jones & Lutz, 1999). The need to expand opportunities for doctoral study continues to be crucial to the advancement of nursing theory and knowledge.

As the number of nurses earning doctorates in nursing increased, so did the demand for nurses holding such degrees. The major focus of the nursing doctorate, as opposed to the non-nursing doctorate, is nursing practice and research. This shift from nursing education and administration to nursing practice and knowledge development provided opportunities for students to conduct their dissertation research on theoretical concepts and propositions, many times based on nursing theories.

As the number of doctoral programs increased, nursing became a more viable discipline in the university community. Faculty qualified for institutional committee assignments and collaborated with faculty in other university disciplines on educational and research projects. This activity called attention to what we now call the body of nursing knowledge and, at the same time, stimulated nurses to examine knowledge and its role in research and practice.

The number of doctoral programs continues to increase. The popular nurse practitioner programs with significant expansion in required credits, some as high as 60, resulted in a call for a doctor of nursing practice (DNP). The DNP is viewed as a practice, not a research, degree. From the time the first DNP program opened in 1975 until 2007, the number of DNP programs has increased to over 50, with even more under development (American Association of Colleges of Nursing, 2007).

Specialized Educational Accreditation for Nursing

As early as the 1920s, nurse leaders began discussing the standards needed for nursing school curricula related to course content, clinical experience, library books, classrooms, and faculty qualifications. In 1952, the National League for Nursing (NLN) was designated as the accrediting agency for baccalaureate and higher education programs in nursing. Separate agencies within the NLN focused on practical nurse, diploma, and associate degree programs. In 1972, the NLN introduced the idea of basing the curriculum on a **conceptual framework,** viewing this action as significant in the growth of nursing theory and knowledge. The conceptual framework provided guidelines for organizing the curriculum, a novel idea at the time that led to widespread discussion and debate. The criterion directed faculty to develop a philosophical plan to govern curricular activities, such as program goals, content selection, and course sequence. A number of schools based the curriculum on a nursing theory.

In 1977, the NLN required the curriculum to be based on a conceptual framework. Faculty recognized the limitations of the framework on educational innovation and creativity and, by 1983, the conceptual framework was deleted from the criteria and the emphasis shifted to a more logically organized and internally consistent nursing curriculum. The deletion of framework-specific criteria after 11 years is a powerful statement about the progress faculty made during this interval to define nursing theory and knowledge and give faculty increased authority to strengthen the body of nursing knowledge.

In 1996, the American Association of Colleges of Nursing proposed a new specialized accrediting agency for baccalaureate and graduate nursing. Today's accreditation standards provide for measuring effectiveness of programs by setting standards and assessing the performance of students and graduates to achieve student learning outcomes (Commission on Collegiate Nursing Education, 2003).

Other Influences on the Growth of Nursing Theory

The growth of nursing theory, knowledge, and research has been influenced by many ideas, events, and activities beyond the control of nurses. A regulatory system for nursing education, individual licensure, and a voluntary accreditation agency for educational programs in nursing were important steps for the acceptance of nursing by higher education. Numerous individuals and a number of events and activities helped lay the groundwork as well. The ideas of Schlotfeldt and Ellis, the allocation of federal funds for nursing, Esther Lucile Brown's study of nursing education, the initiation of scholarly nursing journals, and a variety of other activities contributed to the growth of theory and knowledge.

The Role of Ideas in Nursing Theory

As some nurses began to express ideas about theory and its use in nursing practice, others took important positions related to nursing as a field of study, a body of knowledge, and a nursing science. Rozella M. Schlotfeldt, dean and professor of nursing, and Rosemary Ellis, professor of nursing, both at Case Western Reserve University, Cleveland, were instrumental in establishing nursing as a field of study and inspiring other nurses to focus on the advancement of nursing theory and knowledge.

Although Schlotfeldt developed a health-seeking behavior model that illustrates relationships between nursing practice, research, and education (Fitzpatrick & Whall, 1996), she is better known for her innovative ideas about education and her leadership in theory and knowledge development. She expressed original ideas in the 1960s that are now accepted as fact. These include the need to verify knowledge through systematic inquiry, the effect of systematic inquiry on the knowledge base in nursing, and the use of theory to guide practice (Schlotfeldt, 1960). When you examine these ideas separately, you will recognize how they affect your practice. For example, when you care for a person with diabetes, you become aware that the results of many research studies have verified knowledge about diet, insulin dosage, and the general care of that person. As nurses prepare to care for patients, they recall that systematic inquiry changes what we know about that care. Although nurses' experiences are important, they can never rely solely on their observations and experience.

Several years later, Ellis presented her views on what theory meant and how to determine the significance of a theory (1968). Ellis was quick to identify important, but not necessarily popular, issues, such as the importance of testability in evaluating theory. Ellis believed that the state of knowledge in nursing at that time required more attention to the "elegance and complexity" of the theory than to achieving agreement on precise conceptual definitions for testing. In later writings, Ellis raised the issue of the appropriateness of designing individualized patient care based on the uniqueness of the patient. Her position was in opposition to what were considered at the time the essential theoretical components of theory and science, such as patterning and order (Ellis, 1982; Meleis, 1997). Schlotfeldt and Ellis helped interpret the advancement of nursing as it moved from a group of ideas and principles that served to guide nurses' actions to the use of knowledge verified through clinical research.

Schlotfeldt, Ellis, and the 22 nurse theorists described in the next chapter constitute only a small group of the nurses who contributed to the theoretical and research climate of today. As you continue to study nursing theory, research, and practice, you will hear more about nurses who played critical roles in the advancement of the scholarship of nursing.

Federal Funds

The U.S. Public Health Service (USPHS) was established in 1798, when the country depended upon merchant trade and was concerned about the health of seamen. When the United States became involved in World War I, there was a severe shortage of nurses to care for the wounded. The federal government agreed to support the training of nurses through the establishment of Army schools of nursing outside the university, as well as intensive nursing education for female college graduates in a university setting. This was a milestone in nursing history, but was limited with the beginning of the Great Depression (Miller, 1985).

With today's questions about the viability of the Social Security Administration program, it is interesting to note that the second allocation of federal funds for nursing was included in the first Social Security Act passed in 1935. In addition to establishing retirement benefits for the citizenry, the Act authorized the use of federal funds to develop state and local public health services, including funds to train public health nurses in approved university programs. During the first year of the program, 1000 nurses received funds for education, and between 1936 and 1956, almost 14,000 nurses received government assistance to prepare for public health nursing positions (Kalisch & Kalisch, 2004). These funds made significant contributions to the advancement of nurse education at the time, setting a precedent for nursing as a viable recipient of federal funds. The Bolton Act, which included the Nurse Training Act of 1943, was passed, establishing the U.S. Cadet Nurse Corps; the Corps was terminated at the end of the war.

In 1955, Congress established a Special Nurse Research Fellowship Program in the National Institutes of Health (NIH), Division of Nursing. By 1956, the need for nurses in areas other than public health was evident, and Congress passed the Health Amendments Act, with Title II authorizing traineeships that provided tuition and other financial support to registered nurses for full-time study in administration, supervision, and teaching (Kalisch & Kalisch, 2004). Although the legislation did not specify research training, assisting nurses to obtain advanced degrees was vital to the growth of theory and knowledge. Sixty percent of nurses who received initial traineeships studied at the graduate level, with some earning doctoral degrees (Kalisch & Kalisch, 2004).

In 1964, Congress passed the Nurse Training Act, incorporating many recommendations from the Report of the Surgeon General's Consultant Group on Nursing, including an expanded traineeship program (Kalisch & Kalisch, 2004). The first allocation for traineeships in 1957 was $2 million but increased to more than $7 million by 1964 when the Nurse Training Act replaced it (Kalisch & Kalisch, 2004). By 2004, the traineeship allocation increased to $15 million. Federal **nurse traineeships** are still available for nurses enrolled in master's degree and doctoral programs, now preparing them with a strong **body of knowledge** for future nursing practice and research.

Other important federal legislation includes the Nurse Scientist Graduate Training Grant Program started by the Division of Nursing in the Department of Health, Education, and Welfare in 1962, and the First Nurse Scientist Conference on the Nature of Science in Nursing sponsored by the University of Colorado in 1968.

Although private funds preceded and complemented many of the federal funding programs for nursing, the experience nurses gained from obtaining funds from Congress and the national recognition the nurses received for these efforts helped pave the way for significant funding of nursing education and research today. In addition, each federal program helped nursing improve its standing as a significant player in health care and contributed to the theoretical knowledge base for nursing.

Brown's *Nursing for the Future*

Brown, a sociologist on the research staff of the Russell Sage Foundation, conducted a study for the National Nursing Council in the late 1940s. The purpose of the study was to determine the need for health services in the second half of the 20th century and the role of nurses in filling those needs. Brown made an extensive trip across the United States, visiting some 50 schools of nursing. She looked especially at who was responsible for organizing, administering, and financing professional schools of nursing. The report of her research, *Nursing for the Future*, was published in 1948.

At the time of Brown's study, 1214 schools of nursing submitted statistical data. Only 77, or less than 6.5%, of the schools were located in universities or colleges, and eight of those offered diploma, not baccalaureate, programs (Brown, 1948). In her report, Brown recommended that nursing education be established in colleges and universities and that it adopt policies, customs, and traditions of recognized academic disciplines, including the preparation and status of faculty that would make them comparable to faculty in the rest of the institution (Brown, 1948). Such a move was crucial to the future development of a theoretical body of nursing knowledge, because, at the time, most intellectual work was being developed in colleges and universities. Later, academic health centers, medical centers, and free-standing hospitals began to recognize the need for research departments and the scientific staff to run them. As you study about nurses who made very significant contributions to theory and knowledge in Chapter 7, you will realize that almost all were associated with institutions of higher education.

Unfortunately, interest in changing nursing education was more academic than pragmatic at the time. While many programs accepted Brown's advice and moved to higher education campuses, they remained academically and socially isolated from other academic disciplines. Few nursing programs changed their approach to education, knowledge, or theory from the prevailing **apprenticeship model** in the community hospitals. Faculty defended the way they were doing things and requested exemptions under the assumption that nursing was unique and different from other fields of study. Nevertheless, Brown's work made an important statement for establishing nursing within the intellectual climate of the university and laid the groundwork for developing a body of knowledge comparable to other disciplines in the university.

Many similar studies about nursing education were conducted that contributed to the advancement of theory and knowledge, including Goldmark's *Nursing and Nursing Education in the United States* (1923) and Bridgeman's *Collegiate Education for Nursing* (1953). Each study made important recommendations, some similar to those in *Nursing for the Future,* but the timing of the Brown report, just before the midcentury, was pivotal.

Scholarly Journals

The establishment of scholarly journals played another important role in the advancement of scholarship and research in nursing. *Nursing Research*, the first journal of its kind, began publication in 1952. The first issue was sent to 8500 subscribers around the world and became an indicator of the growth of research development. The content in early issues of the journal tended to focus on areas that were suitable for nursing research, emphasizing the need to support research. Eleven years later, in 1963, *Nursing Science* was established and doubled the opportunity for nurse researchers to share intellectual ideas and research. Additional opportunities became available when *The Journal of Nursing Scholarship* began publishing in 1967, known as *IMAGE* from 1967 to 2000; *The Canadian Journal of Nursing Research* in 1968; *The Western Journal of Nursing Research* in 1979; and *Research in Nursing & Health* and *Advances in Nursing Science* in 1978. In 1988, *Nursing Science Quarterly* was established as the only journal dedicated to nursing theory, requiring that every article be linked to nursing theory (Cody, 1997). These eight journals, some of which are published in Canada and London, disseminate important perspectives and positions about theory, research, and knowledge. Early issues of these peer-reviewed journals provide an excellent history of nursing theory and research.

Some journals, dedicated to the publication of nursing research, increased the number of issues per year, whereas others expanded the number of pages. International and interdisciplinary journals dedicated to research were published, including *Scholarly Inquiry for Nursing Practice: An International Journal, Applied Nursing Research, Journal of Advanced Nursing, Qualitative Inquiry,* and *Qualitative Health Research.*

In addition to increasing the number of journals dedicated to nursing research, nurses became more sophisticated in reading and using research and about the need to publish research results. Faculty also recognized that articles in refereed journals carried more weight when they were being considered for promotion, tenure, or appointment to a new position. A "refereed journal" relies on peers of the author who are experts in the field to review manuscripts and recommend whether or not they should be published. The author and the peer reviewers remain anonymous during the process.

Research Activities

In 1948, after the end of World War II, the federal government, with the encouragement of professional organizations, established the Division of Nursing Resources in the USPHS, to collect data about nursing needs and resources (Gortner, 2000). In 1950, the American Nurses Association began a 5-year study of the functions, standards, and qualifications for practice, ending with the publication of *Twenty Thousand Nurses Tell Their Story* (Hughes, Hughes, & Deutscher, 1958). The findings of these studies focused on nurses, rather than on nursing practice. Although they added little to the body of knowledge expected of a scientific discipline, nurses gained experience about research and its conduct.

In the fall of 1955, Lucille Petry Leone, the chief nurse officer and assistant surgeon general of the USPHS, proposed the types of studies needed in nursing. These included the nursing care most essential to patient recovery, the nature of therapeutic relationships, and the analysis and optimal use of nursing skills in patient care (Leone, 1955). That same year, she was able to obtain one half million dollars for nursing grants from the NIH. About the same time, Virginia Henderson, one of the theorists you will study later, pointed out that nurses were studied 10 times more frequently than nursing practice. She suggested that an essential characteristic of a profession was studying the methodology of the subject matter, not the people comprising the profession. Finally, in 1962, federal funds were given to university schools of nursing for nurse scientist graduate training grants. Many institutions receiving the awards were those who offered doctoral programs in nursing, including Boston University; University of California at San Francisco; Teachers College, Columbia University; the University of Pittsburgh; and New York University.

When Congress approved the National Center for Nursing Research (NCNR) as a unit in the NIH in 1986, overriding a presidential veto, nursing achieved a new level of acceptance among health care professions. The elevation of the NCNR to the National Institute of Nursing Research (NINR) in 1993 and a budget increase from $16.2 million in 1986 to $50 million in 1994 (Polit & Hungler, 1995), $90 million in 2000, $134.76 million in 2004, and over $136 million in 2006 encouraged nursing faculty and doctoral students to focus on studying nursing knowledge, especially as it relates to improved practice. The inclusion of a nursing institute in the NIH stimulated a new commitment to knowledge development.

Periodically, the NINR brings prominent nurse scientists together to set priorities for funding nursing research. The first Conference on Research Priorities (CORP #1) established the following funding priorities through 1994:

- Prevention and care of low–birth-weight infants
- Prevention and care of human immunodeficiency virus (HIV)-positive patients, partners, and families
- Long-term care
- Symptom management
- Nursing information systems
- Health promotion
- Technology dependence across the lifespan

CORP #2 was held in 1993 and set new priorities for a portion of the NINR's funding between 1995 and 1999. The short period of time between the two conferences reflects the increasing level of emphasis on nursing research and knowledge development. The list of priorities in CORP #2 illustrates not only changes in the content of funded projects, but also an increased emphasis on nursing practice over what was evident in the initial list of priorities:

- Developing and testing community-based nursing models
- Assessing effectiveness of nursing interventions in HIV/acquired immunodeficiency syndrome (AIDS)
- Developing and testing approaches to remediate cognitive impairment
- Testing interventions for coping with chronic illness
- Identifying biobehavioral factors and testing interventions to promote immunocompetence

The intent in both conferences was to designate areas that would be considered most important for funding rather than to eliminate pertinent proposals (Polit & Hungler, 1995). After CORP #2, the NINR adjusted its planning process to use more groups that were smaller and involved systematic reviews of its research programs. The NINR selected the following areas of science to support in 2000 to 2004:

- End-of-life/palliative care
- Chronic illness
- Quality of life and quality of care
- Health promotion and disease prevention
- Symptom management
- Telehealth intervention and monitoring
- Implications of genetic advances
- Cultural and ethnic health

A review of the NINR web site in September 2003 confirmed that the NINR continues to work with panels of nursing research experts. These panels have identified Research Themes for the Future. The five themes are:

1. Changing lifestyle behaviors for better health
2. Managing the effects of chronic illness to improve health and quality of life
   a. Health care practice
   b. Self-management of chronic illness symptoms and treatment
   c. Informal (family) caregiving

3. Identifying effective strategies to reduce health disparities

4. Harnessing advanced technologies to serve human needs

5. Enhancing the end-of-life experience for patients and their families

In October 2006, on the 20th anniversary of its inception, the director of the NINR, Dr. Patricia A. Grady, RN, presented a strategic plan that identified four strategies to advance the science of clinical research in nursing:

1. Integrating biology and behavior for better health

2. Adopting, adapting, and generating new technologies for better health care

3. Improving methods for future scientific discoveries

4. Developing scientists for today and tomorrow

Within these objectives, there are the following areas of research emphasis:

1. Promoting health and preventing illness

2. Improving quality of life

3. Eliminating health disparities

4. Setting directions for end-of-life research

All of the above themes encompass certain cross-cutting issues, such as ethnic, cultural, and gender differences; family and community considerations; a multidisciplinary approach; biological and behavioral mechanisms and interrelationships; and cost effectiveness (Grady, 2003). Research funded by the NINR plays a central role in the development of theory and the body of nursing knowledge that nurses use in their practice.

Summary

Scholarly advances during the last 50 to 60 years have enabled the development of theory and the body of nursing knowledge. These advances are closely related. For example, without theory and research, there would be no justification for establishing scholarly journals to publish theories and research results. Without these journals, the dissemination of this crucial information would be impossible. Without a theoretical base in nursing, it is unlikely that nursing would have become an institute in the NIH. At the same time, research that is conducted to verify or disprove theories is enhanced by funding provided by the NINR. The ultimate outcome of theory development and research is the development of a body of nursing knowledge that is used to improve nursing practice.

Only a few individuals, events, and activities that affected theory development are identified in this chapter, but many others played important roles as well. You can pick up an early copy of a scholarly journal and read about ideas that are now apparent in practice. You can explore the influence of wars and economic depressions on nursing progress, for example, or the effects that medical technology and the expansion of the drug industry have had on nursing practice. As the impact of theoretical frameworks and research findings is recognized in daily nursing practice, nurses are more attentive to whether current theories are suitable either as distinct individual theories or as an integrated group. Theory and research are the base for improving practice. They will become increasingly important as you continue on your way to become a nurse.

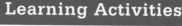

Learning Activities

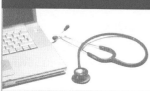

1. A look back and a look forward: Select one of the following events and explore its influence on nursing knowledge. How did it affect nursing practice as you know it?

   a. World War I

   b. The Great Depression of 1929

   c. World War II

   d. The discovery of antibiotics

   e. Your selection of a significant societal event

2. How has scholarship changed? Select one of the scholarly journals mentioned in the chapter. Review an issue from the first year of publication as well as one from the most recent.

   a. What are the major differences in the topics of articles?

   b. What are the educational credentials of the authors?

   c. How many authors received federal funds or private funding for their project?

   d. Identify differences in the language that is used, if any.

   e. Compare the references to theories in the early issue with those in the recent issue.

References

American Nurses' Foundation. (1969). Directory of nurses with earned doctoral degrees. New York City: Author.

Bridgeman, M. (1953). *Collegiate education for nursing*. New York: Russell Sage Foundation.

Brown, E. L. (1948). *Nursing for the future*. New York: Russell Sage Foundation.

Cody, W. K. (1997). Of tombstones, milestones, and gemstones: A retrospective and prospective on nursing theory. *Nursing Science Quarterly, 10,* 3–5.

Commission on Collegiate Nursing Education. (2003, October). *Standards for accreditation of baccalaureate and graduate nursing programs*. Washington, DC: Author.

Doheny, M. O., Cook, C. B., & Stopper, M. C. (1997). *The discipline of nursing: An introduction*. Stamford, CT: Appleton & Lange.

Ellis, R. (1968). Characteristics of significant theories. *Nursing Research, 17,* 217–222.

Ellis, R. (1982). Conceptual issues in nursing. *Nursing Outlook, 30,* 406–410.

Fitzpatrick, J. J., & Whall, A. L. (1996). *Conceptual models of nursing: Analysis and application*. Stamford, CT: Appleton & Lange.

Goldmark, J. C. (1923). *Nursing and nursing education in the United States*. New York: Macmillan.

Gortner, S. R. (2000). Knowledge development in nursing: Our historical roots and future opportunities. *Nursing Outlook, 48*(2), 60–67.

Grady, P. A. (2003). National Institute of Nursing Research, National Institutes of Health. Bethesda, MD: National Institute of Nursing Research, National Institutes of Health. http://www.nih.gov/ninr.htm.

Grady, P. A. (2006). National Institute of Nursing Research, National Institutes of Health. Changing Practice: Changing Lives. Bethesda, MD: National Institute of Nursing Research, National Institutes of Health. http://www.nih.gov/ninr.htm.

Hughes, E. C., Hughes, H. M., & Deutscher, I. (1958). *Twenty thousand nurses tell their story.* Philadelphia: J. B. Lippincott.

Jones, K. D., & Lutz, K. F. (1999). Selecting doctoral programs in nursing: Resources for students and faculty. *Journal of Professional Nursing, 15,* 245–252.

Kalisch, P. A., & Kalisch, B. J. (2004). *American nursing: A history* (4th ed.). Philadelphia: J. B. Lippincott.

Leone, L. P. (1955). The ingredients of research. *Nursing Research, 4,* 51.

Matarazzo, J. D. (1971). Perspective. In *Future directions of doctoral education for nurses: Report of a conference* (pp. 49–105). Bethesda, MD, January 20, 1971 (DHEW Publication No. [NIH] 72–82). Washington, DC: U.S. Government Printing Office.

Meleis, A. I. (1997). *Theoretical nursing: Development and progress.* Philadelphia: Lippincott-Raven.

Miller, P. G. (1985). The Nurse Training Act: A historical perspective. *Advances in Nursing Science, 7,* 47–65.

Polit, D., & Hungler, B. (1995). *Nursing research: Principles and methods.* Philadelphia: J. B. Lippincott.

Roberts, M. M. (1963). *American nursing: History and interpretation.* New York: Macmillan.

Schlotfeldt, R. M. (1960). Reflections on nursing research. *American Journal of Nursing, 60*(4), 492–494.

West, M., & Hawkins, C. (1955). *Nursing schools at the mid-century.* New York: National Committee for the Improvement of Nursing Services.

Nursing Theory

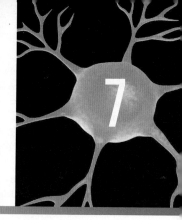

7

Intent: Key elements of the major nursing theorists and their theories from the United States and Canada are presented with examples of how they influenced nursing education, practice, and research. The chapter ends with a look at nursing theory around the globe.

Key Words/Concepts
academic degree
emerita/emeritus
honorary degree

Introduction

The definition of nursing is important to the discussion of nursing theory. Nurses have tried for decades to define nursing, going back to Florence Nightingale's book, *Notes on Nursing: What It Is and What It Is Not* (1859/1992). Numerous nursing scholars (Henderson, 1966; Meleis, 1997; Newman, Sime, & Corcoran-Perry, 1991) and organizations such as the American Nurses Association (1980, 1995) and others have tried to capture the essence of nursing into one global definition. Henderson's definition has probably been distributed to more countries than any other definition, but still there are differences of opinion.

The intent of this book is not to debate what nursing is or is not. However, for the purpose of identifying nursing theory and knowledge, the following definition is used: Nursing is the desire, intent, and obligation to apply knowledge, skills, values, meanings, and experience for, with, or on behalf of those requiring or requesting assistance to achieve and maintain their desired state of health and wellness.

Nurse Theorists and Theories

In this chapter, you will learn about Florence Nightingale, 17 nursing theorists from the United States, 4 from Canada, and the theories they developed. You will meet each theorist, gain basic knowledge about the theory, and learn about the impact it has had on nursing practice, education, and research. Theories selected for inclusion have significance for today's nurse. You may be interested in investigating theories not included, such as Lydia E. Hall, the core, care, and cure model; Joyce Travelbee, the human-to-human relationship model; Ernestine Wiedenbach, the helping art of clinical nursing (or the prescriptive theory of nursing); and Josephine G. Paterson and Loretta T. Zderad, humanistic nursing theory. The chapter ends with a sampling of theories from other countries: Greece, Japan, Sweden, England, and Scotland.

Theories in the book are presented in chronological order beginning with Florence Nightingale in the mid-1800s and then, by decade, from 1950 to 2000. In most cases, these theories are designated by the date they were first published. Although a nurse who is developing a theory may talk to colleagues or distribute written material about that theory, until it is published in nursing literature it is not available for discussion and critique and, therefore, not included here. A few exceptions are made; for example, Dorothy Johnson did most of her theoretical work on the behavioral system model in nursing in the 1950s and 1960s but did not publish the theory until 1980. She presented her theory at a conference at Vanderbilt University in 1968, however, so her model is included with those of the 1960s.

The presentation about each theorist and theory follows a similar pattern. First, personal, educational, and experiential information about the theorist is summarized in a box; a picture of the theorist is also included when available. The theory is described in understandable language to the extent possible and focuses on basic information related to the development of the theory and its meaning. Building blocks related to each theory are summarized, including phenomenon, idea, concepts/internal variables, and examples of propositions, assumptions, and external variables. In selected theories, especially those based on support theories or with a history of repetitive theory testing, examples of facts, principles, and laws are included. Finally, the influence that the theory has had on nursing education, practice, and research is explored, including an example of evidence-based practice, when available.

Florence Nightingale and Nursing Theory

Nursing theory started with Nightingale in 1859, then took a "leave of absence" for almost 100 years, and gradually returned in the middle of the 20th century. When Nightingale wrote *Notes on Nursing: What It Is and What It Is Not* (1859/1992), she was treading new ground. She used data she had collected over a number of years, especially during the Crimean War, to describe her ideas about health care. *Notes on Nursing* was written for "health nurses," those who were responsible for the health of families, as opposed to "proper nurses," who took care of the sick. Both "health" and "proper" nurses were responsible for "putting the patient in the best condition for nature to act upon him" (Nightingale, 1859/1992, p. 133). Nightingale makes a convincing argument for nurses to improve the patient's environment as a means to better health. *Notes on Nursing* was used at the St. Thomas's Hospital school for nurses, has been translated into at least nine languages, and is reprinted periodically. Almost every nursing theorist since Nightingale recognizes the importance of her ideas and beliefs.

Florence Nightingale: Environmental Model—1859
The Theorist

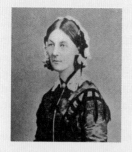

FLORENCE NIGHTINGALE was born May 12, 1820, in Florence, Italy, and died August 13, 1910, in London. At the age of 17 she felt "called" to fill a useful role in society, and at the age of 31, she decided that call was to be a nurse. In 1853 she trained as a nurse in a hospital at Kaiserworth, Germany, for 3 months, the only nurse training she ever had. In November 1854, she led a group of trained nurses to the Crimean War, returning in April 1856. She wrote *Notes on Nursing: What It Is and What It Is Not* in 1859 (reprint in 1992). She wrote 15,000 to 20,000 letters, many in historical collections, and 200 books, reports, and pamphlets on nursing, hospitals, and the military. She was known as the "lady with the lamp" and the "mother of modern nursing."

Florence Nightingale was born while her parents and sister, her only sibling, were on a lengthy tour of Europe. The family returned to England a year later where they had two large estates, Lea Hurst and Embley Park; the latter was located near London, affording the Nightingale daughters opportunities to be involved in the social, intellectual, and political life of England. Nightingale and her sister received a classical education in mathematics, statistics, philosophy, history, economics, government, and several languages. They were extremely well educated compared to other women of their time.

In 1854, the British Secretary of War, who was a family friend, asked her to lead a group of trained nurses to the Crimean War in Scutari, Turkey, to care for wounded soldiers. She arrived at the Barracks Hospital with 38 nurses on November 5, 1854, where she dealt with significant environmental and health problems, such as contamination, filth, poor nutrition, and little or no sanitation (Woodham-Smith, 1951). During her first 2 months, the death rate was 420 soldiers per 1000. Nightingale was able to decrease the rate to 22 soldiers per 1000 within 6 months after her arrival (Woodham-Smith, 1951). She worked at Scutari for 21 months, which was the longest continuous period of time she practiced nursing during her lifetime. During this time, she demonstrated that order, independence, power, and environmental control would reduce mortality and morbidity (Reed & Zurakowski, 1996). Nightingale returned to London in August 1856 when the war ended, ignoring the grand welcome that was planned in her honor.

Nightingale is most famous as the "mother of modern nursing," although mathematicians recognize her as a "passionate statistician." In 1860, she presented a proposed hospital statistical system to the International Statistical Conference. The proposed system contained the idea that is now the widely accepted international classification of diseases (Thompson, 1980). It also referred to concepts that we now call utilization review, evaluation of medical care, cost effectiveness, and cost benefit. Nightingale received many distinguished awards during her lifetime. She was elected a fellow of the Royal Statistical Society in 1858 for her contributions to the British Army and comparative hospital statistics, was made an honorary member of the American Statistical Association in 1874, and in 1907 became the first woman to receive the Order of Merit (Agnew, 1958).

During the last 50 years of her life, Nightingale lived in a small London apartment because of self-described poor health. She seldom left her rooms, but invited friends and colleagues to come and discuss the issues of the day with her. She received groups of physicians and others who were interested in opening schools of nursing in the Nightingale tradition. Although we call the first three nursing schools in America the "Nightingale schools," she never visited this country.

The Theory

Nightingale's environmental model focuses on the manipulation of physical and social factors that affect health and illness. Her book, *Notes on Nursing: What It Is and What It Is Not,* was written for women who were responsible for the health of their family members, not necessarily just for nurses (Nightingale, 1859/1992). Nightingale viewed the physical environment as a critical component in both health and illness. She enumerated the 12 concepts described in Box 7.1. The concepts are consistent with mid-19th-century health care when surgery was performed on kitchen tables in many instances and hospitals primarily housed the dying and the homeless. After almost 150 years, however, Nightingale's model continues to be relevant to the contemporary health care environment, setting a standard for prevention of illness and restoration of health.

Examining the 12 concepts in the model provides an excellent illustration of the current usefulness of the model. Five concepts focus on cleanliness: health of houses, bed and bedding, cleanliness of rooms and walls, personal cleanliness, and ventilation or air purity, which is consistent with cleanliness. Standards in the mid-1800s for water and sanitation were essentially absent, and laundering clothes and changing linens occurred infrequently. Even today, in the 21st century, cleanliness continues to be a problem, and the infection rate for hospitalized individuals is a vital concern. Nightingale shunned germ theory, antiseptics, and bacteriology. She disregarded Lister's theoretical postulations about disease and germs and was deeply concerned that antiseptics and disinfectants would lead people to ignore the importance of good sanitation and cleanliness (Reed & Zurakowski, 1996).

Nightingale also spoke to the social or esthetic environment. She emphasized the importance of a variety of colors and forms in the patient's room to encourage recovery. She cautioned nurses about using "chattering hopes and advices" that would give patients false hope, while she encouraged the use of good news. The environmental model also considers the family, their economic status, and management of the household: These continue to be concerns of nurses today as they work with patients and their families in the community. The remaining concepts—light, noise, nutrition, and observation of the sick—continue to be important to current nursing practice as well. Her ideas about food presentation and variety, assisting patients who were unable to feed themselves, and allowing patients to select foods they liked to eat continue to be important.

Box 7.1   Summary of Nightingale's Environment Model

Phenomenon: The environment affects health and illness of individuals and families.

Idea: Nurses influence health through management of the environment.

Key Concepts/Internal Variables: (Tomey & Allgood, 2002)

Health of Houses: Maintain cleanliness of the house, including pure air, pure water, efficient drainage, cleanliness, and light.

Ventilation and Warming: Maintain ventilation and patient warmth. Measure body temperature through palpation of extremities.

Light: Light, especially direct sunlight and its purifying effect, is second only to fresh air.

Noise: Avoid unnecessary noise, including physical activities that could jar the patient.

Variety: Use various colors, flowers or plants, and rotating paintings in the environment.

Bed and Bedding: Place the bed so patient can see out a window; regularly change damp, soiled, and wrinkled linens.

Cleanliness of Rooms and Walls: A clean room is a healthy room; remove dust with a damp cloth, and have floors that are easily cleaned, with no carpets.

Personal Cleanliness: Frequent, even daily, bathing of patients (which was not the norm at the time). Nurses should also practice cleanliness and wash their hands frequently.

Nutrition and Taking Food: Provide a variety of foods, follow the meal schedule, offer frequent small servings, and ensure the patient avoids distractions while eating.

"Chattering Hopes and Advices": Avoid talking about patients in their presence or giving them false hope. Give good news as appropriate.

Observations of the Sick: Obtain complete and accurate information using precise, specific, and individualized questions.

Social Considerations: Encourage the social environment of the patient, including family, friends, and other visitors.

Examples of Propositions

Managing the environment improves the health of the patient.

Maintaining a clean house, room, bedding, and clothes aids recovery.

Good news has a positive effect on patient recovery.

Examples of Assumptions

Cleanliness of the environment affects the health of individuals and families.

Noise is harmful to patients.

Disease is nature's way to remedy the patient's condition.

Examples of External Variables

Contact with pathological disease-causing organisms

Isolation from other patients

Use of antiseptics

Examples of Facts, Principles, and Laws

Fact: A clean, aesthetic environment aids recovery.

Principle: Cleanliness aids in maintaining health.

Law: The environment influences health.

Nightingale believed that the nurse's function was to put the patient in the best possible situation for nature to act on him or her, projecting the idea that nursing is based on knowledge of people and their surroundings.

Although Nightingale probably would not have described her work as theoretical, today's nurses recognize it as an embryonic scholarly effort that continues to give credibility to basic ideas about nursing theory. Box 7.1 summarizes the basic features of the model.

Influence of Nightingale's Environmental Model

Education. Nightingale's influence on nursing education, practice, and research continues to be significant and her work is included in major discussions of nursing knowledge and health. The establishment of St. Thomas's Hospital school for nurses, the hands-on role of nurses in the military and in hospitals, and her extensive work in the Crimean War attest to the influence of the environmental model on education.

While Nightingale was in Scutari, friends and colleagues established the Nightingale Fund, using it to support the school for nurses (Reed & Zurakowski, 1996). The 15 probationer nurses who comprised the first class received a year's training primarily on the hospital wards with an occasional lecture by a physician; their names were placed on a register as certified nurses when they completed the year. Initially, Nightingale exercised little direct oversight of the school, although at times she was involved with selecting those to be admitted and monitored their progress. By 1872, she was devoting more attention to the school, its students, and its graduates, and she sent groups of trained nurses out with a mentor to establish training schools in other countries, patterned after the Nightingale model. One group traveled as far as Australia to establish a school. Even though she never traveled to other countries, she advised physicians and hospital board members who traveled to London to meet with her in her London apartment. When the first three schools for nurses opened in America in 1873, they were patterned after the Nightingale school model.

Practice. The central focus of Nightingale's *Notes on Nursing* (1859/1992) is practice. She viewed the roles of the nurse and the physician as separate, with the nurse focused on the person and the physician on the person's illness; some of that is still evident today. The centerpiece of the Nightingale school for nurses was practice and, eventually, *Notes on Nursing*, with its practice approach, was used as a textbook. A review of the concepts in her model illustrates that many of her concerns continue to be addressed by nurses in the 21st century.

Research. Nightingale's model preceded the development of theory and research in nursing and is not in testable form by today's standards. Although her theory has not generated the amount of research expected of more modern theories, Nightingale's intellectual curiosity, observational skills, meticulous collection and analysis of data, background in statistics, and gift of written and oral communication made her ultimately prepared to conduct the research that was a high point of her life (Palmer, 1977). The death statistics related to her work in Scutari reported earlier not only illustrate her ability to collect data, but also demonstrate her ability to use those findings to achieve a higher level of care.

An example of the continuing interest in research of Nightingale's model relates to the concept of noise. Pope (1995) conducted a literature review of the significance of noise on patients, examining the effect of noise and the human voice, the effect of music, cultural interpretations, and the implications of noise on the environment. Pope concludes with suggestions for continued research about the noise and unnecessary sounds in the patient environment.

Theory Development in the 1950s

Almost 100 years after Nightingale's *Notes on Nursing* (1859/1992) was first published and 80 years after the first schools of nursing were established in the United States, Hildegard Peplau and Virginia Henderson gave theory an intellectual boost. They set the stage for discussion and debate about nursing knowledge that affected the development of theory in the second half of the 20th century. The theories to be discussed next are:

- Hildegard Peplau's interpersonal relations in nursing in 1952
- Virginia Henderson's definition of nursing in 1956

Hildegard E. Peplau: Interpersonal Relations in Nursing—1952
The Theorist

HILDEGARD E. PEPLAU was born September 1, 1909, in Reading, Pennsylvania, and died March 17, 1999, in California at the age of 89. She graduated from a diploma program in Pottstown, Pennsylvania, and received a bachelor of arts in interpersonal psychology from Bennington College, Vermont, in 1943. She did her graduate work at Teachers College, Columbia University, New York City and earned a master of arts in psychiatric nursing in 1947 and a doctor of education (EdD) in curriculum development in 1953. She worked as a school nurse, a private duty nurse, and a general duty hospital nurse. She served in the U.S. Army Nurse Corps, conducted research, taught nursing, and had a private practice in psychiatric nursing. She taught the first graduate psychiatric course at Columbia University, taught at Rutger's University for 24 years, and retired as professor emeritus in 1974. She served as a visiting professor in the United States as well as abroad.

Hildegard E. Peplau provided a strong role model for nurse educators and scholars beginning in the 1950s by developing and publishing nursing's first theoretical model. Peplau's book, *Interpersonal Relations in Nursing* (1952), broke the scholarship barrier in nursing when she described the therapeutic relationship between nurse and patient as part of the domain of nursing knowledge. Although the book was completed in 1948, it was not published until 1952 because Peplau did not have a physician coauthor or an endorsement from one, which was essential at the time. Peplau's book was the first nursing textbook of its kind.

Peplau was recognized nationally and internationally as a leader in nursing and health care. She served as president and executive director of the American Nurses Association and as a board member of the International Council of Nursing. She received honorary degrees from a number of universities, as well as numerous national and international awards. An **honorary degree** is conferred by a college or university in recognition of distinguished activity, as opposed to an **academic degree,** which is conferred for completing a program of study. She was highly revered by psychiatric nurses around the world, who regarded her as the "mother of psychiatric nursing." Her impact on nursing was much broader than psychiatric nursing, however, and she had a vast following of nurses who were dedicated to her work as an educator, practitioner, scholar, and professional.

The Theory

Peplau's interpersonal relations in nursing theory changed the role of the patient from being the object of the nurse's action to being a partner with the nurse (Box 7.2). Prior to publication of *Interpersonal Relations in Nursing* (Peplau, 1952), the idea of a theory had not been used in nursing.

Peplau's work was grounded in interpersonal theory as well as clinical events that she and her students experienced. She recognized the influence of the work from other disciplines on her theory, such as Harry Slack Sullivan's interpersonal development model and his theory of personality development, and George Hubert Mead's symbolism in communication. After Peplau formulated the idea of a nurse–patient relationship, other nurse scholars built on it until it became an accepted standard in nursing practice. As the first modern nurse theorist, Peplau set high standards for the development of a scientific body of knowledge.

Peplau described the phases of the nurse–patient relationship process, the role for the nurse, and methods for studying nursing. Initially, she identified four steps: orientation, identification, exploitation, and resolution. In 1997, she combined identification and exploitation, resulting in three phases: orientation, working, and termination (Peplau, 1997). The roles that the nurse serves during these phases include:

- Teacher: imports knowledge about a need or problem
- Resource: provides information to understand a problem
- Counselor: helps recognize, face, accept, and resolve a problem
- Leader: initiates and maintains group goals through interaction
- Technical expert: provides physical care through clinical skills
- Surrogate: takes the place of another

In the orientation phase, the nurse works as a counselor to establish a relationship with the patient and family in order to identify actual or potential problems. When a problem is clarified, the nurse becomes a teacher and resource, providing information about the problem and the types of assistance that are available. At the end of the orientation phase, the nurse and patient are no longer strangers and are ready to move to the working phase and begin to resolve problems that have been identified.

As the nurse, patient, and family move into the working phase, the nurse–patient partnership is clarified to determine the level of dependence/independence the patient expects from the nurse. For example, one patient may expect to be completely dependent on the nurse, another may wish to share decision making with the nurse, and a third may seek complete independence, only conferring with the nurse at times of need. As a partner and leader, the nurse is responsible for supporting the patient's ability to deal with the problem and for setting goals to increase independence.

Box 7.2   Summary of Peplau's Interpersonal Relations in Nursing Theory

Phenomenon: Interpersonal relations occur between a nurse and patient.

Idea: A nurse's interaction with a patient is goal directed.

Key Concepts/Internal Variables

Interpersonal relationship: The interaction between two or more individuals with a common goal. In nursing, the goal provides the incentive for a therapeutic process in which the nurse and patient respect each other as individuals and partners.

Interpersonal process: The development of an interpersonal relationship between nurse and patient occurs in three phases that overlap, interrelate, and vary in duration as the process evolves: orientation, working, and termination.

Examples of Propositions

Every professional contact between a nurse and patient is an opportunity for education.

The nurse assists the patient to advance through the interpersonal process.

The nurse—patient relationship evolves through stages based on the needs of the patient and family.

Examples of Assumptions

Both nurse and patient want an interpersonal relationship.

The nurse's experience reflects on the therapeutic relationship with the patient.

Interpersonal relations between nurse and patient enhance maturity and self-fulfillment of both.

Examples of External Variables (Peplau, 1997)

Conflicting self-interests of the nurse or patient

Competition between family members

Expectations of behavioral changes

Examples of Facts, Principles, and Laws

Fact: Interpersonal interactions occur in phases.

Principle: Interactions between a nurse and patient are intentional and designed to be therapeutic.

Law: Therapeutic interactions influence patient outcomes.

The termination phase occurs when the problem is resolved and the patient needs to regain independence from the nurse. The nurse may serve as the leader in the evaluation of the process and may assist the patient to set new goals for achieving independence.

Influence of Peplau's Interpersonal Relations in Nursing Theory

Education. Peplau, the first nurse to publish a theory, had a significant impact on nursing education. Her ideas stemmed in part from her work with students and spoke to the need for a more organized approach in the identification of nursing subject matter. She was a pioneer in developing both undergraduate and graduate courses, as well as programs in psychiatric nursing that were based on her theory. She was the stimulus for other theorists, such as Henderson, Johnson, and King, to become involved in identifying nursing subject matter for other fields of nursing.

Practice. From the start, Peplau's theory had a significant influence on psychiatric nursing practice, giving it structure, foundation, and visibility. Her work on nurse–patient relationships is so well known globally that it continues to influence how nursing practice is viewed and evaluated. Peplau derived her theory from an empirical study of human interaction that enabled nurses to assist patients in understanding their responses to experiences related to health and illness (1997).

Research. Peplau's theory influenced the study of clinical practice and the development of a body of nursing knowledge (Sills, 1977). Her contributions to research provided the means to evaluate and validate the theory (Tomey & Alligood, 2002). At first, research generated by the theory focused on patient problems, then shifted to a social system point of view within a broader set of relationships between patients, families, groups, and communities. More recently, theoretical concepts, such as pattern recognition, formed the basis for study of the theory. For example, Beeber and Caldwell (1996) studied clinical data from six young women who were depressed. The analysis revealed that there were patterns in the interactions between nurses and their clients. In another study, the importance of the interpersonal therapeutic relationship in 10 nurse–patient dyads was reaffirmed in nursing practice (Forchuk, Westwell, et al., 1998).

Virginia Avenal Henderson: Definition of Nursing—1955
The Theorist

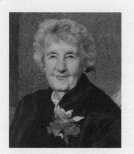

VIRGINIA HENDERSON was born November 30, 1897, in Kansas City, Missouri, but spent her formative years in Virginia. In 1924, she graduated from the Army School of Nursing in Washington, DC, a federally funded diploma program to help overcome a nurse shortage. She earned a bachelor's degree in 1932 and a master's degree in 1934 from Teachers College, Columbia University, in New York City. She served on the faculty there from 1934 to 1948. Over the ensuing years, she revised the *Textbook of the Principles and Practice of Nursing* and published *Basic Principles of Nursing* for the International Council of Nursing (ICN). She then joined the Yale University faculty, where she continued to work after she retired until her death on March 9, 1996, at the age of 98.

Henderson is known around the world for creating a definition of nursing. She also made major contributions to the development of nursing knowledge through a study of nursing research. Beginning in 1953, Henderson and social anthropologist Leo Simmons conducted a survey and assessment of nursing research for the National Committee for the Improvement of Nursing Services under the auspices of Yale University School of Nursing. Their work resulted in two significant publications, *Nursing Research: A Survey and Assessment* (Simmons & Henderson, 1964) and *Nursing Studies Index,* four volumes (Henderson, 1963, 1966, 1970, 1972). Throughout her lifetime, Henderson continued to support theory development and expansion of the scientific knowledge base in nursing, as well as education of future generations of nurse scientists. Her impact on nursing has been so great that she has been called "the first lady of nursing," "the first truly international nurse," "the mother of modern nursing," and the "American Florence Nightingale." In her eulogy, she was called "the best loved nurse in the world."

Henderson, as so many other nurse theorists did, gave a lifetime to nursing and made enormous contributions as a nurse, teacher, author, researcher, and friend of students, faculty, and practicing nurses. Many undergraduate and graduate students and faculty were honored to be in her presence and to have the opportunity to meet and talk with her. Henderson entered the Connecticut Hospice in Bradford about 7 weeks before her death; she died on March 19, 1996, in a peaceful death.

The Theory

During the revision of the *Textbook of the Principles and Practice of Nursing* (Harmer & Henderson, 1955), Henderson was concerned that state nurse practice acts at the time did not clearly define what nursing was and therefore failed to ensure safe and competent care to the public. Although she did not believe that her work was a theory, the profession recognized that her definition of nursing helped identify the boundaries of the nursing knowledge domain.

Henderson's definition, with some minor changes, reads:

> *The unique function of the nurse is to assist the individual, sick or well, in the performance of those activities contributing to health, or its recovery, or to a peaceful death that he would perform unaided if he had the necessary strength, will, or knowledge and to do this in such a way as to help him gain independence as rapidly as possible (Henderson, 1966, p. 15).*

The definition of nursing was subsequently adopted by the ICN and distributed around the world. When Henderson (1966) updated *The Nature of Nursing: A Definition and Its Implications for Practice, Research, and Education,* she stressed the function of the nurse more than she did originally (Henderson, 1991). Henderson identified 14 components of nursing consistent with the definition. These components are listed in the summary as major concepts/internal variables.

Henderson's definition of nursing carries significant meaning for theory development, its concepts, and its propositions. In addition, elements of Henderson's definition are evident in Orem's self-care deficit theory, Orlando's nursing process model, and other nursing theories (see Box 7.3).

Influence of Henderson's Definition of Nursing

Education. As a teacher, Henderson knew that a nursing curriculum needed to be organized around the unique functions of the nurse, whether they were related to activities of daily living, recovery from disease, or achieving a peaceful death. Her definition of nursing was instrumental in stimulating curricular change in North America and around the world. When the ICN translated her definition into 25 or more languages for global distribution, the impact on nursing education was significant.

Henderson supported Nightingale's idea of a different role for the nurse and physician when she stated that the nursing "curriculum must be organized around the nurse's major functions rather than that of the physician" (Henderson, 1964, p. 67). She advocated the development of assessment skills, independent professional practice, and moving schools of nursing from hospitals to colleges and universities (Henderson, 1964). These were some of the topics she loved to discuss with students and faculty on campuses around the country and around the world; they responded to her with enthusiasm and challenging ideas.

Practice. Henderson wrote three classics: *Basic Principles of Nursing Care* (1960), *The Nature of Nursing* (1966), and *Principles and Practice of Nursing* (1978). These books have been best-sellers around the world. They offer nurses an understandable and coherent philosophy, as well as a syn-

Box 7.3 Summary of Henderson's Definition of Nursing

Phenomenon: A definition of nursing will help set boundaries for nursing knowledge.

Idea: A definition of nursing functions protects the safety of the public.

Key Concepts/Internal Variables (14 components of nursing)

Breathe normally.

Eat and drink adequately.

Eliminate body wastes.

Move and maintain desirable postures.

Sleep and rest.

Select suitable clothing—dress and undress.

Maintain normal body temperature by adjusting clothing and modifying the environment.

Keep the body clean and well groomed and protect the integument.

Avoid dangers in the environment and avoid injuring others.

Communicate with others in expressing emotions, needs, fears, or opinions.

Worship according to one's faith.

Work in such a way that there is a sense of accomplishment.

Play or participate in various forms of recreation.

Learn, discover, or satisfy the curiosity that leads to normal development and health using available health facilities.

Examples of Propositions

The definition of nursing guides nursing action.

Nursing actions are designed to protect the public.

The components of nursing establish areas of competency for nurses.

Examples of Assumptions

The goal of nursing is to maintain or restore the individual's independence to satisfy fundamental needs.

Nurses help patients meet specific needs that others cannot provide.

One definition can describe what nursing is and does.

Examples of Facts, Principles, and Laws

Fact: Nursing assists patients in different ways.

Principles: The components of nursing guide nursing action.

Law: Nursing is defined by what it does.

thesis of research and expert opinion about current nursing practice and individualized care. Henderson's definition of nursing affected not only education, but also nursing practice. Read the definition again and try to match some of your recent clinical activities with her succinct statements.

Research. Henderson's definition of nursing carries significant meaning for theory development and its concepts and propositions. As you study other nursing theories, you will find evidence of Henderson's definition in many of them. While the definition may not lend itself to the type of research expected of grand theories, Henderson was an avid supporter of nursing research. As indicated earlier and deserves repeating, for 19 years, she worked with Leo Simmons on the four-volume *Nursing Studies Index* (1963, 1966, 1970, 1972), reading and indexing all the related nursing literature published in English between 1890 and 1959—all done by one nurse and a colleague. It demonstrates her commitment to developing a body of nursing knowledge and strengthening the ability of nurses to conduct research and improve the practice of nursing.

Sigma Theta Tau International Library, located in Indianapolis, was named in honor of Virginia Henderson, because of her devoted advocacy of nursing libraries around the world. Her desire was to provide practicing nurses with current resources wherever they were.

Nursing Theory in the 1960s

Peplau and Henderson provided the foundation and possibly the stimulus for theory development in the 1960s and later. The basis of the theories identified with the 1960s are diverse: a typology of 21 nursing problems, a nursing process discipline theory, conservation of energy in health care, and a behavioral model based on general systems theory. The theories from the 1960s to be discussed are:

- Faye Abdellah's patient-centered approaches theory in 1960
- Ida Jean Orlando's nursing process model in 1961
- Dorothy Johnson's behavioral system model for nursing in 1968
- Myra Levine's four conservation principles in 1969

Faye Glenn Abdellah: Patient-Centered Approaches Theory—1960
The Theorist

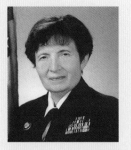

FAYE ABDELLAH was born in New York City in 1919. She graduated from Fitkin Memorial Hospital School of Nursing in 1942 and earned three degrees at Teachers College, Columbia University, New York City: a bachelor of science in nursing in 1945, a master of arts in 1947, and an EdD in 1955. After early positions as staff nurse, head nurse, faculty member, and public health nurse, Abdellah began working in the U.S. Public Health Service (USPHS) in 1949. In 1970, she was appointed Chief Nurse Officer of the USPHS, and in 1982, she was the first woman and first nurse to hold the position of Deputy Surgeon General. She retired from the USPHS in 1989 and, in 1993, was appointed dean and professor of nursing at the Uniform Services University of the Health Sciences (USUHS) graduate school of nursing in Bethesda, Maryland. She retired in 2002 and currently lives in Maryland.

Abdellah's distinguished career in practice, education, and research has led her to be recognized as one of the leading researchers in health and public policy in the nation, as well as an international expert on health problems. Abdellah has been involved in health care activities and consultation in many countries, including France, Israel, Japan, New Zealand, The People's Republic of China, Portugal, the Soviet Union, and Yugoslavia. Her global publications, presentations, and service are immeasurable in terms of their impact on nursing practice, health care, and research. She has received numerous awards, medals, honorary degrees, and memberships, nationally and internationally.

The Theory

Abdellah's doctoral dissertation focused on improving clinical teaching in nursing (1955). At the time, she was a member of the National League for Nursing subcommittee to develop a clinical evaluation tool for undergraduate nursing programs. She realized that nursing had to develop a strong scientific base of knowledge in order to gain full professional status in its own right. Using the results of several studies, Abdellah and Levine (1954) classified medical diagnoses in small hospitals into 58 categories representing nursing problems. With the assistance of faculty from 40 schools of nursing, the subcommittee developed the typology of 21 nursing problems, identified in Box 7.4. These problems became the basis for Abdellah's theory. The typology indicates that each type of problem comprises other problems. For example, the 11th problem states: "To facilitate the maintenance of sensory functions." Knowing that there are five senses—hearing, sight, smell, taste, and touch—the nurse could compile a lengthy list of problems to consider for each of these senses. What may have seemed a rather simple approach to problem solving initially became more complex. The theory, which has also been called a framework, was published in *Patient-Centered Approaches to Nursing* (Abdellah, Beland, Martin, & Matheney, 1960). Abdellah updated the framework in 1973 (Abdellah, Beland, Martin, & Matheney, 1973) and further refined it in 1994 (Abdellah & Levine, 1994).

In addition to the 21 problems, Abdellah identified 11 nursing skills to assist in developing a treatment typology, including observing health status, applying knowledge, teaching patients and families, planning and organizing work, using resource materials, problem solving, directing work of others, and therapeutic use of self (Abdellah et al., 1960). Abdellah viewed the 21 nursing problems and 11 skills as a unique body of nursing knowledge, an idea that was very important as nursing sought to move from a medical to a nursing model (Box 7.5).

Influence of Abdellah's Patient-Centered Approaches Theory

Education. Abdellah's framework was developed in the 1950s to provide a clinical record for nursing students, thereby lending structure to the nursing curriculum. The patient-centered approach that resulted from her efforts supported and facilitated the move from the medical model that was used at the time to a nursing model. In her book, *Patient-Centered Approaches* (Abdellah et al., 1960), three chapters comprising more than 50% of the book focus on implementing the model in baccalaureate, associate degree, and diploma nursing programs. Abdellah's work and her worldwide reputation have been instrumental in disseminating the patient-centered approach to educational programs around the world.

Practice. As the education of nurses improves, nursing practice improves as well. Abdellah's typology of 21 nursing problems has been updated to focus on the patient and nursing diagnosis. The typology helps the practicing nurse to organize the administration of care and provides a scientific base for making decisions. As a theorist who is actively involved in nursing and health care

---

Box 7.4   Abdellah's Typology of 21 Nursing Problems (Abdellah, et al., 1960, pp. 16–17)

To maintain good hygiene and physical comfort

To promote optimal activity: exercise, rest, sleep

To promote safety through prevention of accident, injury, and other trauma and through the prevention of the spread of infection

To maintain good body mechanics and prevent and correct deformity

To facilitate the maintenance of a supply of oxygen to all body cells

To facilitate the maintenance of nutrition of all body cells

To facilitate the maintenance of elimination

To facilitate the maintenance of fluid and electrolyte balance

To recognize the physiologic responses of the body to disease conditions

To facilitate the maintenance of regulatory mechanisms and functions

To facilitate the maintenance of sensory functions

To identify and accept positive and negative expressions, feelings, and reactions

To identify and accept the interrelatedness of emotions and organic illness

To facilitiate the maintenance of effective verbal and nonverbal communication

To promote the development of productive interpersonal relationships

To facilitiate progress toward achievement of personal spiritual goals

To create and maintain a therapeutic environment

To facilitate awareness of self as an individual with varying physical, emotional, and developmental needs

To accept the optimum possible goals in light of physical and emotional limitations

To use community resources as an aid in resolving problems arising from illness

To understand the role of social problems as influencing factors in the cause of illness

---

internationally, Abdellah gives credence to the use of the model and is an advocate of applying new knowledge to improve practice.

Research. The selection of the 21 problems was based on several significant research studies. The framework continues to stimulate research about the role and responsibilities of the nurse (Abdellah & Strachan, 1959). The broad nature of the concepts in Abdellah's framework offers few opportunities to identify directional relationships, although some may be derived from the concepts. At least some of the value of the theory stems from its effect on related areas, such as the body of nursing knowledge, the improvement of nursing education, and the structure of the curriculum.

Box 7.5   Summary of Abdellah's Patient-Centered Approaches Theory

Phenomenon: A clinical evaluation tool strengthens undergraduate nursing education.

Idea: Nurses solve health problems through their knowledge of nursing problems derived from medical diagnoses.

Key Concepts/Internal Variables

Nursing: The application of intellectual competencies and technical skills along with the attitude, desire, and ability to help people cope with their needs whether ill or healthy

Health: A dynamic pattern of functioning with continued interaction with internal and external forces that results in the optimal use of resources

Nursing Problem: A health condition that the nurse assists a patient or family to resolve through the performance of professional functions

Problem Solving: Identifying overt and covert nursing problems and interpreting, analyzing, and selecting appropriate courses of action to solve them

Examples of Propositions

The nurse uses a dietary plan to assist the patient to obtain adequate nutrition.

The nurse's early awareness and treatment of pain increases the patient's relaxation.

The nurse's knowledge of community resources facilitates patient/family decision making.

Examples of Assumptions

A body of nursing knowledge is identified by designating common patient problems.

Common patient problems are useful for teaching and evaluation of practice.

Nurses can be taught to identify common patient problems and facilitate their resolution.

Examples of External Variables

Medical diagnosis

Nurses who are unacquainted with specific health problems

Physicians who do not relinquish patient problems to the nurse for resolution

Ida Jean Orlando (Pelletier): Nursing Process Theory—1961

The Theorist

Over the years, Orlando has presented numerous workshops and lectures about her theory, and served as a consultant. Her nursing process discipline theory resulted from an analysis of 2000 nurse–patient contacts she recorded to demonstrate a shift in the focus of nursing from tasks and functions to the role of the individual patient in nursing actions. Initially, the theory was called "the theory of effective nursing practice" (1961), then "deliberative nursing process" (1972) and, in 1990, "nursing process discipline theory."

IDA JEAN ORLANDO was born August 12, 1926. She received a diploma in 1947 from New York Medical College, Flower and Fifth Avenue Hospital School of Nursing; a bachelor of science in public health nursing in 1951 from St. John's University; and a master of arts from Teachers College, Columbia University, New York City. She was research associate and principal investigator of a federal project at Yale University School of Nursing from 1954 to 1958 to integrate mental health concepts into the undergraduate curriculum. In 1961, she married Robert K. Pelletier and moved to Massachusetts. From 1962 to 1972, she was a clinical consultant to a private psychiatric hospital and implemented the theory she developed and published in 1961. She held a variety of positions before retiring in 1992. She lives in Massachusetts.

Orlando raised questions about elements of effective care and nursing actions. She linked effective care to the nurse's knowledge of patient needs that are validated by the patient response. Orlando's theory focuses primarily on individuals who are ill and under the care of physicians. Although the theory of nursing process discipline resembles the nursing process you may use in practice, it is not the same. Orlando's theory requires more comprehensive interaction between the nurse and patient and more involvement of the patient in his or her care. Orlando's process is reflexive and circular, occurring during encounters with patients, not the linear process taught in the nursing classroom (Rittman, 2001).

Orlando believes nursing is unique and independent from medicine. The uniqueness and the nursing licensure give nurses the authority to work independently. She also believes that the primary concern of nursing is to resolve the individual's need for help, using an interactive discipline process that is gained through training. Her interpretation of the nursing process is broader than the one generally advocated in undergraduate nursing curricula (see Box 7.6).

Influence of Orlando's Nursing Process Theory

Education. Orlando's theory of nursing process has influenced nursing education in North America and abroad, although in some instances, the emphasis on the process itself may have detracted from the broader intent of the theory to increase the interactions between patient and nurse. Orlando defines the actual role of the nurse as seeing the patient as an individual. Students, and possibly some faculty, are unaware that the original intent of Orlando's theory was to provide a theory of effective practice, not a tool to guide the nurse's actions. Orlando's theory is used to teach students in Germany, Japan, and Sweden, as well as in North America (Tomey & Alligood, 2002).

Practice. Orlando maintains that the usefulness of the nursing process theory is dependent on careful training of nurses. As a clinical consultant to a private psychiatric hospital, Orlando initiated programs to train staff nurses to use the nursing process discipline in their contacts with patients and train clinical nurse supervisors to use the discipline in their supervisory contacts. Orlando obtained federal funds to study the effectiveness of the training program. An extensive report of the study is in her second book (Orlando, 1972). Although nursing process is used across practice fields, her influence on psychiatric nursing is particularly important. Note the use of the word "training" rather than "educating."

Research. Orlando was the first to test the nursing process discipline theory, and numerous other studies provided evidence of the validity of the theory. In a study in Sweden, nurse researchers explored the attitudes and interests of first-year student nurses about geriatric and nursing home care. Two phenomena about the elderly were identified: the patients' helplessness and

Box 7.6   Summary of Orlando's Nursing Process Theory

Phenomenon: A process that assists the nurse to consciously identify and respond to patient needs.

Idea: Identifying patient needs enables the nurse to provide better health care.

Key Concepts/Internal Variables

Professional Nursing: Meeting the patient's needs for health care

Presenting Behavior of the Patient: The immediate or internal response of the patient

Nursing Process Discipline: A requirement or need of the patient that the nurse can relieve or diminish

Examples of Propositions

Nurses using the nursing process are better able to identify patient needs.

The nursing process provides the means to identify problems and monitor health care progress.

Patients who perform adequate self-care have an improved sense of well-being.

Examples of Assumptions

Patients respond to health problems on an individual basis.

Both patient and nurse influence nursing actions.

Interactions between the patient and nurse are important in the selection of appropriate actions.

Examples of External Variables

Hospital procedures and policies

Patient and family response to treatments

Automatic response of the nurse to the patient's problem

---

the nurses' identification or nonidentification with the elderly. Students who were able to describe the helplessness of elderly patients for whom they had cared during a 4- to 8-month period prior to the study were moved by the experiences. They did not understand why staff treated patients in certain ways and were upset by the failure of staff to identify patients as individuals. This relationship between the nurse or student and the elderly patient is of particular interest in Orlando's nursing process theory, although it would not be so in the common nursing process used by many nurses. The study planned to determine the long-term effect on students (Fagerberg & Ekman, 1997). Over the years, Orlando's theory continued to be tested by graduate students and nurse researchers.

Dorothy E. Johnson: Behavioral System Model for Nursing—1968

The Theorist

Johnson wrote four books and many articles. She received an award for excellence in nursing from Vanderbilt University School of Nursing, where she presented her theory; the Faculty

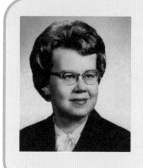

DOROTHY E. JOHNSON was born August 21, 1919, in Savannah, Georgia, She earned a bachelor of science in nursing from Vanderbilt University in Nashville, Tennessee, in 1942, and a master's of public health at Harvard University, Boston, in 1948. She taught briefly at Vanderbilt and then was appointed to the nursing faculty at the University of California in Los Angeles (UCLA). She served as a pediatric nursing advisor at Christian Medical School of Nursing in southern India. Johnson retired from UCLA in 1978 as professor emeritus and moved to Florida to continue her interest in systems as a shell collector (Parker, 2001). She died on February 4, 1999.

Award from the UCLA graduate students; the Lulu Hassenplug Distinguished Achievement Award from the California Nurses Association; and numerous other awards.

The Theory

While Johnson was a faculty member at UCLA in the 1950s, she raised questions about the knowledge base that nurses needed for practice. Her early publications focused on a science of nursing (1959) and a conceptual basis for nursing care (1961). In the latter article, Johnson proposed that nursing must clearly specify the purpose of nursing "to provide a basis for practice and give direction to nursing research" (1961, p. 64). The nursing community soon realized that Johnson was helping to identify boundaries for theory and knowledge development in nursing, not just conducting isolated exercises for selecting class content.

Although Johnson did not publish her behavioral system model in nursing until 1980, she was instrumental in setting the stage for response, discussion, and debate about nursing knowledge, clearly affecting the development of theory and knowledge for years to come. She presented her model in a lecture at Vanderbilt University in 1968 (unpublished). By this time, she had inspired doctoral students at UCLA, among them Sister Callista Roy, Betty Neuman, and Evelyn Adam, to think about conceptual and theoretical models for nursing. Roy's adaptation model was published in 1970, Neuman's health care systems model in 1974, and Adam's conceptual model for nursing in 1979/1980. These three theories are discussed later in this chapter.

Johnson's behavioral system model, based on von Bertalanffy's open system theory, which is discussed in Chapter 5, focuses on the person's response to the stress of illness. Reviewing his theory will demonstrate the significant effect it has had on Johnson's work and its acceptance in nursing.

Johnson identifies two major components: the person and nursing. The person is a system with seven subsystems, four structural characteristics, and three functional requirements. When one or more of the subsystems is in disequilibrium, the person reacts in patterned, purposeful, repetitive ways. The goal of nursing is to help the person return to a state of balance and stability (see Box 7.7).

Influence of Johnson's Model

Education. While it is possible to design a curriculum using Johnson's behavioral system model, it is difficult because of the lack of clearly articulated propositions, the level of abstraction of the model, and multiple concept definitions that are difficult to understand. Johnson must be given credit, however, for differentiating the subject matter for the education of undergraduate and graduate levels. Her ideas about the body of nursing knowledge helped change the focus of graduate education in nursing from preparing administrators and teachers to preparing clinical nurse specialists and nurse practitioners.

Box 7.7   Summary of Johnson's Behavioral System Model for Nursing

Phenomenon: Patients respond to the stress of illness in different ways.

Idea: The nurse helps foster behavioral patterns in patients to achieve homeostasis after a health event produces disequilibrium.

Key Concepts/Internal Variables

Behavioral System: Patterned, repetitive, and purposeful ways of behaving

Patient Behavioral System:

attachment and affiliation	ingestion
dependency	aggression
elimination	achievement
sexuality	

Structural Characteristics:

drive	choices
set	observable behaviors

Functional Requirements:

protection

nurturance

stimulation

Nursing: A distinctive service provided to a person who is ill; the concern of nursing is to assist the patient to cope when the stress of illness exists or threatens.

Examples of Propositions

Johnson does not clearly articulate interrelationships among concepts/internal variables; however, propositions can be deduced from her work as well as systems theory.

A change in one subsystem affects other subsystems.

Nursing assists the patient to return to a state of equilibrium or balance.

Patient assessment should focus on the subsystem involved in the health problem.

Examples of Assumptions

The individual has two major systems, the biological system and the behavioral system

Nursing focuses on the behavioral system; medicine on the biological system.

Patients regain equilibrium with the assistance of the nurse.

Examples of External Variables

The lack of clear definitions and propositions makes it difficult to identify external variables; the following have been projected from her work.

A fluctuating or unpredictable environment

(continued)

> ### Box 7.7   Summary of Johnson's Behavioral System Model for Nursing (Continued)
>
> The nurse's value system
>
> A high level of stress
>
> **Examples of Facts, Principles, and Laws**
>
> **Facts:** Human subsystems exhibit observable behaviors that lead to specific outcomes.
>
> **Principles:** Patterns of behavior are reactions to stressors.
>
> **Laws:** Systems seek to achieve a balance among internal and external forces.

Practice. Dee (1990) reports on the implementation of Johnson's model on the child and adult psychiatric services in one hospital over a period of a decade. Some benefits of using the model include a comprehensive and systematic method of patient assessment; a plan for prioritizing care based on subsystem interactions; and a framework for nurses to explain, predict, and control clinical phenomena. Most of the individuals involved in the use of the model demonstrated long-term or chronic illnesses.

Research. The late dissemination of Johnson's behavioral system model has limited the amount and variety of issues related to the model. Research includes caring for visually impaired children (Small, 1980), developing a research tool to measure patient indicators of nursing care (Majesky, Brester, & Nishio, 1978), visits of elementary school children to the nurse's office (Stamler, 1971), and control of metastatic bone pain (Coward & Wilkie, 2000; Wilkie, Lovejoy, Dodd, & Tesler, 1988).

Myra Estrin Levine: Conservation Principles: A Model for Health—1969
The Theorist

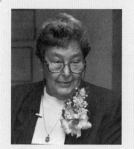

MYRA ESTRIN LEVINE was born in Chicago in 1920. She received a diploma from Cook County Hospital School of Nursing in 1944, a bachelor of science in nursing from the University of Chicago, and a master's of science in nursing from Wayne State University, Chicago, in 1962. She enrolled in postgraduate work at the University of Chicago. She held numerous positions, including professor at four schools in Chicago and visiting professor at two schools of nursing in Israel. She retired from the University of Illinois in 1987 as professor emerita, remaining active in theory development until her death on March 20, 1996, at the age of 73.

Levine held positions, primarily in the Chicago area, as a private duty nurse, supervisor, administrator, civilian nurse in the U.S. Army, and professor. She taught in four schools of nursing in Chicago: Cook County Hospital School of Nursing, Loyola University, Rush University, and the University of Illinois. She served as visiting professor at two schools of nursing in Israel:

Box 7.8   Summary of Levine's Conservation Model

Phenomenon: Every nurse–patient contact results in a puzzle that needs to be solved.

Idea: Nursing actions help the patient conserve energy and other resources needed to recover.

Key Concepts/Internal Variables (Tomey & Alligood, 2002)

Wholeness/Holism: An open system in which there is mutuality between diversified functions and parts of the whole; the boundaries are open and fluent.

Adaptation: A process that is a consequence of person-environment interaction by which individuals maintain their wholeness/integrity in response to environmental challenges.

Conservation: Keeping together the wholeness of the individual, ensuring the ability to confront change appropriately, retaining a unique identity. The nurse's role is to help the patient achieve a balance of energy supply and demand.

Conservation of Energy: Balancing the patient's source of energy with the use of energy to maintain life activities, such as healing and aging.

Conservation of Structural Integrity: Facilitating the healing process to a new level of adaptation by restoring structural and functional integrity of the patient.

Conservation of Personal Integrity: Encouraging a sense of self-worth and a sense of identity by respecting a patient's personal integrity through providing privacy, valuing possessions, supporting defenses, and teaching.

Conservation of Social Integrity: Health is socially determined and gains meaning through social communities. The nurse's role is to conserve the patient's social integrity.

Examples of Propositions

Assisting a patient to ambulate conserves energy.

Encouraging the patient to select a good diet increases healing.

Teaching a patient about dealing with a disability aids in long-term self-worth.

Examples of Assumptions

A person is only understood in the context of his or her environment.

A self-sustaining system monitors behavior by conserving resources required to define its identity.

Human beings respond in a singular, integrated fashion.

Examples of External Variables

Ineffective redundancy

Unexpected stress

Ethical values of the social system

Tel Aviv University and Ben-Gurion University of the Negev. She received an honorary doctorate from Loyola University and a number of other awards.

The Theory

Levine's conservation principles model was not intended to be a nursing theory. Her model was developed to provide a graduate curriculum in medical-surgical nursing that would incorporate all major nursing concepts into the program and be able to generalize the content and focus on maintaining the patient's ability to adapt. At the same time, she wanted to move away from the procedurally oriented process that was in common use at the time. Some of Levine's ideas came from other theories, such as Selye's stress and adaptation, von Bertalanffy's open system, and Erickson's developmental theories. Her conservation principles were initially published in 1969 and updated in 1989.

The model includes four principles: the conservation of energy, the conservation of structural integrity, the conservation of personal integrity, and the conservation of social integrity. Levine defines conservation as guarding and protecting the individual's wholeness by balancing resource expenditures. She uses the word integrity to mean wholeness. Although Levine labeled these as principles of conservation, in this discussion they are considered concepts and defined in Box 7.8.

Influence of Levine's Conservation Model

Education. As indicated earlier, Levine's model was developed to provide a curriculum that would reorganize medical-surgical coursework for a graduate curriculum. Levine believed that a professional nursing practice could only be achieved at the graduate level, although the conservation model has been integrated into both undergraduate and graduate curricula. Frequent publications about the model and presentations by Levine have helped nurse educators become acquainted with the model, but it has not achieved the widespread acceptance in education as some other models have.

Practice. Levine extends the ideas of Orlando by addressing the reasons nurses carry out designated activities (Parker, 2001). Her model has been used with hospitalized elderly (Foreman, 1989), patients with congestive heart failure (Schaefer & Potylycki, 1993), and in various clinical settings, such as the operating room, critical care, long-term/extended care, and the emergency room. The model has been used at all developmental levels from infant to the frail elderly and has been introduced into community-based care for individuals, families, and groups (Parker, 2001).

Research. Levine's model has been the focus of research in a variety of areas over the years. Parker (2001) identifies broad areas of conservation that have been tested to show the significance in nursing practice, such as breathing in labor, conservation of energy in newborns, oxygen consumption during bed making, the fatigue of ventilator patients, and the conservation of energy in the very sick. Three theories have been developed based on Levine's conceptual model: the theory of redundancy, the theory of conservation, and the theory of therapeutic intention (Parker, 2001).

Nursing Theory in the 1970s

The pace of theory development increased in the 1970s with the introduction of nine theories, including two from Canada:

- Martha Rogers' science of unitary man in 1970
- Sister Callista Roy's adaptation model in 1970
- Dorothea Orem's self-care deficit theory in 1971
- Imogene King's theory of goal setting in 1971
- Betty Neuman's systems model in 1974
- The University of British Columbia's directions for practice model in 1976
- Evelyn Adam's conceptual model for nursing in 1979
- Margaret Newman's model of health in 1979
- Jean Watson's theory of human caring in 1979

Martha E. Rogers: Science of Unitary Human Beings—1970
The Theorist

MARTHA E. ROGERS was born May 2, 1914, in Dallas, Texas, on the anniversary of Florence Nightingale's birthday. She attended the University of Tennessee, Knoxville, in 1931 for 2 years and then entered Knoxville General Hospital School of Nursing, graduating in 1936. She earned a bachelor of science in public health from George Peabody College in 1937, a master of arts in public health supervision from Teachers College, Columbia University, in 1945, and a master in public health in 1952 and doctor of science (ScD) in 1954 from Johns Hopkins University, Baltimore, Maryland. She died March 15, 1994, 2 months before her 80th birthday.

During the period between her undergraduate and graduate education, Rogers worked in rural Michigan in public health nursing and in Connecticut in a visiting nurse agency. She established the first visiting nurse agency in Phoenix, Arizona. Immediately after completing the doctorate, Rogers became professor and head of the division of nursing education at New York University, New York City, a position she held until 1975. She continued as professor until 1979, when she retired as professor **emerita.**

Rogers lectured across the country and around the world. She received honorary degrees from a number of universities and numerous awards for her leadership and intellectual contributions to nursing. The Society of Rogerian Scholars, established in 1988 by scholars and doctoral students involved in research of Rogers' theory, publishes a newsletter, *Rogerian Nursing Science News.* The Society also publishes an annual refereed journal, *Visions: The Journal of Rogerian Nursing Science.*

The Theory

In the 1960s, Martha Rogers began to explore why nurses needed to be educated in colleges and universities (Rogers, 1961, 1964). She concluded that nurses did not need to attend college to "do" nursing, but that college was necessary to "know" nursing. The idea of nursing knowledge eventually brought Rogers to propose that nursing science was a distinct body of knowledge, and using this knowledge was the way to help people improve health.

The theory Rogers introduced in 1970, the science of unitary man, was very abstract, and few nurses understood the direction of her thinking. She was ahead of most nurses when she discussed space-time continuum, energy fields, and patterning. In the past 30 years, nursing and nurses' knowledge have changed. Nurse scientists have increased their knowledge and understanding, and changes in world travel and access to other countries and cultures have affected the worldview of many practicing nurses. At the same time, Rogers' theory has become more understandable, and many of her early ideas are now accepted and implemented. Rogers changed the name of her theory in 1983 to the science of unitary human beings but did not change the theory.

Rogers viewed human and environmental energy fields as integral and unable to be separated, an idea that differed with Nightingale's view of the environment, but was consistent with von Bertalanffy's open system theory. Rogers also disagreed with the bio-physio-psycho-sociocultural background that is frequently used in nursing. She believed that a person and his or her environment are one unit and need to be studied together. When she says that humans are integral with their environments, she is saying that a human does not adapt to the environment nor does the environment cause something to happen to the human. Rather, humans and their environments evolve, change, and move ahead together.

After a change occurs, neither humans nor their environments can return to their former state. For example, when you entered the nursing major, you were innocent and un-aware of many aspects of the human system and the health care environment. Regardless of what you do in the future, your perspective of individuals, groups, and communities and their health care has changed and you cannot return to your former innocent state. You now view people and health care in new and different ways than you did in the past. Your family and friends view you and your environment in a different way. They may ask you different questions, discuss different topics, and seek your opinion about different issues than they would if you were studying to be a chemist or an accountant rather than a nurse. When you study Rogers' theory of unitary human beings, expect to confront this type of change in pa-tients as well as yourself.

Rogers' conceptual model is based on scientific knowledge. Although she gives few specific examples about that model, she is adamant when she says, "Nursing exists to serve people". . . in their "entirety and wholeness". . ."for the realization of maximum health potential" (1970, p. 122). A few pages later she adds, "Nursing's conceptual model provides the frame of reference for perceiving and interpreting diagnostic data" (1970, p. 125). The goals of Rogers' model are nursing diagnosis, intervention, maintaining and promoting health, preventing illness, and reha-bilitation (1970). Each of these has equal relevance whether an individual is sick or well, just as you would expect from Rogers.

Two common toys help illustrate Rogers' theory: a Slinky and a kaleidoscope. Each of these toys demonstrates the constant interaction in a human/environment process. The Slinky illus-trates the openness, rhythm, motion, balance, and expanding nature of life and the human life process that is continuously innovative and evolving (Fig. 7.1). The kaleidoscope, which she in-troduced later, illustrates changing patterns that appear to be infinitely different. You cannot re-turn to a previous pattern, but only go forward to new ones.

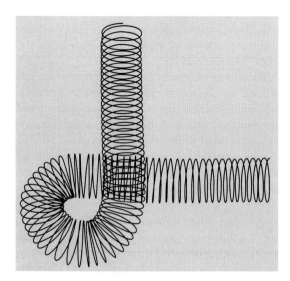

Figure 7.1 The Slinky, illustrating openness, motion, and innovation. (Used with permission of Poof-Slinky, Inc. © 2004. Slinky is a registered trademark of Poof-Slinky, Inc.)

Rogers introduces other concepts, such as resonancy, helicy, and integrality, that you will encounter in your education and future practice. The summary of Rogers' theory in Box 7.9 provides additional ideas and information to integrate into your theoretical knowledge.

Influence of Rogers' Science of Unitary Human Beings Theory

Education. In 1970, Rogers published *An Introduction to the Theoretical Basis of Nursing*, in which she declared that nursing was a science and a discipline with a unique body of knowledge specific to nursing. This challenged the ways of thinking about nursing and nursing education at

---

Box 7.9   Summary of Rogers' Science of Unitary Human Beings

Phenomenon: Human beings are in constant interaction with the environment.

Idea: Identifiable patterns in the human/environment connection are identifiable and influence nursing actions.

Key Concepts/Internal Variables

Energy Field: The fundamental unit that is unique for each person. Each energy field is infinite, that is, without boundaries, and dynamic. *Energy* is the dynamic moving and flowing of humans and their environments that leads to change. *Field* unites the human and the environment.

Pattern: The distinguishing characteristic of an energy field. The pattern changes continuously while giving identity to the human-environment process.

Unitary Environment: The environment is considered a whole with its own identity and pattern that is integral with a human being.

Unitary Human Being: A person, group, family, or community that is a unified whole, that can be studied and understood only as a whole, not body parts (heart or liver) or body systems (cardiovascular or neurological).

Examples of Propositions

Unitary human beings/environments are dynamic fields of energy.

A positive human/environment energy field decreases anxiety and tension of patients.

A nurse who identifies patterns of human/environment energy fields will provide individualized care.

Examples of Assumptions (Rogers, 1970, pgs. 46, 54, 59, & 65)

Human beings are more than and different from the sum of their parts.

Man and environment are continuously exchanging matter and energy with one another.

The life process evolves irreversibly and unidirectionally along the space-time continuum.

Pattern and organization identify man and reflect his innovative wholeness.

Examples of External Variables

Technical skills

Laboratory results.

Medical diagnoses.

that time. Rogers viewed humans and their environments as constantly changing and evolving and viewed nursing as knowing, as well as doing. In two earlier books, *Educational Revolution in Nursing* (1961) and *Reveille in Nursing* (1964), Rogers spoke about the impact of theoretical knowledge on higher learning, the curriculum, and the education of the nurse.

Rogers' theory was developed in part from her efforts to improve the nursing curriculum at New York University (NYU), where she was professor and head of nursing. Her theory, the science of unitary human beings, became the base for the curriculum at NYU, as well as other programs in the United States and abroad. Rogers' writings continue to stimulate students to think about nursing and health care.

Practice. The nursing curriculum in the 1970s advanced the idea that skills were the base for practice. At the time, there were few nursing theories and even less theoretical knowledge to consider. Rogers' theory and other publications stimulated nurses to begin to rethink practice. For example, she advocated higher education, creativity, and a search for knowledge for the nursing curriculum. However, she also used concepts and language that deterred many nurses from using her theory in their practice. Looking at the increasing clarification and acceptance of Rogers' theory during the past 30-plus years suggests that the science of unitary human beings will continue to have an impact in the future.

Research. Rogers advocated using both qualitative and quantitative research methods to test her theory but felt that neither was completely adequate. Researchers have designed a number of tools to facilitate the measurement of patterns; time dragging, time racing, and timeliness; dream experiences; and other concepts (Parker, 2001).

A significant effect of any theory is its ability to stimulate the development and design of additional theoretical work. Rogers' theory has accomplished that very effectively, especially through the development of nurse scholars and doctoral students who have formed the Society of Rogerian Scholars. A number of theories have spun off of the science of unitary human beings, including a theory of perceived dissonance, a theory of sentience (the capability to think, feel, and perceive), and a theory of healthiness (Parker, 2001). In addition, Rogers' theory has influenced the development of theories by Newman and Parse that are discussed later in this chapter.

Sister Callista Roy: Adaptation Model—1970
The Theorist

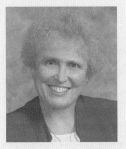

SISTER CALLISTA ROY was born October 14, 1939, in Los Angeles, California. She entered the Sisters of Saint Joseph of Carondelet after high school. She received a bachelor of arts in nursing from Mount Saint Mary's College in Los Angeles in 1963, a master of science in nursing from UCLA in 1966, and a master's and a doctor of philosophy (PhD) in sociology from UCLA in 1973 and 1974, respectively. She was a Robert Wood Johnson postdoctoral fellow at the University of California at San Francisco (1983–1985). She held faculty and administrative positions at Mount St. Mary's College and the University of Portland, Oregon, and was Dean of Nursing at Boston College. She is a professor and nurse theorist at the college; she published her third book on the adaptation model in 2008.

In 1989, a group of researchers, using Roy's model as a guide for their work, formed the Boston-Based Adaptation Research in Nursing Society (BBARNS) to advance nursing practice. The name of the group was changed to Roy Adaptation Association (RAA) in 2001. RAA provides scholarly colleagueship and networks, promotes the development of expert nurse scientists, and publishes a newsletter, *Roy Adaptation Association Review*, twice a year.

Roy received numerous awards and honors and is a prolific writer and speaker. She is active in many nursing organizations and may be the most widely recognized name in nursing worldwide (Parker, 2001). Her work has been used in practice, education, administration, and research in America as well as abroad.

The Theory

As a graduate student at UCLA in 1964, Roy was challenged by Dorothy E. Johnson, known for her behavioral systems in nursing theory, to develop a conceptual model for nursing. As a pediatric nurse, Roy was aware of the ability of children to confront and adapt to their illnesses. She used her observations to develop an adaptation model. Later, as chair of nursing at Mount Saint Mary's College, she operationalized the model, refining it to include adults. The College faculty adopted the framework for the nursing curriculum the same year it was published in *Nursing Outlook* (Roy, 1970). In the 1970s and 1980s, many baccalaureate programs used the Roy model as a curricular framework in preparation for accreditation (Roy, 1975).

Roy views the individual as a system that adapts to health and illness problems. Her major concepts—nursing, health, and environment—are interrelated with the concept of adaptation. The role of nursing is to bring about changes in the environment that free the patient to respond or adapt to other stimuli. This is accomplished within four modes: basic physiological needs, self-concept, role mastery, and interdependence. The nurse assesses the state of the patient's health to determine how the four adaptive modes are affected. For example, a patient with a recent diagnosis of diabetes may have physiological needs related to adjusting the amount of insulin required, self-concept needs related to injections, role mastery needs related to diet limitations, and interdependence needs related to telling friends about diabetes. The nurse's interventions in the environment may vary from education about the disease and teaching injection skills to providing an opportunity for the patient to join a support group.

Over the years, Roy has been active in the continuing development of the model. When she spoke about the future of the adaptation model in the late 1990s, she proposed some changes (Roy, 1997). The original definition of adaptation was changed in 1997 to the one in the summary in Box 7.10.

Influence of Roy's Adaptation Theory

Education. While Roy was developing the adaptation model, it was used as an organizing framework for an undergraduate curriculum. The model was introduced as a "conceptual framework," which was consistent with the language used in accreditation criteria at the time (Roy, 1970). The following year, Roy published a second article that spoke to the additional value of the model in nursing practice (Roy, 1971).

Roy's adaptation model has had widespread use by baccalaureate programs in the United States and elsewhere. In some cases, every course in a program included the term "adaptation" in its title. Even in programs that do not establish a theoretical base, adaptation may be a prominent concept in didactic and clinical courses.

Practice. The adaptation model influenced nursing practice early in its inception (Roy, 1971). An early attempt to test the model in practice focused on adapting an assessment tool and using it in actual patient settings (Wagner, 1976). Five graduate students decided to test whether Roy's

Box 7.10   Summary of Roy's Adaptation Model

Phenomenon: Children demonstrate adaptability and resilience to illness.

Idea: People adapt to illness in predictable ways.

Key Concepts/Internal Variables (Tomey & Alligood, 2002)

Adaptation: The process and outcomes of individuals and groups who use conscious awareness, self-reflection, and choice to create human and environmental integration.

System: A set of parts that functions as a whole for a specific purpose. A system has inputs, outputs, control, and feedback processes.

Adaptation Level: The condition of life processes on three graduated levels: integrated, compensatory, and compromised. The level is constantly changing consistent with the patient's ability to respond.

Adaptation Problems: Broad areas of concern related to the adapting person or group.

Examples of Propositions

Nursing actions promote effective adaptive responses by the patient.

Nursing actions decrease ineffective adaptive responses.

Nursing actions improve patient–environment interactions.

Examples of Assumptions

The person is in constant interaction with a changing environment.

Adaptation occurs when the patient responds positively to environmental change.

Positive adaptive responses promote the patient's return to health.

Examples of External Variables

Health promotion and maintenance

Unconscious patients

Psychological problems

Examples of Facts, Principles, and Laws

Fact: Human beings are able to adapt to physical and psychological stress.

Principle: Adaptation is an attempt to achieve or maintain homeostasis.

Law: Human beings vary in their ability to adapt.

model could be used in practice. Each nurse selected one patient to observe for an undesignated period of time. The group then evaluated the results and concluded that the model was useful but difficult to implement in practice.

Research. In 1999, BBARNS published *Roy Adaptation Model-Based Research: 25 Years of Contributions to Nursing Science.* The book reported that 116 of the 163 studies that had been conducted on the Roy model met the criteria of linkages between model concepts and research variables, the model and empirical measures, and the findings and the model (Fawcett, 2002). Five Canadian nurse researchers examined a group of studies conducted on Roy's model to identify theoretical propositions. Stress, conflicts, and coping mechanisms were linked directly or indirectly to adaptation in the self-concept mode (Levesque, Ricard, Ducharme, Duquette, & Bonin, 1998).

Dorothea E. Orem: Theory of Self-Care Deficit—1971
The Theorist

DOROTHEA E. OREM was born in 1914 in Baltimore, Maryland. She earned a diploma in nursing in the early 1930s from Providence Hospital School of Nursing in Washington, DC, a bachelor of science in nursing education in 1939, and a master of science in nursing education from Catholic University of America (CUA), Washington, DC. She held numerous positions in nursing and taught at CUA from 1959 to 1970, serving a term as interim dean. She retired in 1984 and lived in Savannah, Georgia, until she died June 22, 2007, at the age of 92.

Orem held nursing positions in practice, education, management, and administration. She worked at the Indiana State Board of Health from 1949 to 1957; the U.S. Department of Health, Education, and Welfare (HEW, the predecessor of the U.S. Department of Health and Human Services) from 1957 to 1959; and CUA from 1959 to 1970, where she taught and subsequently served as interim dean. She left CUA for full-time consultation and retired in 1984. She continued to work individually and with colleagues to refine the self-care deficit theory. Orem's theory is used worldwide. She received several honorary degrees and other honors and awards and was described as one of America's foremost nursing theorists (Tomey & Alligood, 2002).

The Theory
Orem conceived of the concept of self-care during the time she was at the Indiana State Board of Health working to upgrade the quality of nursing in Indiana hospitals. She moved to HEW in 1957 as a curriculum consultant for a project to improve practical nurse training through better selection of nursing subject matter. During this project, she explored the reasons why nurses were needed to care for patients.

Two years later, when she was appointed professor at CUA, she continued to develop the concept of self-care, working as an individual and with a faculty committee, called the Nursing Models Committee. In 1971, a year after she left CUA, Orem published *Nursing: Concepts of Practice*, a book that has been revised and updated five times, the latest in 2001. Orem provided the leadership for another group that was formed in 1968 and was known as the Nursing Development Conference Group (NDCG). The work of this group was published in 1973 (NDCG, 1973). Orem's theory is regularly reviewed and upgraded.

Orem's general theory of self-care deficit nursing delineates when patients are unable to care for themselves, even with the assistance of family members. When the patient or family members are unable to provide the necessary care, there is a self-care demand that can be met by a nurse. The general theory is composed of three interrelated theories: the theory of self-care, the theory of self-care deficit, and the theory of nursing systems. The theory of self-care explains why people care for themselves and includes the concepts of self-care agency, basic conditioning factors, and therapeutic self-care demand. Self-care requisites are also incorporated into the theory and provide the basis for undertaking self-care. The three classifications of requisites are universal self-care requisites or activities of daily living, such as eating, resting, sleeping, and social interaction; developmental requisites associated with adjusting to events, such as attending college, getting a job, marriage, and old age; and health deviation requisites, such as trauma, surgical interventions, and the need for crutches after fracturing a leg.

The theory of self-care deficit describes and explains when people need nursing care. Orem specifies five methods that nurses use to help meet the self-care needs of the patient: acting for or doing for another, guiding and directing, providing physical or psychological support, providing and maintaining an environment that supports personal development, and teaching (Orem, 2001). The first method may include the three requisites mentioned above—universal, developmental, and health deviation—while the other four methods relate only to health deviation requisites.

Finally, the theory of nursing systems describes and explains the three systems that can be used to meet the self-care requisites of the patient. The system selected depends on the nurse's assessment of the patient's abilities to perform self-care activities. In the wholly compensatory system, the patient is unable to perform any self-care actions and depends on the nurse to perform them; this would include comatose patients and people in late stages of Alzheimer's. In the partially compensatory system, both patient and nurse perform self-care actions with the major role shifting from the nurse to the patient as the self-care demand changes. This system is evident in patients who have had recent surgery or are recovering from serious trauma. As the patient regains the ability to perform self-care, the need for nursing care is diminished.

The third nursing system is the supportive-educative system. In this system, the nurse's role is to promote the patient as the self-care agent. The patient has the ability to carry out self-care, but cannot do so without assistance from the nurse in decision making and acquiring knowledge and skill. For example, patients with newly diagnosed diabetes are able to eat, but need assistance in selection of an appropriate diet. They also need knowledge about foot care and skills for testing blood sugar and administering insulin, with the goal of being able to fulfill all these self-care demands in the future. As they learn and use the knowledge and skills, they move toward being able to care for their own health care needs.

As the balance shifts from self-care abilities to self-care demands, nursing agency is needed. The definitions of many of Orem's concepts are in Box 7.11.

Influence of Orem's Theory

Education.   Orem is among the most widely known and accepted of the nurse theorists in the United States and globally. Her theory was adopted by significant numbers of schools of nursing as an organizing framework for curricula during the 1970s when accreditation criteria required a theoretical framework. Many schools of nursing continue to use frameworks such as Orem's, even though they no longer are required, because they are readily understood and easily implemented. Some schools discontinued using the framework because it focused primarily on hospitalized individuals, although the most recent editions of *Nursing: Concepts of Practice* include the patient at home and groups of people (Orem, 2001).

Practice.   A brief review of several research projects that focused on Orem's self-care deficit theory of nursing illustrates the use of the theory in nursing practice. Three nurses from Thailand conducted a study of elderly people concerning their life satisfaction. The study was based on Orem's definition of well-being and self-care behaviors. Two teams of 73 participants between the ages of 60 and 94 years who attended elderly clubs were matched according to their level of life satisfaction. Findings revealed that individuals who participated to a greater extent in daily positive health practices, or self-care, showed higher levels of satisfaction than those who did not. Some practices, such as drinking milk and exercising 30 minutes a day, received little attention by either group (Othaganont, Sinthuvorakan, & Jensupakarn, 2002). The researchers thought it was important

Box 7.11   Summary of Orem's Self-Care Deficit Theory in Nursing

Phenomenon: Human beings have varying abilities to care for themselves during illness.
Idea: Nurses use different approaches based on the patient's ability to care for self.

Key Concepts/Internal Variables

Self-Care: Activities that individuals initiate and perform that contribute to their continuing health and well-being.

Self-Care Agency: An individual's acquired ability to engage in self-care that meets the requirements for human functioning and development. The ability is affected by basic conditioning factors such as age, developmental stage, cultural factors, and patterns of living.

Self-Care Demand: All the care measures that are needed at a specific time or for a period of time to meet an individual's self-care requisites using appropriate methods and related actions.

Self-Care Deficit: An event that delineates when nursing is needed. For example, a patient newly diagnosed with diabetes needs information about the disease, blood sugar, insulin, diet, foot care, and other areas. When the nurse provides the knowledge and skill training, the patient is able to resume the responsibility for self-care.

Therapeutic Self-care: Activities needed to meet all the individual's self-care requisites for existing conditions and circumstances that are provided by the nursing agency.

Nursing Agency: The knowledge and abilities of nurses that enable them to act, know, and help patients in a legitimate interpersonal relationship to meet their self-care demands.

Nursing Systems: Three classifications of actions that nurses perform consistent with a patient's actions that are wholly compensatory, partially compensatory, and supportive-educative.

Examples of Propositions

The individual is capable of providing self-care to meet some health needs.

The nurse compensates for the patient's inability to engage in self-care by providing care.

The patient resumes self-care actions as he/she regains ability to do so.

Examples of Assumptions

Humans require continuous, deliberate self-care for health, development, and well-being.

Individuals have the power to make decisions about their self-care by identifying needs and taking specific actions.

Nurses maintain an individual's capacity for self-care and assist when he/she is unable to do so.

Examples of External Variables

The patient is discharged from the hospital early.

The environment inhibits the patient from ambulating.

The family encourages dependency.

(continued)

> ## Box 7.11 Summary of Orem's Self-Care Deficit Theory in Nursing (Continued)
>
> ### Examples of Facts, Principles, and Laws
>
> **Fact:** Some illnesses interfere with a patient's ability for self-care.
>
> **Principle:** Individuals have varying abilities to care for themselves.
>
> **Law:** Self-care is therapeutic.

that Thai elders become aware of these uncommon practices and that nurses and other health care professionals promote their use to ensure a more satisfying life.

In a study of homeless adults, the relationship between self-care agency, self-care, and well-being were studied. Structured interviews were conducted with 150 homeless people, with 75% men and 25% women. The group was 25% Caucasian and 75% African American. Low self-esteem and dependence on alcohol and drugs were predictors of self-care agency; however, gender and race were not. Strengthening the homeless person's self-care agency was important in increasing self-care measures and well-being (Anderson, 2001).

Research. During an interview in 2000, Orem revealed that she was identifying "a base from which researchers could raise questions for investigation," but leaving identification of specific research methods to others to design (Fawcett, 2002, p. 37). A doctoral student conducted a philosophical inquiry into Orem's theory and concluded that descriptive, descriptive-correlational, quasi-experimental, and case study methods are most consistent with the theory (Tomey & Alligood, 2002).

Research on Orem's theory has been limited to hospitalized individuals; however, some studies are expanding to groups and the community. Mosher and Moore (1998) demonstrated relationships between self-concept and self-care, dependent care, and basic conditioning factors in 74 children with cancer and their mothers. Soderhamn and Cliffordson (2001) conducted a secondary analysis of 125 elderly subjects who responded to a questionnaire that included the Appraisal of Self-Care Agency scale, the Self-Care Ability scale for the elderly, and other questions about health, self-care, and conditioning factors. The analysis showed consistency between the self-care structure and the self-care deficit theory.

Imogene M. King: Theory of Goal Attainment—1971

The Theorist

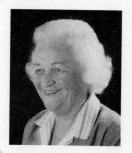

IMOGENE M. KING was born January 30, 1923. She earned a diploma from St. John's Hospital School of Nursing, St. Louis, Missouri, in 1945; a bachelor of science in nursing education and a master of science in nursing from St. Louis University in 1948 and 1957, respectively; and an EdD from Teachers College, Columbia University, in 1961. She completed postdoctoral study in systems research, advanced statistics, research design, and computers. She was director and professor at Ohio State University in the 1960s, and professor at the University of South Florida, where she retired as professor emeritus. She died December 24, 2007.

King was involved in the Florida Nurses Association as well as Sigma Theta Tau International, Inc., Honor Society of Nursing, as a Virginia Henderson Fellow. In addition, she lectured on theory and research and enjoyed serving as a curriculum consultant. She participated in scholarly activities related to her theory and its use in practice, education, research, and administration. She loved to talk with students and authors of books related to theory and research.

The Theory

King published her conceptual framework, *Toward a Theory for Nursing: General Concepts for Human Behavior*, in 1971. In preparing to write her book, she raised questions about nursing goals, functions, and knowledge and the difficulty that nurses had in selecting and using content to deal with specific situations. Using systems analysis and general system theory literature, she identified questions about nursing decision making related to essential information and alternative actions (1971). King, as well as a number of other theorists, was involved in identifying the knowledge base for nursing curricula at the undergraduate and graduate levels. She identified 15 concepts in her conceptual framework that were related to personal, interpersonal, and social systems that represented basic theoretical knowledge for nurses (Fig. 7.2).

In 1981, King published *A Theory of Goal Attainment: Systems, Concepts, Process*. She developed a theory of goal attainment from her conceptual framework in which she selected 10 of the concepts. Within her theory, she derived a transaction process model. When nurses use the transaction process, in which mutual goal setting is the critical variable, goals, as outcomes, are achieved in almost every situation. When documented in the patient's record, it presents evidence-based practice. In addition, the recorded goals provide research data for future study (Box 7.12).

Influence of King's Theory of Goal Achievement

Education. King's conceptual framework and theory have served nursing education since she began to think about and develop a graduate curriculum. She extended that contribution when she

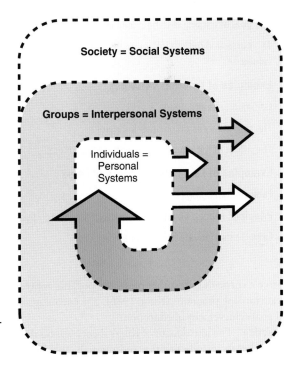

Figure 7.2 Dynamic interacting systems. (Adapted from King, I. M. [1971]. *Toward a theory for nursing* [p. 20]. New York: Wiley. Copyright © 1971, by John Wiley & Sons, Inc. Used with permission.)

Box 7.12   Summary of King's Theory of Goal Achievement

Phenomenon: Human behavior involves goal-directed actions that lead to outcomes that represent evidence-based nursing practice.

Idea: Interactions that lead to transaction between the nurse and the patient result in goal achievement; that is, outcomes.

Key Concepts/Internal Variables

Health: Dynamic life experiences implying continuous adjustment to stressors from the internal and external environment. The individual achieves maximum potential through the optimal use of his/her resources.

Nursing: A process of action, reaction, interaction, and transaction between the nurse and client by sharing information about perceptions of the nursing situation.

Self: The person's inner world as distinguished from other people and things. The self comprises thoughts, feelings, and awareness of existence and includes ideas, attitudes, values, and commitments.

Examples of Propositions

Transactions between nurse and patient enable mutual goal setting and actions.

When nurse and patient transact, goals are achieved.

When goals are achieved, effective goal-directed nursing occurs.

Examples of Assumptions

Humans are open systems in constant interaction with their environment.

The goal of nursing is to help individuals and groups maintain health.

The nurse and patient influence the interaction process with their perceptions, goals, needs, and values.

Examples of External Variables

Community health needs

The role of stress on positive behavior

The effect of the environment on health problems

Examples of Facts, Principles, and Laws

Fact: Human beings have goals.

Principle: Human beings can work together to achieve health-related goals.

Law: Goals motivate health behavior.

wrote a curriculum text that presented possible approaches to both associate degree and baccalaureate nursing programs (King, 1986). She encouraged theoretical research and refining the theory of goal achievement in education.

Practice. The initial focus of King's theory was on the basic and advanced education of nurses, but expanded to include practice and research. In 1981, King designed the Goal Oriented Nursing

Record (GONR) to monitor goals and outcomes. The GONR facilitates the development of care plans with the input of patients and provides for the documentation of effectiveness of care. Nurses in almost every area of patient care have been able to use King's theory. In addition, King's theory is recognized globally and has a substantial publication history documenting its use and testing.

Research. King's framework and theory have generated considerable interest and research around the world over a long period of time. Frey and Sieloff (1995) edited a book with over 30 authors, including some from Canada, Japan, and Sweden, describing the use of King's work in their research as well as practice with adults, children, and families. Discussions on subjects as diverse as the concept of space, family health, adult orthopedic nursing, and organizational structure help illustrate the usefulness of nursing theory in empirical testing of intellectual products and knowledge development.

A number of nurses have used King's framework as a base for further theory development, including Frey's theory of families, children, and chronic illness; Sieloff's theory of departmental power; and Wicks' theory of family health (Frey & Sieloff, 1995). King (2003) continued to update the assessment of goals and measuring of nursing outcomes.

Betty Neuman: Neuman Systems Model—1974

The Theorist

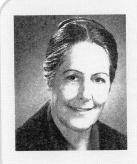

BETTY NEUMAN was born in 1924 on a farm near Lowell, Ohio. She earned a diploma in 1947 from Peoples Hospital School of Nursing, Akron, Ohio, now General Hospital. She earned a bachelor's in nursing, public health, and psychology and a master's in mental health and public health consultation from UCLA in 1957 and 1966, respectively. She earned a PhD in clinical psychology from Pacific Western University, San Francisco, California, in 1985. She practiced as staff, head, school, and industrial nurse and served as professor at UCLA. She lives in Ohio and maintains an active private practice as a licensed clinical marriage and family therapist.

Neuman is known around the world and participates in numerous international activities. She serves as a consultant to educational and practice institutions and to the Neuman systems model. An incorporated group for the model meets biennially to sponsor an international symposium to foster the work of the theory. Unanimous agreement of the trustees is required for changes in the Neuman systems model diagram (George, 2002).

The Theory

When Neuman taught at UCLA, she was responsible for developing the community mental health clinical specialist postgraduate program. Students entering the graduate clinical program requested an overview course for breadth of understanding about nursing variables, rather than depth. The model that Neuman developed in 1970 in response to this request became known as the Neuman systems model. At the time, she described what she did as a teaching tool, not a model. The model was first published in 1972 (Neuman & Young, 1972).

The Neuman systems model (1995) focuses on the response of the client to environmental stressors. These stressors may be actual or potential and may be physical, such as an elevated temperature;

psychological, a denial of diagnosis; or sociocultural or economic, such as inadequate nutrition. The nurse can use primary, secondary, and tertiary nursing prevention interventions to maintain or attain the goal of optimal client system wellness. Primary prevention is the general knowledge the nurse applies to promote wellness and stability through the prevention of stressors and the reduction of risk factors. Secondary prevention is the development of prevention as an intervention typology, and tertiary prevention relates to the adaptive process as the client returns to optimal wellness.

The Neuman systems model illustrates characteristics of open system theory. For example, the elements in nursing practice interact with each other, and the organization of nursing can respond to change. Clients include individuals, groups, and communities and their interactions with the environment. The systems perspective recognizes the client as a whole but values the interactions of the parts. Neuman views the major components of the model as stress and the reaction to stress with the goal to achieve optimal client stability (1995) (Box 7.13).

Box 7.13   Summary of Neuman's Systems Model

Phenomenon: Physiological, psychological, sociocultural, developmental, and spiritual stressors influence the patient.

Idea: Nurses interact with individuals, families, and communities in an interrelated and goal-directed manner.

Key Concepts/Internal Variables

Wholistic Client Approach: A unifying focus for nursing problem definition and for understanding the client in interaction with the environment.

Wholistic Concept: Clients are wholes whose parts are in dynamic interaction. All variables, such as physiological, psychological, sociocultural, developmental, and spiritual, are best considered simultaneously.

Wellness: Wellness exists when the parts of the client system interact in harmony and system needs are met.

Examples of Propositions

Nurses can increase the client's level of wellness by supporting client strengths.

Patients unconsciously create an intrapersonal environment that assists in coping with stressors.

The patient's normal line of defense enables a return to a state of wellness.

Examples of Assumptions (Neuman, 1995)

Nursing clients are dynamic with both unique and universal characteristics.

Clients present a normal range of responses to the environment that represent wellness and stability.

Stressors attack flexible lines of defense, normal lines of defense, and lines of resistance.

Nurses' actions are focused on primary, secondary, and tertiary prevention.

Examples of External Variables

Environmental changes

Extrapersonal stressors

Neuman continues to clarify, refine, and expand her model, which focuses on a wholistic approach to nursing care and provides a clear direction for nursing interventions (George, 2002).

Influence of Neuman's Systems Model

Education. The Neuman systems model is one of the three most widely used nursing models in existence (Reed, 1993), with an extensive body of literature coming from nurses in 17 or more countries. Baccalaureate and associate degree programs in nursing in the United States have made extensive use of Neuman's model as a framework for the curriculum (Neuman, 1989). Many found the model consistent with their philosophy and major concepts. The model has also been used by educational institutions around the world. George (2002) enumerates over three pages of continents and countries where the theory is being used, including Africa, Asia, Australia, Europe, the Pacific Islands, Scandinavia, and the United Kingdom.

Practice. Neuman's model is used worldwide in practice in a wide variety of settings. Bowman (1997) conducted a descriptive study of 43 elderly patients undergoing unplanned or planned hip surgery. Pain and sleep satisfaction were assessed for 5 days postoperatively. The author concluded that additional study should focus on effectiveness of pain management and prevention through reduction of relevant stressors. Picot, Zauszniewski, Debanne, and Holston (1999) based their study about the relationship between mood and blood pressure in African American caregivers and noncaregivers on the Neuman model. The study examined how stressors affected caregivers' and noncaregivers' mood symptoms and blood pressure. The two groups were equivalent on hypertension risk. The Neuman systems model has also been used in diverse administrative and case management settings (Parker, 2001).

Research. Until recently, Neuman's model has had much less impact on research than on education and practice (Meleis, 1997). A number of nurse scholars have suggested guidelines and methods to stimulate the interest and increased research development (Fawcett, 1995; Gigliotti, 1997; Meleis, 1997; Smith & Edgil, 1995). Gigliotti (2003) describes plans to develop the Institute for the Study of the Neuman Systems Model. The work of the institute would be to formulate and test the credibility of middle-range theories derived from the Neuman systems model.

The University of British Columbia (UBC) Model for Nursing—1976

The Theorists

Several faculty members at the University of British Columbia (UBC) School of Nursing, some of whom were students of Dorothy Johnson at UCLA, were inspired by her behavioral system model. These faculty members, along with other UBC colleagues, are considered the theorists of the UBC model for nursing.

Theory

The UBC model for nursing, first published in 1976, was inspired by Johnson's model and provides a structure for combining general knowledge about human health and illness with specific knowledge about individual patients. The UBC model broadened the view of human experience and considered the behavioral system to be composed of nine basic human needs (Fig. 7.3). Each of these needs is shaped by the psychological and sociocultural environment in which it is expressed (Campbell, Cruise, & Murakami, 1976).

Each need was considered to be universal and fundamental to basic human experience. The achievement of need-related human behavior was directed by goals and strategies that are

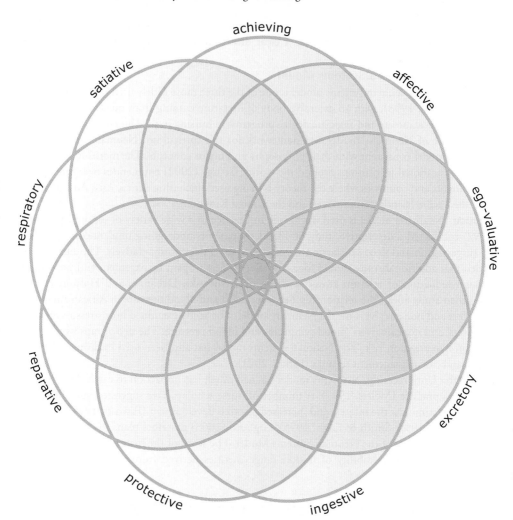

Figure 7.3 The University of British Columbia (UBC) model for nursing. (Courtesy of Sally Thorne, UBC School of Nursing.)

unique to the individual and his or her particular physiological, psychological, or social circumstances (Thorne, Jillings, Ellis, & Perry, 1993). The UBC model provides a structure by which general knowledge about human health and illness is combined with particular knowledge about each individual patient. In accordance with general systems theory, the goal of nursing is to achieve balance in the behavioral system. The nurse fosters, protects, sustains, and teaches the patient (Campbell, 1987) and thereby brings about balance, stability, and optimal health (Box 7.14).

Influence of UBC Model for Nursing

The UBC model for nursing was the foundation for the undergraduate curriculum at the University of British Columbia during the 1970s and 1980s. The model was used in clinical agencies on the UBC campus, primarily to study client assessment. Graduates of the program were expected to incorporate concepts of the model into their practice.

Box 7.14   Summary of the University of British Columbia Model for Nursing

Phenomenon: The nurse's knowledge about health and the patient affects the achievement of optimal health care.

Idea: Combining general knowledge about human health and illness with particular knowledge about the individual patient creates a balanced, goal-directed system.

Key Concepts/Internal Variables

Nine Basic Needs: Universal requirements based on nine subsystems that comprise the behavioral system. Each need is shaped by the psychological and sociocultural environment.

Goals: Individualized for each patient based on his or her needs. The ultimate goal is optimal health.

Critical Periods: Maturational and unpredictable events in the life cycle that require nursing interventions to achieve optimal health.

Examples of Propositions

Nurse assists clients to define and pursue optimal health.

Nurse focuses on the development of new coping behaviors of the client.

Nurse engages client during pregnancy (maturational event).

Examples of Assumptions

Basic human needs are universal.

When basic needs are satisfied, the system is in balance.

Optimal health is the highest level of system stability.

Examples of External Variables

Psychomotor skills

Medical orders

Family interference in care

Evelyn Adam: Conceptual Model for Nursing—1979 (French) and 1980 (English)

The Theorist

EVELYN ADAM was born on April 9, 1929, in Lanark, Ontario, Canada. She graduated from Hotel Dieu Hospital School of Nursing in Kingston, Ontario. She earned a bachelor's from the University of Montreal in 1966 and a master's in nursing from UCLA in 1971. She taught at the University of Montreal from 1982 to 1989, when she retired and was named professor emeritus. She lives in Montreal.

When Adam was enrolled in the UCLA graduate nursing program, she met Dorothy Johnson, who developed the behavioral systems model discussed earlier. Adam described Professor Johnson as "the most important influence" on her professional life (Tomey & Alligood, 2001). Adam served as visiting professor at several universities and continues to consult, speak, and write. She has received numerous awards, including an honorary doctorate.

The Theory

Adam's conceptual model for nursing was influenced by Johnson and Virginia Henderson; however, her work focuses primarily on the development of models and theories (1991). She used Johnson's behavioral systems model and applied Henderson's definition of nursing to her assumptions, values, and fundamental needs. Adam's work has contributed to theory development by clarifying the earlier models of Johnson and Henderson. For example, by establishing a structural model for Henderson's writing, Adam was able to extend its usefulness in nursing. The connection between Adam's model and Henderson's definition is evident in the summary (see Box 7.15).

Box 7.15   Summary of Adam's Conceptual Model for Nursing

Phenomenon: The nurse is responsible for meeting the patient's fundamental needs.

Idea: Nursing facilitates the patient's independence in meeting basic health needs.

Key Concepts/Internal Variables

Helping Relationship: Interactions that aid the patient to live more freely. An interpersonal exchange in which the nurse demonstrates qualities such as empathy and respect.

Need: A requirement common to all human beings, either well or ill, that may be specific, particular, or personal to an individual and is derived from a fundamental need.

Independence Nursing: The nature of the nurse's contribution to the large and complex areas of health services.

Examples of Propositions

The nurse assists the patient to identify fundamental needs.

Nursing interventions assist patients to meet fundamental needs.

Patients benefit from a helping relationship with the nurse.

Examples of Assumptions

Every individual strives for and desires independence.

Every individual is a complex whole, made up of fundamental needs.

When a need is not satisfied, the individual is not complete, whole, or independent.

Examples of External Variables

Nurses and others who prefer dependent patients.

Family members who encourage dependency in the patient.

Psychological illness that excludes nursing involvement.

Throughout the description of the conceptual model of nursing, Adam (1991) focuses on the nurse's independent contribution to health services, which she calls independence nursing. The nurse is responsible for knowing what independence nursing is and for explaining it to others (Adam, 1991). In the appendix of her book, Adam provides three clinical examples and an assessment tool, which focuses on Henderson's 14 basic human needs.

Influence of Adam's Conceptual Model of Nursing

Education. Adam identifies educational goals, objectives, and nursing content for educational programs at baccalaureate, master's, and doctoral levels, with each level building on the prior one. Because this was one of the first theories developed by a Canadian nurse, one would anticipate that it would influence the educational system. The clinical examples and the assessment tool presented in the book's appendix support the idea that the model has educational value (Adam, 1980).

Practice. Although the literature does not include articles about using the model in the practice setting, the values, assumptions, and basic needs are closely related to Henderson's work and to common nursing practice. The clinical examples and the discussion of collecting data for identified patient needs are practice oriented, as is the assessment tool. Examples include a 58-year-old woman with a neurological condition, a 22-year-old man with depression, and a postpartum patient with cystitis. The assessment tool would be useful in all of these instances, as well as many other practice settings.

Research. While Adam's model has been viewed very favorably, it has generated little research as determined by the literature. Adam poses questions that would be relevant for research and indicates that some master's theses have been based on the model. In 1988, Adam indicated that there was increasing interest in the model, especially in teaching and research (Tomey & Alligood, 2001).

Margaret A. Newman: Theory of Health as Expanding Consciousness—1979
The Theorist

MARGARET A. NEWMAN was born on October 10, 1933, in Memphis, Tennessee. She earned a bachelor's in home economics and English at Baylor University, Texas, in 1954; bachelor's in nursing from the University of Tennessee, Mephis, in 1962; a master's in medical-surgical nursing and teaching from the University of California, San Francisco, in 1964; and a PhD in nursing science and rehabilitation from New York University (NYU) in 1971. Newman selected NYU to work with Martha Rogers and her theory on the science of unitary human beings, which we discussed previously. Newman was on the faculties of the University of Tennessee, New York University, Pennsylvania State University, and the University of Minnesota. She retired in 1996 as professor emeritus and lives in Minneapolis.

Newman has received numerous awards and honors and has presented papers and conducted workshops in 11 or more countries around the world.

The Theory

As a recent college graduate in home economics, Margaret Newman was the primary caregiver of her mother, who had amyotrophic lateral sclerosis (ALS, or Lou Gehrig's disease). Although she had not entered nursing at the time, Newman became interested in nursing and health care. She explored relationships between time, movement, and space and how they were related to health and illness. She credits Martha Rogers and the science of unitary human beings for influencing her work. At first she questioned Rogers' proposition that "health and illness are simply expressions of the life process—one no more important than the other" (Marchione, 1993, p. 3). Later, Newman recognized that Rogers was correct and introduced the idea into her theory. Newman presented the basic assumptions of her theory at a national conference in New York City in 1979. Her first major publication was in 1986.

The theory of health as expanding consciousness considers health and illness as components of a unitary process that Newman calls the pattern of wholeness. Therefore, both health and disease are part of the pattern. The major concepts in Newman's theory are consciousness, movement, space, and time. She views these concepts through pattern, pattern recognition, and expanding consciousness. Understanding each of these concepts, unfortunately, does not always yield understanding of the entire theory.

Newman views the role of the nurse as forming relationships with patients and facilitating their ability to recognize patterns in their lives and health. These patterns then identify the individual as

---

Box 7.16   Summary of Newman's Theory of Health as Expanding Consciousness

Phenomenon: Physical or social immobility alters one's perception of time.

Idea: During a period of illness or disease, the individual's perspective of time changes.

Key Concepts/Internal Variables

Health: A fusion of disease and nondisease. Health is the evolving pattern of the person and the environment and is viewed as a pattern of the whole.

Pattern: Characteristics of an individual as a particular person, such as the genetic pattern, the voice pattern, and the movement pattern.

Pattern Recognition: Meaning and understanding that speed up the evolution of consciousness.

Consciousness: A manifestation of an evolving pattern of person-environment interaction, including cognitive and affective awareness and interconnectedness of the system.

Expanding Consciousness: Moving toward increasing complexity of the living system, that is, health.

Examples of Propositions

Time and space have a complementary relationship.

Movement is a reflection of consciousness.

Time is a function of movement and a measurement of consciousness.

Examples of Assumptions

Health and disease are parts of the same whole and are interrelated in space, time, movement, and pattern development.

Disease is a manifestation of the underlying pattern of the person.

Health is the expansion of consciousness.

Examples of External Variables

Treatment outcomes, unrelated to evolving consciousness

Therapeutic nursing interventions, not related to healing

Disease, in the traditional sense of the word

a particular person. When an individual confronts a disease, for example, the interaction of the person with the disease enhances the person's energy and power in the situation.

As Newman cared for her mother, she came to realize that long-term illness can be dealt with if the person's consciousness is expanding. This is exhibited by deeper appreciation for life and having more meaningful relationships (Yamashita & Tall, 1998) (Box 7.16).

Influence of Newman's Theory

Education. Newman's theory focuses on health, which she defines as including both health and disease. Although this definition provides content in a model called The Healing Web, it is not consistent with the undergraduate curriculum in most institutions (Bunkers et al., 1992). On the other hand, a health-oriented graduate program provides a coordinated education, practice, and research theme. Newman's theory is useful when viewing nursing practice and research as a whole, but less useful in nursing education.

Practice. Newman's nurse is responsible for establishing a primary relationship with the client for the purpose of identifying health care needs and facilitating the client's action potential and decision-making ability. Newman's theory has been used in various practice settings. For example, in Japan, the theory was used as a basis to understand the experience of primary family caregivers of clients who were afflicted with schizophrenia (Yamashita & Tall, 1998). The occurrence of pattern identification and subsequent action helps deepen the relationship between client and family.

Research. Newman views the role of research as testing theory and establishing a scientific knowledge base from which professional practice takes place. She promotes the idea of research as praxis, that is, the integration of theory into practice. Research of the theory has focused on a variety of topics, such as the relationship between music and chronic pain (Schorr, 1993) and comparing expansion of consciousness of caregiving in Canada and Japan (Yamashita, 1999). As you read other reports of research about Newman's theory, you will be able to increase your understanding of the relationships of time, movement, and space.

M. Jean Watson: Theory of Human Caring—1979

The Theorist

Watson joined the faculty of the CU School of Nursing in 1973. While she was dean, she founded and directed the Center of Human Caring at CU Health Science Center, now called the International Center for Integrative Caring Practices. She holds the Endowed Chair in Caring Science at the CU School of Nursing. She has received many awards and honorary degrees and is recognized worldwide. She received a Fulbright Research and Lecture Award in Sweden and an International Kellogg Fellowship in Australia.

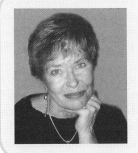

M. JEAN WATSON was born and raised in West Virginia. She earned a diploma from Lewis Gayle School of Nursing in Roanoke, Virginia; a bachelor of science in nursing in 1964 from the University of Colorado (CU), Boulder; a master of science in psychiatric-mental health nursing in 1968 from the CU Health Sciences Center; and a PhD in educational psychology and counseling in 1973 from CU, Boulder. She served as dean of the CU School of Nursing from 1983 to 1990 and currently serves as distinguished professor of nursing. She is recognized worldwide.

The Theory

Watson published *Nursing: Human Science and Caring,* describing her theory of human caring, in 1979 with later editions in 1985, 1988, and 1999. She described her first book as a treatise for undergraduate nursing students (1979) and designed her second one especially for use by graduate students (1985). The initial book's reference to a philosophy and science of caring in nursing (Watson, 1979) was changed to human science and human care in later books (1985).

Watson defines 10 "carative" factors as the core of nursing. The core is intrinsic to the nurse–patient process as opposed to the "trim," which she describes as the practice setting and the procedures, techniques, and terminology of nursing (1979). Trim exists in relation to the caring relationship. Carative factors vary considerably in structure and nature, for example, from altruistic values to scientific problem solving and from sensitivity to others to expressions of negative feelings. The 10 carative factors are listed in Box 7.17.

The nurse who adopts Watson's theory intends and is committed to caring for the patient. Caring is a way of being for this nurse with the intention of going above and beyond, or transcending, human-to-human contact. In other words, the nurse and patient become aware of the other person's frame of reference and share perceptions emotionally and spiritually. This self-awareness and spiritual evolution focuses on the soul of human beings. In a transpersonal caring relationship, nurse and patient reveal the spirit and humanity of the professional experience through human-to-human contact with the goal of restoring the patient's inner harmony, or wellness.

To Watson, nursing is both a science and an art that assists the patient to obtain greater harmony or agreement among the mind, body, and spirit. The nurse and patient explore the meaning of their health–illness experiences through human-to-human transactions. Watson speaks of the values of respect, reverence for the spiritual, and human autonomy. The ultimate, guiding value of the model, however, presents caring "as the moral ideal of nursing, with a concern for the preservation of humanity, dignity, and fullness of self" (1985, p. 74).

In 1999, Watson incorporated the paradigm of postmodern nursing into her theory. She describes this as an expanded view of consciousness that is holistic and embraces energy and spirit. Postmodern nursing explores the nature of healing relationships, with the use of nursing and self-knowledge in the healing process coming from the discovery of facts, principles, laws, and technology that stem from the sciences. Modernism and postmodernism are discussed in Chapter 9.

Influence of Watson's Theory of Human Caring

Education. The theory of human caring has been used to develop new frameworks for nursing curricula. The nursing doctorate (ND) at the University of Colorado and entry-level nursing programs across the country are based on the theory of human caring. As a worldwide traveler and speaker, Watson has influenced nursing programs in Australia, Scandinavia, and the United Kingdom. These programs have adopted the theory of human caring as an organizing framework for the curriculum or included significant elements into their programs. At this time, her theory appears to have more acceptance abroad than it has in America. Some nursing faculty are concerned that the theory does not emphasize pathophysiological aspects sufficiently. Watson views pathophysiology as an element of the trim, which she considers necessary but less important than the core as defined by the carative factors.

Practice. Watson's theory is accepted as a holistic view of nursing care in the practice field. The focus on human caring is particularly appealing to individuals and institutions that are committed to a holistic approach to care, and they are more willing to adopt the theory. The Caring Center at the University of Colorado, founded by Watson, provides high-quality health care for people with human immunodeficiency virus (HIV) infections or acquired immunodeficiency

Box 7.17 Summary of Watson's Theory on Human Caring

Phenomenon: Human caring encompasses "spirit rather than matter, flux rather than form, inner knowledge and power rather than circumstance."

Idea: To provide a philosophical perspective that offers an alternative to technology, science, and the disease-cure model.

Key Concepts/Internal Variables (Tomey & Alligood, 2002)

Caring: The essence of nursing practice that is intrinsically related to healing; a moral ideal rather than a task-oriented behavior

Ten Carative Factors:
Humanistic-altruistic system of values
Faith-hope
Sensitivity to self and to others
Helping-trusting, human care relationship
Expression of positive and negative feelings
Creative problem-solving caring process
Transpersonal teaching-learning
A supportive, protective, and corrective mental, physical, sociocultural, and spiritual environment
Human needs assistance
Existential-phenomenological-spiritual forces

Examples of Propositions

Caring occurs when both nurse and patient participate in a transpersonal relationship.

Human-to-human contact enhances the patient's capacity for self-healing.

Healing takes place and health is realized through the patient's self-discovery and self-awareness.

Examples of Assumptions (Selected from eleven assumptions [Watson, 1985]).

Caring for the self is a prerequisite for respecting and caring for others.

Caring is the central unifying focus of nursing practice—the essence of nursing.

Only through interpersonal relationships can human care be effectively demonstrated and practiced.

Examples of External Variables

Technology

Short individual exposure to another person

Pathophysiology

syndrome (AIDS) under the belief that understanding, love, and concern foster healing. Watson's theory provides the model for the purpose, organization, and evaluation of the work of the Center. The adoption of Watson's theory refocuses nursing from a biomedical model to a healing, caring process. Nurses who value the caring/healing emphasis may also hope to retain the physical aspects of care as well.

Research. There has been little research supporting Watson's theory. The abstract framework of the theory has raised questions about the type of research techniques that could be used to generate useful findings. Watson believes that traditional research methods are inadequate for knowledge development about human caring. She suggests that using qualitative-naturalistic-phenomenological methods and descriptive phenomenological approaches are more useful (1985).

Nursing Theory in the 1980s

The emphasis of new nursing theories in the 1980s was primarily on care and caring, with each theory helping to open the way for nurses to revisit basic characteristics of nursing and then contemplate nontraditional approaches to practice. This is illustrated by the following four theories:

- Rosemarie Parse's theory of human becoming in 1981
- Patricia Benner's skill acquisition model in 1984
- Madeleine Leininger's theory on culture care diversity and universality in 1985
- McGill University's practice-based model in 1987

Rosemarie Rizzo Parse: Theory of Human Becoming—1981

The Theorist

ROSEMARIE RIZZO PARSE earned a bachelor of science in nursing from Duquesne University, Pittsburgh, and both a master of science in nursing and PhD from the University of Pittsburgh. She was a faculty member of the University of Pittsburgh, dean of nursing at Duquesne University, and professor and coordinator of nursing research at Hunter College, City University of New York. She served as professor at Loyola University in Chicago as the Marcella Niehoff Chair until she retired as professor emeritus. Parse is the founding editor of *Nursing Science Quarterly*, a scholarly journal that requires every article to be linked to theory.

The Theory

In 1981, Parse introduced the man–living–health theory that deals with man's total experience with health. In 1992, she changed the name to the theory of human becoming in response to a change in the meaning of "man" from mankind to a gender designation. She revised some of the assumptions at that time, but other aspects of the theory were not changed. Initially Parse relied on Rogers' work that viewed the person as an energy field; now Parse sees the person as an open being. While Rogers defined health as a value, Parse views it as a process (Bunting, 1993). Parse classifies nursing as a human science in which the nurse relates to the person and family on a one-to-one basis without offering advice, opinions, or a canned approach to care (Parse, 1987).

Parse designed the theory to consider the person as a whole, not in the traditional way that focuses on systems or fragments of the whole. She poses two world perspectives. In one, the person is a total being that is a combination of bio-psycho-social-spiritual aspects who interacts with and adapts to the external and internal environment. She describes this view as an applied science that draws from natural sciences. In the other world perspective, the person is more than and different from the sum of his or her parts. The person is free to choose and has mutual interchanges with the environment. This perspective is considered a basic science with its own body of knowledge (George, 2002). These perspectives are called the totality worldview and simultaneity worldview, respectively. These ideas will be important in the discussion below about the influence of the theory on nursing practice.

Parse identified three theoretical structures or propositions, fortunately stating them in more concrete terms so they could guide nursing practice. The first theoretical structure, powering emerges with the revealing-concealing of imaging, can be stated as "struggling to live goals discloses the significance of the situation" (Parse, 1987, p. 170). An example of this might be when family members meet to discuss thoughts and feelings about selecting a nursing home for their grandmother. The following topics may arise and be discussed: distance to the facility, financial matters, the grandmother's wishes, and how other family members and friends will react. As members reveal their opinions about these topics, the meaning of the situation changes for family members, as well as for the family as a whole.

The second theoretical structure is originating emerges with the enabling-limiting of valuing. Parse restates this as "creating anew shows one's cherished beliefs and leads in a directional movement" (Parse, 1987, p. 170). As family members share thoughts about their grandmother's care, additional ideas are identified with individuals agreeing or disagreeing. For example, a family member suggests a temporary stay in an assisted-living facility that is in the immediate neighborhood as a stepping stone to nursing home care. This suggestion encourages other family members to think about other alternatives.

The final theoretical structure is that transforming emerges with the languaging of connecting-separating. The interpretation of this statement is "changing views emerge in speaking and moving with others" (Parse, 1987, p. 170). The family meeting to decide on a nursing home changes when the discussion shifts to other, possibly interim, alternatives. The family may find the alternative more appealing, and the group of family members may come together around the new approach. The goal of nursing in the theory of human becoming is quality of life of the person and the person's family. Think about whether that goal in the above example is achieved.

As you see, Parse's approach to nursing practice and her use of language differs from more traditional nursing language. At times, it is difficult to understand what she means, and it may take considerable effort to describe how nurses can use it.

Parse proposes nine concepts of human becoming: languaging, valuing, imaging, revealing-concealing, enabling-limiting, connecting-separating, powering, originating, and transforming. Parse formulates these concepts as participles to emphasize the process orientation of the theory. You have seen how several of these concepts are used in the above example. As you continue to study the theory of human becoming, explore possible meanings for other concepts of human becoming (Box 7.18).

Influence of Parse's Theory

Education. An unusual feature of Parse's theory is its use by the South Dakota Board of Nursing (SDBON) as the theoretical foundation for its regulatory model for decisioning; the Board's values and tenets of public policy making are also used. A 3-year study that began in 1995 revealed that the nursing licensing examination focused only on the totality paradigm in nursing, which is based on the natural sciences. The SDBON agreed to recognize graduates of programs embracing the simultaneity paradigm as well; this paradigm is based on nursing science. This will obviously have an impact on educational programs in the state (Damgaard & Bunkers, 1998) and possibly elsewhere.

Until recently, the theory has been used primarily at the graduate level. The 1981 introduction of the theory presented a sample curriculum for a master's in nursing; the curriculum plan was updated in 1998.

Box 7.18   Summary of Parse's Theory of Human Becoming

Phenomenon: Humans who change the priorities of their values change their health patterns as well.

Idea: The interrelationship between the nurse and the patient /family depends on lived experience.

Key Concepts/Internal Variables (Parse, 1998)

In addition to the nine concepts mentioned above, Parse uses the following:

Meaning: The linguistic and imagined content of something and the interpretation that one gives to something. The ultimate meaning or purpose in life and the meaning in moments of everyday living.

Rhythmicity: The paced, paradoxical patterning of the human–universe mutual process. Parse suggests that the patterning can be visualized as the ebb and flow of waves coming into shore.

Transcendence: Reaching or going beyond the possibles; that is, the hopes and dreams and shifting views people have about their lives.

Human Becoming: Human beings' participative experience with the world—past, present, and yet to come. Unique unfolding, which is health.

Examples of Propositions (See theoretical structures above)

Struggling to live goals discloses the significance of the situation.

Creating anew shows one's cherished beliefs and leads in a directional movement.

Changing views emerge in speaking and moving with others.

Examples of Assumptions (George, 1998)

The human is open, freely choosing meaning in situation, bearing responsibility for decisions.

The human is unity, continuously coconstituting patterns of relating.

The human is transcending multidimensionality with the possibles.

Examples of External Variables

Medical diagnosis

Prescriptive rules

Traditional nursing interventions

Practice. Parse's theory was developed to provide a model for nursing practice and has been used in the United States and worldwide. The theory has been used in a community-based nursing practice (Bauman, 1997), hospitals (Daiski, 1996), and long-term care (Mitchell, 1997), as well as in the acute psychiatric setting described below.

An evaluation of the theory in an acute psychiatric setting yields some interesting findings (Northrup & Cody, 1998). Three units were selected: a minimally secure forensic inpatient unit; a small neuropsychiatric inpatient unit for people with progressive disorders of the nervous system, such as Parkinson's disease; and a geriatric psychiatry inpatient unit primarily for assessment and treatment of affective disorders or dementia. Data were collected through taped interviews, written questionnaires, and chart audits. Subjects included nurses, patients, unit managers, and hospital supervisors. The changes that nurses reported included shifting views of human beings, thinking about patients as people, having closer relationships, heightened awareness of the patient's perspective, and looking beyond labels. While some nurses had difficulty learning Parse's theory, most adopted it and were able to benefit from its approach.

Research. Like Watson, there has been little research conducted on this theory. Parse does not believe that the theory of human becoming can be tested in the usual manner, because it is not a predictive, or cause-and-effect, theory. The focus of research is to uncover the essences of lived phenomena to gain further understanding of universal human experiences. Understanding evolves from connecting the descriptions from people to the theory, thus making the real meaning of humans more explicit.

Although Parse uses language that can be confusing, she has been meticulous in constructing the theory and has provided new insights into aspects of health. The theory is rooted in the human sciences and responds best to qualitative research, such as descriptive and ethnography.

Patricia Benner: Model of Skill Acquisition in Nursing—1984

The Theorist

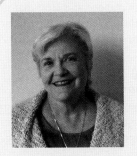

PATRICIA BENNER was born in 1942 in Hampton, Virginia, and spent her childhood in California. She earned a bachelor of arts in nursing from Pasadena College in 1964; a master's from University of California, San Francisco (UCSF) in 1970; and a PhD from University of Carlifornia, Berkeley, in 1982. She was a research assistant as a graduate student and a postdoctoral nurse researcher for 12 years at UCSF. She worked in acute medical-surgical, critical care, and home health. She is a prolific writer and well known for *From Novice to Expert: Excellence and Power in Clinical Nursing Practice* (1984). Currently she directs the Carnegie National Nursing Education Study, the first national study of nursing education in 30 years that will compare six professions: teaching, clergy, engineering, law, nursing, and medicine.

Benner has received awards and honors nationally and internationally for leadership in research and education, as well as contributions to nursing science and research. She is a tenured professor at UCSF, teaching at the master's and doctoral levels. She continues to lecture and lead workshops worldwide.

The Theory

Benner developed the model of skill acquisition in nursing based on a study of the acquisition and development of skills by chess players and airline pilots in emergency situations (Dreyfus & Dreyfus, 1980). In her model, students pass through five levels of skill acquisition: novice, advanced beginner, competent, proficient, and expert (Benner, 1984). As individuals progress through these levels, they demonstrate changes in four performance areas. First, they move from relying on abstract principles to using concrete experiences. Second, they move from analytic, rule-based thinking to intuition. Third, their perception changes from a situation composed of equally relevant parts to a complex whole in which certain parts are more relevant than others. Finally, they move from a detached observer to an actively involved performer (Benner & Wrubel, 1989).

Whether you look at chess players, pilots, or nurses, it is clear that skill acquisition includes interventions and judgment skills, not just psychomotor skills. In nursing, this refers to the application of nursing skills in actual clinical situations. The findings of Benner's study that were based on interviews with 51 nurses and observations of 26 of these subjects provide intriguing information about clinical nursing knowledge. Benner also identified seven domains of nursing practice: the helping role, the teaching–coaching function, the diagnostic and patient-monitoring function, effective management of rapidly changing situations, the administration and monitoring of therapeutic interventions and regimens, monitoring and ensuring the quality of health care practices, and organizational and work-role competencies (Benner, 1984) (Box 7.19).

Benner and Wrubel (1989) extended the model of skill acquisition in nursing by introducing caring as the necessary response to stress, illustrating the process through exemplars of practicing nurses. The book attracted significant attention for depicting nursing practice as nurses know it, demonstrating how a nurse thinks and how thinking and reasoning change with significant experience.

In her original research, Benner's goal was to "uncover meanings and knowledge embedded in skilled practice" (Benner, 1984, p. 218). From the findings discussed above, it is clear that she achieved her goal. As she continues to study and expand the model, the knowledge about skill acquisition expands as well (Benner, Hooper-Kyriakidis, & Stannard, 1999; Benner, Tanner, & Chesla, 1996; Benner & Wrubel, 1989).

Influence of Benner's Model of Skill Acquisition in Nursing

Education. In the 20 years since Benner's book, *From Novice to Expert*, was published, educators and practitioners have adopted it as a model for understanding the knowledge of practice and how it should be taught (Benner, 1984). The model touches both undergraduate and graduate students, as well as the practicing nurse. Descriptions of the expectations of learners and the changes that occur at each level are useful to teachers and students.

A series of practical applications are included in *From Novice to Expert*. One application describes the use of a curriculum planning and evaluation method for graduate programs that had yielded more problems than solutions (Fenton, 1984). When faculty adopted Benner's approach, there were many advantages, such as sharing ideas, validating educational practices, and narrowing the gap between practice and education.

Practice. Continuing education and career development departments use the Benner model extensively, as does nursing management, preceptors, and clinical interns. Nurses who are exposed to the model early in their professional careers respond with excitement and interest. Fenton (1984) reports that the model has been used successfully for developing clinical ladders, new graduate orientation, and clinical symposia.

Research. Benner's (1984) model of skill acquisition for nursing is based on descriptive research. She and her cohorts listened to nurses who were making a positive difference in the care of patients and reported their descriptions. Nurse researchers have continued this approach. Two examples illustrate the type of research being conducted. Brykczynski (1989)

Box 7.19   Summary of Benner's Model of Skill Acquisition

Phenomenon: The stage or level of skill acquisition a nurse achieves is based on his or her experience.

Idea: Nurses move through distinct phases as they develop clinical expertise.

Key Concepts/Internal Variables

Competence: A feeling of mastery; the ability to cope with and manage the contingencies of clinical nursing; conscious, deliberate planning to achieve efficiency and organization.

Skill Acquisition: Development and implementation of nursing interventions and clinical judgment skills. It does not include context-free psychomotor skills or other enabling skills.

Experience: An active process of refining and changing preconceived theories, notions, and ideas when confronted with actual situations.

Theoretical Knowledge: "Knowing that" or theoretical explanations; establishing causal relationships between events.

Practical Knowledge: "Knowing how" is the acquisition of skills. Individuals are able to practice these skills before developing a theoretical explanation.

Examples of Propositions

The nurse's critical thinking ability is related to professional nursing experience.

The length of experience a nurse has in a specific nursing specialty affects his or her stage of competence.

The acquisition of skills occurs in actual clinical situations.

Examples of Assumptions (Benner, 1984)

"All practical situations are more complex than can be described by formal models, theories and textbook descriptions" (p. 178).

"The clinician's knowledge is embedded in perceptions rather than precepts" (p. 43).

"Expert nurses depend on discretionary judgment and need only limited rules" (p. 202).

Examples of External Variables

Policies, procedure books, and other regulations

The stage of competence of other nurses in the work setting

The intellectual capability of the nurse

analyzed 199 clinical situations to identify the knowledge and clinical judgment that experienced nurse practitioners use in their practices. Three major themes were identified in the study: discretionary judgment, background knowledge, and practical skills. Maynard (1996) used Benner's model to examine the relationship between a nurse's critical thinking ability and professional competence.

Madeleine M. Leininger: Culture Care: Diversity and Universality Theory—1985
The Theorist

MADELEINE M. LEININGER was born in Sutton, Nebraska. She received a diploma in 1948 from St. Anthony's Hospital School of Nursing in Denver and served in the Cadet Nurse Corps while pursuing her basic nursing education. She earned a bachelor's in biological science from Benedictine College in Kansas in 1950 and, after completing advanced study in nursing at Creighton University in Omaha, a master's in psychiatric nursing from Catholic University of America in Washington, DC. She was the first nurse to study anthropology at the doctoral level, earning her PhD from the University of Washington, Seattle, in 1965. She currently lives in Omaha, Nebraska.

In the mid-1950s, when Leininger was working in a child guidance home in Cincinnati, she discovered that staff did not understand the cultural factors that influenced the behavior of children. She concluded that nursing decisions and actions did not help children adequately. This experience stimulated her to pursue doctoral study in anthropology. Her early writings, beginning in the late 1970s, focused on caring and transcultural nursing. She continued to write about these areas before publishing her theory on culture care diversity and universality in its entirety (Leininger, 1985, 1988).

Leininger has held positions in nursing education and administration, serving as dean of nursing at the Universities of Washington and Utah. She was director of the Center for Health Research at Wayne State University in Michigan until she retired as professor emeritus. In addition to studying in New Guinea during her doctoral study, she has studied 14 other cultures in depth. She is the founder and leader of the field of transcultural nursing and has served as a consultant about transcultural nursing and her theory of culture care around the globe. She established the *Journal of Transcultural Nursing* in 1989 and served as editor for 6 years. She has numerous honorary degrees and other national awards and has served as visiting professor or lecturer in 10 or more countries.

The Theory

The conceptual and theoretical framework for Leininger's culture care diversity and universality theory was laid out in her early writings about transcultural nursing, but was not published until 1985. Initially, Leininger focused on the importance of caring in nursing and became aware of the special needs of children with different cultural backgrounds. Transcultural nursing, as this subfield of nursing practice and research is known, focuses on the cultural values, beliefs, and practices of individuals and groups with the goal of providing culture-specific care (George, 2002). Both the nurse and the client are considered.

Leininger's theory includes 14 concepts, 10 labeled as major and 4 as "other." The concepts she shares most frequently with other theorists are care, caring, health, and nursing, but those that are most distinctive to her theory are culture care, diversity, universality, worldview, and ethnohistory. Leininger developed the sunrise model to help nurses visualize the components of the culture care theory. The model is a cognitive map that moves from the most abstract to the least abstract and provides a holistic and comprehensive conceptual picture of the important factors in the theory. The top of the map provides the worldview and social system level, which directs the study of perceptions of the world outside of the culture (Fig. 7.4).

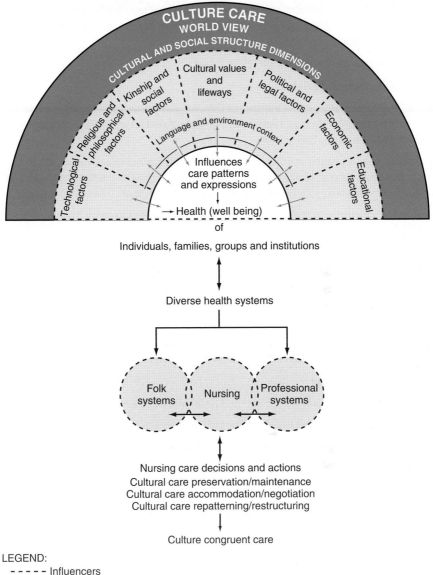

Figure 7.4 Leininger's sunrise model depicts dimensions of culture care diversity and universality. (From Leininger, M. M. [Ed.]. [1991]. *Culture care diversity and universality: A theory of nursing* [p. 43]. New York: National League for Nursing Press. Used with permission.)

Leininger continues to revise and refine her theory and is actively involved in identifying concepts and phenomena for study. She assists graduate students and others to use her framework for designing their research. Although nurses credit Watson with inventing the caring movement, Leininger played a significant role in bringing the caring concept to the nursing community in the mid-1960s (Leininger, 1977) (Box 7.20).

Phenomenon: Every individual and group belongs to a culture or subculture that has specific beliefs and values that influence nursing care.

Idea: Effective nurses provide culturally relevant care.

Key Concepts/Internal Variables

Culture: "The learned, shared, and transmitted knowledge of values, beliefs, norms, and lifeways of a particular group that guides an individual or group in their thinking, decision, and actions in patterned way" (Leininger, 1985, p. 210).

Culture Care: The subjectively and objectively learned and transmitted values, beliefs, and patterned lifeways that assist, support, facilitate, or enable an individual or group to maintain well-being and health, to improve the human condition and lifeway, or to deal with illness, handicaps, or death.

Diversity: The variables and/or differences in the ways that cultures perceive, know, and practice health and nursing care.

Universality: The commonalities in the ways that cultures share the perceptions, knowledge, and practices related to health and nursing care.

Worldview: The way people look at the world or the universe, and form a "picture or value stance" about the world and their lives (Leininger, 1985, p. 105).

Ethnohistory: "Past facts, events, instances, and experiences of individuals, groups, cultures, and institutions that are primarily people-centered (ethno) and that describe, explain, and interpret human lifeways within a particular culture over periods of time" (Leininger, 1985, p. 106).

Examples of Propositions

Culture-specific caring actions lead to improved health and well-being of individuals.

Economics, religion, and kinship ties of a culture influence health care patterns.

Nursing and health care that is culturally congruent has a favorable impact on health and well-being.

Examples of Assumptions

Health care is shaped by the individual's or group's cultural values, beliefs, and practices.

The central purpose of nursing is to serve human beings worldwide.

Beneficial, healthy, and satisfying culturally based nursing care contributes to the well-being of individuals, families, groups, and communities within their environmental context.

Examples of External Variables

The use of universal procedures and techniques

Health care that is shaped by textbooks

Mass production of health care

Examples of Facts, Principles, and Laws

Fact: Human beings belong to different cultures and subcultures.

Principle: Cultures have specific values and beliefs about health and health care.

Law: Cultural values and beliefs influence health behavior.

Influence of Leininger's Culture Care: Diversity and Universality Theory

Education. The impact of culture care preceded the 1985 introduction of Leininger's theory. In 1966, Leininger introduced the concepts of cultural care at the undergraduate level and in 1977, at the master's and doctoral levels. There are few, if any, nursing programs that do not recognize the impact of culture on nursing care, even though they may not give credit to the theory. Leininger's theory has made an enormous impact on how nursing is taught around the world; however, she is concerned that few programs use it as a major focus. Her global influence on education has been significant, with presentations and consultations on every continent and in innumerable counties (Tomey & Alligood, 2002).

Practice. As the world becomes smaller and populations shift, neighborhoods become more diverse, and there is a need to consider cultural backgrounds of patients in your decisions about nursing care. When you travel outside the country or even your community, you will be exposed to ideas that are different than those you learned and practiced as a child. When you look at patients, you see things you would not have noticed prior to Leininger's work. Your patients may look different, speak a different language, eat different foods, worship different gods, wear different clothes, use different standards of daily hygiene, and care for the ill and elderly in different ways. For example, in some countries, a family member sleeps on a mat under the patient's hospital bed; in others, family members provide the food the patient eats. The culture care diversity and universality theory has been applied universally and affects nursing care significantly worldwide, including in Australia, Canada, Germany, India, Japan, Sweden, New Zealand, and the United Kingdom. In the United States, transcultural practice has included such culturally diverse communities as African American, African American elderly, the deaf, Hispanic, Japanese American, Lithuanian American, Mexican American, Navajo, and Vietnamese (George, 2002).

Research. Leininger's theory has enjoyed global recognition in terms of research. The development of the theory over a long period of time has allowed it to be tested in many cultures. It is the only theory that speaks specifically to cultural needs with a research method to examine the theory, ethnonursing. By 1995, over 100 cultures and subcultures had been studied, with many more in progress (Tomey & Alligood, 2002). Two examples illustrate the type of research and results.

An ethnographic study was conducted of family vigilance in two acute care neurological units. Informal, semi-structured interviews and participant observation of family members were used to collect data. All subjects stayed with the family member for 24 hours, except one. Participants were asked to talk about their reasons for staying. Data were compiled into five categories: commitment to care, emotional upheaval, dynamic nexus (changing family relationships), transition, and resilience. The findings affirm substantive knowledge that expands the understanding of vigilance as a caring expression and contributes to the body of knowledge about culture care (Carr, 1998).

The purpose of the second study was to identify and analyze the care expressions, practices, and patterns of elderly Anglo American and African American residents in a long-term care institution using the ethnonursing qualitative research method. Data were gathered from 40 participants, including residents and nursing staff, and provided four themes: maintenance of preadmission lifestyles, professional care that was beneficial and satisfying to residents, major differences between apartment and nursing home residents, and an institutional culture that reflected patterns and practices of care. The findings are useful to the residents and professional staff, as well as elaborating on the culture care diversity and universality theory (McFarland, 1997).

Moyra Allen: McGill Model, Canada:
A Practice-Derived Model in Nursing—1986
The Theorists

MOYRA ALLEN developed the McGill model with the faculty, students, and nurses in the community practice setting in the McGill University area. The model is also referred to as the Allen model (Gottlieb & Rowat, 1987) or the developmental health model. The effort was stimulated in part by the adoption of a universal health care system in Canada. This change in health care delivery challenged nurses in Canada to redefine the role of the nurse to provide available, accessible, and responsive health care to all Canadians.

The Theory

The McGill practice-derived model of nursing evolved over a 20-year period. The model speaks to the prevalence of health problems tied to family lifestyles and health habits, leading to the conclusion that the role of the nurse should be primary promoter and facilitator of family health. The family, therefore, would be involved increasingly in bringing about healthier lifestyles of its members. In an article originally published in 1977, Allen (1999) compares the replacement and complementary functions of the expanded role of the nurse. The complementary functions focus on the health of the family unit as an open system that actively participates in decisions about health care. The model that was developed 10 years later emphasizes these elements.

The intent of the model was to describe, monitor, and evaluate the full function of nursing wherever it was practiced. Model elements were tested in various settings to clarify, refine, and further develop them. The testing demonstrated that nursing comes from the practice setting, stresses health promotion, and focuses on health, family, and family goals and strengths, rather than emphasizing illness, treatment, the individual, nursing goals, and family deficits.

Using a grounded theory approach to the study of actual nursing situations, called situation-responsive nursing, Allen and others created a way of thinking about nursing that was oriented toward promoting health. Because they recognized that many health problems and concerns faced by clients were most effectively approached through changes in lifestyle and longstanding habits, their attention focused on the individual in the context of his or her family. Like Nightingale, the McGill model presents nursing as being complementary to medicine. The primary characteristics of the model include "a focus on health rather than illness and treatment, on all family members rather than the patient alone, on family goals rather than on those of the nurse, and on family strengths rather than deficits" (Gottlieb & Feeley, 1999, p. 194) (Box 7.21).

Influence of McGill Practice-Derived Model in Nursing

Education. The McGill model serves as the framework for the McGill University nursing curriculum at the undergraduate and graduate levels. At each level of the program, the four major concepts—health, family, collaboration, and learning—are key threads. As students complete the program, they enter different sectors of the working world and show evidence of the model and its usefulness. The faculty is actively involved in testing the implementation of the model.

Practice. Two examples illustrate the use of the model on practice, one in an ambulatory care setting and the other with chronically ill children. In the first example, the model for nursing was tested in an existing pediatric ambulatory care setting where nurses were dissatisfied with

Box 7.21   Summary of McGill University's Practice-Derived Model

Phenomenon: The health of individuals is related to family lifestyles and health habits.

Idea: Nursing influences family health by promoting and facilitating healthy lifestyles and habits.

Key Concepts/Internal Variables

Health: A dynamic, multidimensional construct encompassing a number of processes including coping and development.

Family: An open system in constant interaction with one another and with other systems in their environment, that is, the community. The family is the unit of concern to the nurse.

Collaboration: The person/family and nurse share all aspects of the situation, with the person taking the lead and the nurse serving as facilitator and motivator.

Learning: Structured experiences that facilitate meeting the health needs, goals, and problem-solving styles of the individual or family.

Coping: Problem-oriented efforts to deal with specific situations, such as family relationships, pain, immobility, and death.

Development: Recognizing, mobilizing, maintaining, and regulating the potentials and resources of the family to achieve life goals.

Examples of Propositions

Health problems are frequently linked to lifestyle health habits of the family.

Nurses are primary promoters and facilitators of family health.

Health is fostered through situation-responsive nursing.

Examples of Assumptions

The health of the nation is its most valuable resource.

Individuals, families, and communities aspire and are motivated toward better health.

Health is best learned through active participation and personal discovery.

Examples of External Variables

Medical interventions

Nursing rather than family goals

Illness and treatment

the underutilization of their professional knowledge and skills in promoting healthy coping in families. The use of assessment skills, a review of relevant literature, and the expansion of a nursing knowledge base enabled nurses to change their practice to be more available to families, deal with changes in the nurse–physician relationship, and demonstrate the benefits of using the model for nursing (Feeley & Gerez-Lirette, 1992).

Another example was a yearlong intervention focused on children who were undergoing psychosocial adjustment to chronic disease. Some children improved with the use of the model, some already had adjusted to their illnesses and remained at the same level, and others remained unadjusted or deteriorated. A profile analysis was conducted of the first and third groups to help explain the outcomes. The findings support the use of flexible interventions that are tailored to the unique needs and characteristics of each family and the need to extend the period of intervention to at least 1 year (Feeley & Gottlieb, 1998).

Research. After the initial idea of expanding family health services was accepted, the practice-derived model was tested, refined, and further developed through a series of demonstration projects funded by the Canadian government (Gottlieb & Rowat, 1987). Some projects had a built-in research component. Although the model was developed in the community, it was intended to be broad based.

Graduate nursing students at McGill University conduct research related to the model to meet the requirements for a master's degree. One student focused on health and health behaviors of children without disabilities (O'Conner-Francoeur, 1982), while another examined health and health behaviors of physically disabled children (Starr, 1984). McGill faculty and others in the nursing community participate in testing hypotheses and implementing results. These include the two mentioned above as well as a study of the concept of readiness to change (Dalton & Gottlieb, 2003). This study examined the perspectives of five patients who were adjusting to illness and disability over a period of 7 months. The findings identified indicators to assess the degree of readiness and ways to support patients to become ready. The development of the model continues to bring together nurses in the university and practice settings who are committed to the continued growth of the model for its use in education, practice, and research.

Nursing Theory in the 1990s and 2000

As the 20th century was closing down, there was less emphasis on developing new nursing theories but continuing efforts to revise and update theories from the 1970s and 1980s. One theory in 1993 and another in 2000 are discussed:

- Anne Boykin and Savina Schoenhofer's nursing as caring in 1993
- Prince Edward Island's conceptual model for nursing in 2000

Anne Boykin and Savina Schoenhofer: Theory of Nursing as Caring—1993
The Theorists

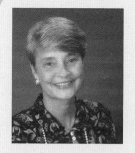

ANNE BOYKIN was born in 1944. She earned a bachelor of science in nursing at Alverno College, Wisconsin; a master of science in adult nursing from Emory University, Georgia; and a PhD in higher education administration from Vanderbilt University, Tennessee. She practiced in acute and community health settings and served on the faculty at Clemson University, Valdosta State College, and Marquette University. Currently, she is professor and dean of nursing at Florida Atlantic University (FAU). She is active in the International Association of Human Caring and serves as the director of the Christine E. Lynne Center for Caring at FAU.

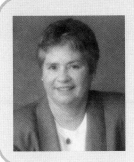

SAVINA SCHOENHOFER was born in 1940. She earned a bachelor of arts in psychology; a bachelor of science in nursing; a master's in education, guidance, and counseling; and a master's in nursing, all from Wichita State University, Kansas. She earned a PhD in higher education administration from Kansas State University. She practices in mental health and migrant health care settings and held faculty and administration positions at Texas Tech, Wichita State, and Florida Atlantic Universities and at the University of Mississippi. She currently is professor of nursing at Alcorn State University, Mississippi.

The Theory

Boykin and Schoenhofer worked for 10 years before presenting their theory in 1993 of nursing as caring. The foundation of the theory is that "all persons are caring" (Boykin & Schoenhofer, 1993, p. 3). They define the focus of nursing, as both a discipline and a profession, as the nurturing of persons as they are living their caring and growing in caring. The nurse attempts to know the nursed as a caring person and focuses on nurturing that person as he or she lives and grows in caring. Nurses enter into the world of the nursed with the intention of knowing that the person they care for is also a caring person. The discipline of nursing attends to the discovery, creation, structuring, testing, and refinement of knowledge that is needed for the practice of nursing. The profession of nursing then attends to the use of that knowledge in response to specific calls for caring (Boykin & Schoenhofer, 1993).

Boykin and Schoenhofer view the theory of nursing as caring as a personal, not an abstract, theory. A nurse is able to nurture another person when that nurse grows in knowing self as a caring person and grows in expressing caring effectively. The major themes of the theory of nursing as caring are to see the other person as caring, enter the world of the other person with the intention of knowing that person, recognize the person's call for nurturance, and respond in ways that enhance personhood.

Many traditional nursing theories are modeled after medicine and focus on nursing as a problem, a need, or a deficit. The goal of Boykin and Schoenhofer's theory is not to explain how nursing can correct the wrong, meet the need, or ease the deficit. The theory of nursing as caring is based on interconnectedness and collegiality between the nurse and the nursed, not on esoteric knowledge and technical expertise. The theory is a model of helping, supporting, and celebrating the human person in the fullness of his or her being a caring person (Boykin & Schoenhofer, 1993) (Box 7.22). The relationship between nurse and nursed is depicted as a dance of caring people (Fig. 7.5). The circle represents caring and valuing others, with each making a contribution. Dancers may leave the circle, and others may join. Dancers connect by holding hands or by eye contact.

Influence of Boykin and Schoenhofer's Theory of Nursing as Caring

Education. Nurse faculty members need to know themselves as caring people in deepening and broadening ways and to demonstrate that caring to students. Knowing self as caring enhances knowing others as caring, while knowing others as caring contributes to discovery of the caring self. Teaching/learning strategies, such as storytelling, provide possibilities for nurses to understand nursing as nurturing people who live caring and grow in caring. Boykin and Schoenhofer advocate storytelling and dialogue between teacher and student to elaborate nursing as caring. The book *Living a Caring-Based Program* could be a source of support for an educational program centered in caring in nursing. Boykin and Schoenhofer and nine other authors explore various parts of the

Box 7.22   Summary of Boykin and Schoenhofer's Theory of Nursing as Caring

Phenomenon: A relationship between the nurse and the nursed is personal and unique in each situation.

Idea: Caring is the central element of nursing and the relationship between the nurse and the nursed.

Key Concepts/Internal Variables

Although Boykin and Schoenhofer do not identify the following as concepts, they have integral relationships within the theory that meet the common definition.

Nursing: The response of a caring nurse to the needs of an individual to be supported as a caring person.

Nursing Actions: Cultivation of opportunities for the person to grow and live as a caring individual.

Nursing Situation: A shared lived experience in which the caring between nurse and nursed enhances personhood. All nursing knowledge is created and resides within the nursing situation (Boykin & Schoenhofer, 2001).

Call for Nursing: The call for nurturance through personal expressions of caring.

Caring: An altruistic, active expression of love, and the intentional and embodied recognition of value and connectedness. Caring is the central value in nursing.

Personhood: Living grounded in caring. Personhood is the universal human call.

Examples of Propositions

Nurses must experience caring to care for and nurture others.

Nurses respond to patient need through caring.

Caring influences through connectedness and collegiality between the nurse and nursed.

Examples of Assumptions (Boykin & Schoenhofer, 2001)

Persons are caring by virtue of their humanness.

Persons are whole or complete in the moment.

Nursing is both a discipline and a profession.

Examples of External Variables

Health care problems

Nurses who believe they are not nurturing

Nursing procedures

---

undergraduate and graduate curricula in nursing to illustrate courses, evaluation, knowledge, objectives, philosophy, practice, and teaching-learning (Boykin, 1994).

Practice. The assumption that all people are caring is relevant to practice for both the nurse and the patient. Boykin and Schoenhofer view instances in which caring is difficult as a challenge for the practicing nurse to increase efforts to know and nurture the patient. They do not view nursing as a process with a number of steps, but rather as a process that the nurse guides as it unfolds.

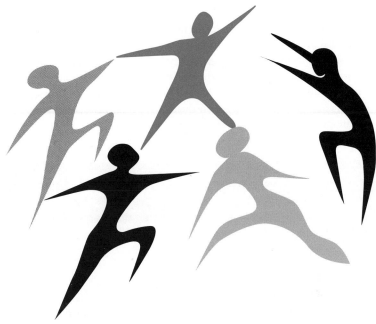

Figure 7.5 The dance of caring persons. (Used with permission from Boykin, A., & Schoenhofer, S. O. [© 2001]. New York: NLN Press.)

Research. The theory of nursing as caring can be tested qualitatively, but not quantitatively. Research questions can be generated, but not research hypotheses (George, 2002). Boykin and Schoenhofer speak to the need of developing a research methodology for the theory.

A number of methodologies grounded in nursing as caring have been used. For example, Schoenhofer, Bingham, and Hutchins (1998) examined the phenomenon of caring as the giving of oneself on behalf of another. As these methodologies become more evident, the research generated will gain increased credibility.

University of Prince Edward Island (PEI), Canada: Conceptual Model for Nursing: A Perspective of Primary Health Care—2000
The Theorists

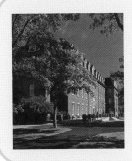

PEI CONCEPTUAL MODEL: Eight faculty members from the University of Prince Edward Island and a nurse consultant from the Canadian Department of Health and Social Services developed the conceptual model for nursing for the theory called conceptual model for nursing: a perspective of primary health care. It is also called the PEI model for Prince Edward Island.

The Theory

The Prince Edward Island conceptual model for nursing, also called the PEI model, is congruent with the international movement toward primary health care. It evolved in part from the need to provide students with guidelines for nursing practice based on primary health care.

Health is conceptualized in terms of the social, economic, and political environments in which nurses practice and health care takes place. The model features a nurse–client partnership with the goal of encouraging clients to act on their own behalf because they have a right and a duty to participate in the course of their health care.

Box 7.23   Summary of The University of Prince Edward Island's Conceptual Model for Nursing: A Perspective of Primary Health Care

Phenomenon: Clients who assume responsibility for personal health practices improve their health outcomes.

Idea: Nurses and patients form health partnerships.

Key Concepts/Internal Variables (Munro, et al., 2000)

Primary Health Care: A philosophy and a method of delivering health care. Philosophy: Health is a product of individual, social, economic, and political factors that support a social framework built on the ability of individuals, families, groups, and communities to control their own health. *Delivery method:* A commitment to essential health care and equitable distribution of care to all populations, with optimal individual and community involvement.

Nurse-Client Partnership: An agreed-upon sharing of power between health professional and client to enhance the capacity of the client to act more effectively on his or her own behalf.

Environment: The internal and external context in which one lives, plays, and works with emphasis on the sociopolitical factors that affect the health of individuals, families, groups, and communities.

Examples of Propositions

Patients influence and are influenced by interaction with the environment.

Health is influenced by the sociopolitical environment and the determinants of health.

Nurses work in partnership with patients to achieve wellness.

Examples of Assumptions (Munro, et al., 2000)

Patients want to be partners in designing their health care.

Wellness promotion is relevant regardless of the current state of health.

Primary health care is the most effective means of achieving wellness.

Examples of External Variables

Nursing orders

Client dependency

Significant others

The initial publication of a theoretical model in the nursing literature provides assumptions, principles, concept definitions, and implications for nursing education, practice, and research. Because this is the most recent theoretical model in the book, the resources and information about the model are limited. This may make you wonder why the theory is included. At some point, each of the other 20 theories you have just read about was new, with only a few publications. This gives you an opportunity to participate in the development of a theory. One of the learning activities at the end of the chapter will assist you in that direction. The PEI theorists extend an invitation to their colleagues to "dialogue, critique, and test" the model and, therefore, help refine it (Munro et al., 2000, p. 53). Think about this as you review the summary (Box 7.23).

Influence of the University of Prince Edward Island's Conceptual Model for Nursing: A Perspective of Primary Health Care

Education. The model provides guidelines for curriculum design and implementation. A partnership is established between students and faculty. Teaching strategies are selected that support the participation of students in their own education. The philosophy and principles of primary health care are used to direct the selection of subject matter content.

Practice. The model describes the components of primary health care and provides guidelines for identifying the dimensions of the client and the environment. Students are introduced to the model early in their education to enhance the implementation of the model at the time of graduation.

Research. Research is proposed to test new concepts of the model as they are identified, relationship statements linking the concepts, and a newly derived set of propositions for validation. Also, a project determines how the principles interact with and influences the implementation of the nursing process. Other studies could focus on communication skills and the participation of clients in the partnership. The recent publication of the model has not allowed for testing and presentation of findings.

A Global View of Nursing Theory

As transportation, communication, and technology continue to improve, the world grows smaller and more accessible. Rather than wait days or even weeks for letters or postcards to arrive from friends who are traveling abroad, you can send an e-mail message and receive a response almost instantaneously. Many international and national meetings provide an Internet café, with access only limited by the number of computers available and the conference attendees who choose to "check their e-mail" at any time.

The world of nursing theory has also expanded beyond the border of the United States, although nurses from other countries continue to use American theories. The following information from other countries provides a beginning introduction to a global view of nursing theory. Collecting information about nursing theory from other countries requires access to library resources and language translation. Fortunately, many theories have web sites and provide translations. These web sites are listed in the Internet Sites for Nursing Theory, Nurse Theorists, and Related Information in Appendix A of the book.

The name of the theorist/theory and a descriptive title are listed alphabetically by country, along with information about the theorist and his or her theory when available. These theories come from five countries. They will expand and enhance your knowledge about nursing theory and the body of nursing knowledge.

Greece

The Evolving Essence of the Science of Nursing: A Complexity Integration Nursing Theory: Ionnis A. Kalofissudis and Sharon V. Van Sell

This theory was developed in June 2001 by combining the following two theories into one:

- The theory of nursing knowledge and nursing practice: Ioannis A. Kalofissudis (Greece). Kalofissudis' theory emphasized building blocks for the complexity integration necessary for the individual to develop not only as a professional nurse, but also for individual self-development.

- Holistic conceptual development model of nursing science: Sharon L. Van Sell (United States). Van Sell's model was a mathematical formulation that provided conceptualization to describe, explain, and predict nursing practice. The results offered common ground for nursing education, nursing administration, and clinical practice nurses to dialogue, which could then facilitate the education of the nursing professional.

Complexity integration of the two theories demonstrated an evolutionary pathway to the introduction of a paradigm shift in the essence of the science of nursing. Kalofissudis and Van Sell believe this is necessary to be able to accept, implement, and evaluate the global vision for health for all.

Japan

Nursing of Dying Patients: Sister Matuno Teramoto

Sister Matuno Teramoto was born in 1916. She was educated at a nurse training school at Kumamoto Medical School Hospital and served in the Japanese military in the 1930s. Sister Teramoto is a professor at Seibo Women's Junior College.

The theory of nursing of dying patients focuses on the long tradition of respect that the Japanese have for the dead. Nurses perform elaborate postdeath nursing procedures consistent with this respect.

Scientific Nursing: Hiroko Usui

Hiroko Usui was born in 1931 and was educated at Ochanomizu Women's College and Tokyo University. She served as a nursing researcher for the Japanese Medical Association. She is the president of Miyazaki Prefectural Nursing College.

She conducted empirical/quantitative research over a 5-year period to support the position that nursing is a true profession. She emphasized the importance of "scientific thinking" because no word for "science" existed in the Japanese language until the mid-19th century. Her theory was influenced by Nightingale's ideas on human health and nursing.

Humanistic Nursing: Masako Suzuki

Masako Suzuki was born in 1940. She was educated at Osaka University Nurse Training School, Medical School Hospital, Osaka Kosei Gakuen, Keio University, and Tokyo International University. Before becoming an educator, she worked in both public health and hospital nursing. She is a nursing professor at Hiroshima University.

The theory of humanistic nursing focuses on the communication between a nurse and patient. She discovered that many Japanese patients have poor communication skills and seldom relate their needs to the nurse, even when their lives are at risk. Patients expect nurses to understand their needs as mothers understand the needs of their babies and children. The theory of humanistic nursing explains how nurses are able to bring out crucial medical information from patients by creating contexts favorable for communication.

Social Aspects of Nursing: Midori Kawashima

Midori Kawashima was born in 1931 and was educated at Japan Red Cross Nurse Training School. She was inspired by Henderson's definition of nursing and her argument for the importance of nurses' working conditions. She was among the first nurses who left the hospital to join the early 1960s labor movement to improve nurse wages and working conditions and was the leader of a grassroots movement to provide nurses with continuing education. She promoted safe, comfortable nursing for patients. She is the director of nursing at Kenwakai, a clinical nurse training center.

Sweden

The SAUC Model for Confirming Nursing: Barbro Gustafsson, Ania M. Willman, and I. Porn

The sympathy-acceptance-understanding-competence (SAUC) model focuses on the nurse's self-concept and is supported by the theory of self-relation support. The nurse compares his or her ideal nursing self with actual nursing self and goes through the four stages of the self-relation process: self-assessment, self-determination, self-integration, and self-realization. Using the process, nurses assess their actions and then set and incorporate goals and attain those goals for their nursing practice. The process was tested to determine its usefulness in the care of the elderly.

England

The Tidal Model (Mental Health): Brian E. Hodges and Dr. Phil Baker

The tidal model emerged from a 5-year study of the need for psychiatric nursing. The model extends and develops some traditional assumptions about the centrality of interpersonal relations in nursing practice. It also helps support the process for re-empowering the person who is disempowered by mental distress, psychiatric services, or both.

The tidal model is based on a few simple ideas about being human and helping one another. Some think the idea is too obvious to address the complexity of mental distress. The theorists believe, however, that complex problems do not always need complex solutions. Nurses can learn what others experience when they have various kinds of mental distress. You may never have to experience this firsthand, but by learning something about such experiences, you may come to understand them better.

The theorists compare this to a walk on the moon when they say, "There is much Neil Armstrong could teach me about moon-walking, even if I have no intention of following in his footsteps."

Scotland

The Elements of Nursing: A Model for Nursing Based on a Model of Living: Nancy Roper, Winifred Logan, and Alison K. Tierney

The Theorists

Nancy Roper was born in the United Kingdom on September 29, 1918. She studied at a hospital for sick children for 3 years and became a registered sick children's nurse (RSCN). During World War II, she moved into a general hospital and was qualified as a registered general nurse (RGN). In 1950, she gained London University's Teaching Diploma and taught for 13 years. She became self-employed as a writer in 1964, the first British nurse to do so.

After Winifred W. Logan received a master of arts degree from the University of Edinburgh, she qualified as a nurse at the Royal Infirmary, Edinburgh. In 1966, she completed a master's in nursing and allied fields at Columbia University in New York City. She has held nursing positions in the United Kingdom, Canada, and the United States. Her nursing experience includes a diabetic unit, thoracic and general surgery, and care of Eskimos with tuberculosis. She was the course coordinator for the first basic nursing course at the University of Edinburgh in 1962. She also served as an officer for education and research; executive director of the International Council of Nursing in Geneva, Switzerland; and head of the department of health and nursing at Glasgow Caledonia University.

Alison J. Tierney decided to become a nurse at an early age and entered the University of Edinburgh in 1966 as a student in the department of nursing studies where Winifred Logan was a professor. She graduated with distinction in 1969 and became an RGN in 1971. She completed requirements for a doctorate in 1976, one of the first nurses in the United Kingdom to receive this research degree.

The Theory. Roper received a fellowship to the University of Edinburgh to investigate whether patients provided a core of nursing experiences for student clinical assignment. She defined the core and the model for living and the model for nursing that were published in 1980. The early Roper models were based on an extensive literature review and on research. Using a case-study approach, data about activities of daily living (ADLs) were collected about 774 patients on general, psychiatric, and maternity units in a hospital and in 12 community districts. The study focused on the nature of nursing and where students should practice.

Roper invited Logan and Tierney to help refine and develop the models. The elements of nursing: a model for nursing based on a model of living, or the R-L-T model, was developed and published in 1980. The R-L-T model is used throughout Europe in education, practice, and research and has been translated into eight or more languages. The model has been introduced to students in beginning nursing courses, to practice formulating patient care plans related to ADLs, and later to link classroom and clinical activities (McCaugherty, 1992). In another study, 12 nurses, working as coresearchers, used the model to analyze underlying problems and assumptions about traditional nursing practices that resulted in increased confidence of practitioners and stronger relationships within a multidisciplinary team.

Summary

The rise of contemporary nursing theory began in the 1950s with Peplau and Henderson. More recently published theories, including those of Parse, Leininger, Watson, Benner, and Boykin and Schoenhofer, all focus on care and caring. Many theorists, such as Leininger, Neuman, and Parse, continue to revise, refine, and update their work. While it is always interesting to hear about the development of new theory, testing of theory, also an active field, is very important to theory and knowledge development.

A great deal of time and effort goes into developing theory. Until a theory is published, preferably in the nursing literature, it has little impact on nurses and nursing outside the theorist's immediate locality. Whenever intellectual work is published, it becomes available for discussion, critique, and testing. Most theories described in this chapter have been in the nursing domain for a number of years. There are probably many others in development that will eventually be in the public domain for nurses such as you to study, discuss, and test. If you are interested in expanding your knowledge about some theories, the references at the end of the chapter and Internet sites in Appendix A will help you.

The nurse theorists and theories discussed in this chapter provide a broad view of how knowledge has expanded during the past half-century. Although only brief information about these theorists is provided, the nursing literature is overflowing with books and articles about them. Increasingly, the Internet contains information as well. As you become better acquainted with one or more nurse theorists, you will say, as many students have said before, "I use these concepts in my practice all the time. I just did not know that they were part of theory."

Learning Activities

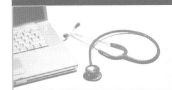

1. Who is your favorite nurse theorist? Select a nurse theorist and explore the following:

   a. What was it about this theorist that made you select him or her?

   b. How would a nurse who adopts this theory act?

   c. What is the most difficult aspect of the theory to understand?

   d. Describe a recent patient experience that you would handle differently now that you are familiar with the theory.

   e. How would you change the theory to make it more attractive to other nurses?

2. Who gets to be your nurse? Select two nurse theorists with different views about theory, for example, Rogers and Watson or Johnson and Orem. You can select any two you wish. Then answer the following questions:

   a. Describe their greatest areas of difference.

   b. Describe areas of similarity, if any.

   c. Compare the impact that each theorist/theory has had on nursing.

   d. If you met each of them, what would you ask about his or her theory?

   e. If you were sick or injured, which of the two theorists would you rather have care for you and why?

3. Participate in the development of a theory. Study the Prince Edward Island (PEI) conceptual model for nursing again and respond to the following questions. You will need to obtain a copy of the article by Munro et al. (2000).

   a. What are the distinguishing features of the model compared to others you have read about?

   b. Review the definition of primary health care. Would the ordinary health care user understand what it means? Rewrite it in a manner that you think more people would understand.

   c. What other concepts should be added and how would you define them?

   d. Discuss the appropriateness of the title or write a new title for the model and discuss why it should be changed.

   e. Select one of the propositions or write one of your own and then suggest how to test the proposition.

References

Abdellah, F. G. (1955). Models of determining covert aspects of nursing problems as basis for improved clinical teaching. Unpublished doctoral dissertation. New York Teachers College, Columbia University.

Abdellah, F. G., Beland, I. L., Martin, A., & Matheney, R. V. (1960). *Patient-centered approaches to nursing.* New York: Macmillan.

Abdellah, F. G., Beland, I. L., Martin, A., & Matheney, R. V. (1973). *New directions in patient-centered nursing.* New York: Macmillan.

Abdellah, F. G., & Levine, E. (1954). Work samplings applied to the study of nursing personnel. *Nursing Research, 3*(1), 11–16.

Abdellah, F. G., & Levine, E. (1994). *Preparing for nursing research in the twenty-first century: Evolution, methodologies, challenges.* New York: Springer.

Abdellah, F. G., & Strachan, E. J. (1959). Progressive patient care. *American Journal of Nursing, 59,* 5.

Adam, E. (1979). *Être infirmière.* Toronto, Ontario. W. B. Saunders.

Adam, E. (1980). *To be a nurse.* Toronto, Ontario: W. B. Saunders.

Adam, E. (1983). Frontiers of nursing in the 21st century: Development of models and theories on the concept of nursing. *Journal of Advanced Nursing, 8,* 41–45.

Adam, E. (1991). *To be a nurse* (2nd ed.). Toronto, Ontario: W. B. Saunders.

Adam, E. (1999). Conceptual models. *Canadian Journal of Nursing, 30*(4), 103–114.

Agnew, L. R. C. (1958). Florence Nightingale—statistician. *American Journal of Nursing, 58,* 664–665.

Allen, F. M. (1999). Comparative theories of the expanded role in nursing and implications for nursing practice: A working paper. *Canadian Journal of Nursing Research, 30*(4), 83–89.

American Nurses Association. (1980). *Nursing: A social policy statement.* Kansas City, MO: Author.

American Nurses Association. (1995). *Nursing's social policy statement.* Washington, DC: Author.

Anderson, J. A. (2001). Understanding homeless adults by testing the theory of self-care. *Nursing Science Quarterly, 14*(1), 59–67.

Bauman, S. (1997). Contrasting two approaches in a community-based nursing practice with older adults: The medical model and Parse's nursing theory. *Nursing Science Quarterly, 10*(3), 124–130.

Beeber, L., & Caldwell, C. (1996). Pattern integrations in young depressed women: Part II. *Archives of Psychiatric Nursing, 10*(3), 157–164.

Bellman, L. M. (1996). Changing nursing practice through reflection on the Roper, Logan and Tierney model: The enhancement approach to action research. *Journal of Advanced Nursing, 24,* 129–138.

Benner, P. (1984). *From novice to expert: Excellence and power in clinical nursing practice.* Menlo Park, CA: Addison-Wesley.

Benner, P., Hooper-Kyriakidis, P., & Stannard, D. (1999). *Clinical wisdom in critical care: A thinking-in-action approach.* Philadelphia: W. B. Saunders.

Benner, P., Tanner, C., & Chesla, C. (1996). *Expertise in nursing practice: Caring, clinical judgment, and ethics.* New York: Springer.

Benner, P., & Wrubel, J. (1989). *The primacy of caring: Stress and coping in health and illness.* Menlo Park, CA: Addison-Wesley.

Bowman, A. M. (1997). Sleep satisfaction, perceived pain and acute confusion in elderly clients undergoing orthopaedic procedures. *Journal of Advanced Nursing, 26,* 550–564.

Boykin, A. (Ed.). (1994). *Living a caring-based program.* New York: National League for Nursing Press.

Boykin, A., & Schoenhofer, J. (1993). *Nursing as caring: A model for transforming practice.* New York: National League for Nursing.

Boykin, A., & Winland-Brown, J. (1995) The dark side of caring. *Journal of Gerontological Nursing, 21*(5), 13–18.

Brykczynski, K. A. (1989). An interpretive study describing the clinical judgment of nurse practitioners. *Scholarly Inquiry for Nursing Practice, 3*(2), 75–104.

Bullough, V. L., Church, O. M., & Stein, A. P. (1988). *American nursing: A biographical dictionary.* New York: Garland Publishing, Inc.

Bunkers, S. S., Bendtro, M., Holmes, P. K., et al. (1992). The healing web: A transformative model for nursing. *Nursing and Health Care, 13,* 68–73.

Bunting, S. (1993). *Rosemarie Parse: Theory of health as human becoming.* Newbury Park, CA: Sage Publications.

Campbell, M. A. (1987). *The U.B.C. model for nursing: Directions for practice.* Vancouver: The University of British Columbia School of Nursing.

Campbell, M. A., Cruise, M. J., & Murakami, T. R. (1976). A model for nursing: University of British Columbia School of Nursing. *Nursing Papers, 8*(2), 5–9.

Carr, J. M. (1998). Vigilance as a caring expression and Leininger's theory of cultural care diversity and universality. *Nursing Science Quarterly, 11*(2), 7478.

Coward, D. D., & Wilkie, D. J. (2000). Metastatic bone pain: Meanings associated with self-report and self-management decision making. *Cancer Nursing, 23*(2), 101–108.

Daiski, I. (1996). Staff nurses' perspectives of hospital power structures. *The Canadian Nurse, 92,* 26–30.

Dalton, C. C., & Gottlieb, L. N. (2003). The concept of readiness to change. *Journal of Advanced Nursing, 42*(2), 108–117.

Damgaard, G., & Bunkers, S. S. (1998). Nursing science-guided practice and education: A state board of nursing perspective. *Nursing Science Quarterly, 11*(4), 142–144.

Dee, V. (1990). Implementation of the Johnson model: One hospital's experience. In M. Parker (Ed.), *Nursing theories in practice* (pp. 33–44). New York: National League for Nursing.

Dreyfus, S. E., & Dreyfus, H. L. (1980). A five-stage model of the mental activities involved in directed skill acquisition. Unpublished report, University of California at Berkeley.

Fagerberg, I., & Ekman, S. (1997). First year Swedish nursing students' experiences with elderly patients. *Western Journal of Nursing Research, 19*(2), 177–189.

Fawcett, J. (1995). *Neuman's systems model: Analysis and evaluation of conceptual models of nursing* (3rd ed., pp. 217–275). Philadelphia: F. A. Davis.

Fawcett, J. (1999). *The relationship of theory and research* (3rd ed.). Philadelphia: F. A. Davis.

Fawcett, J. (2002). The nurse theorists: Callista Roy. *Nursing Science Quarterly, 15*(4), 308–310.

Feeley, N., & Gerez-Lirette, T. (1992). Development of professional practice based on the McGill model of nursing in an ambulatory care setting. *Journal of Advanced Nursing, 17,* 801–808.

Feeley, N., & Gottlieb, L. N. (1998). Classification systems for health concerns, nursing strategies, and client outcomes: Nursing practice with families who have a child with a chronic illness. *Canadian Journal of Nursing Research, 30*(1), 45–59.

Fenton, M. V. (1984). Identification of the skilled performance of master's prepared nurses as a method of curriculum planning and evaluation. In P. Benner (Ed.), *From novice to expert: Excellence and power in clinical nursing practice* (pp. 262–274). Menlo Park, CA: Addison-Wesley.

*Fitzpatrick, J. J., & Whall, A. L. (1996). *Conceptual models of nursing: Analysis and application.* Bowie, MD: Brady.

Forchuk, S. (1983). *Hildegard Peplau: Interpersonal nursing theory.* Newbury Park, CA: Sage.

Forchuk, S., Beaton, J., Crawford, L., Ide, L., Voorberg, N., & Bethune, J. (1989). Incorporating Peplau's theory and case management. *Journal of Psychosocial Nursing, 27*(2), 35–38.

Forchuk, S., Westwell, J., Martin, M., Azzapardi, W. B., Kosterewa Tolman, D., & Llux, M. (1998). Factors influencing movement of chronic psychiatric patients from the orientation to the working phase of the nurse-client relationship on an inpatient unit. *Perspectives in Psychiatric Care: The Journal for Nurse Psychotherapists, 34*(1), 36–44.

Ford-Gilboe, M. V. (1994). A comparison of two nursing models: Allen's developmental health model and Newman's theory of health as expanding consciousness. *Nursing Science Quarterly, 7*(3), 113–118.

Foreman, M. D. (1989). Confusion in the hospitalized elderly: Incidence, onset, and associated factors. *Research in Nursing and Health, 12,* 21–29.

Frey, M. A., & Sieloff, C. L. (Eds.) (1995). *Advancing King's systems framework and theory of goal attainment.* Thousands Oaks, CA: Sage Publications.

*George, J. B. (2002). *Nursing theories: The base for professional nursing practice.* Norwalk, CT: Appleton & Lange.

Gigliotti, E. (1997). Use of Neuman's lines of defense and resistance in nursing research: Conceptual and empirical considerations. *Nursing Science Quarterly, 19*(3), 136–143.

Gigliotti, E. (2003). The Neuman Systems Model Institute: Testing middle-range theories. *Nursing Science Quarterly, 16,* 201–206.

Gottlieb, L. N., & Feeley, N. (1999). Nursing intervention studies: Issues related to change and time in children and families. *Canadian Journal of Nursing, 30*(4), 193–212.

Gottlieb, L. N., & Rowat, K. (1987). The McGill model of nursing: A practice-driven model. *Advances in Nursing Science, 9*(4), 51–61.

Gustafsson, B., & Willman, A. M. (2003). Nurses' self-relation—Becoming theoretically competent: The SAUC model for confirming nursing. *Nursing Science Quarterly, 16*(3), 265–271.

Harmer, B., & Henderson, V. (1955). *Textbook of the principles and practice of nursing* (5th ed.). New York: Macmillan.

Henderson, V. (1960). *Basic principles of nursing care.* Geneva, Switzerland: International Council of Nursing.

Henderson, V. (1963, 1966, 1970, 1972). *Nursing studies index.* Philadelphia: J. B. Lippincott. [Vol. I, 1890–1929, published 1963; Vol. II, 1930–1949, published 1966; Vol. III, 1950–1956, published 1970; Vol. IV, 1957–1959, published 1972.]

Henderson, V. (1964). The nature of nursing. *American Journal of Nursing, 64*(8), 62–68.

Henderson, V. (1966). *The nature of nursing: A definition and its implications for practice, research, and education.* New York: Macmillan.

Henderson, V. (1991). *The nature of nursing: A definition and its implications for practice, research, and education: A reflection after 25 years.* New York: National League for Nursing. Macmillan.

Henderson, V., & Nite, G. (1978). *Principles and practice of nursing.* New York: Macmillan.

Johnson, D. E. (1959). The nature of a science in nursing. *Nursing Outlook, 7,* 292–294.

Johnson, D. E. (1961). The significance of nursing care. *American Journal of Nursing, 61,* 372–377.

Johnson, D. E. (1980). The behavioral system model of nursing. In J. Riehl and C. Roy (Eds.), *Conceptual models for nursing practice* (2nd ed., pp. 207–216). New York: Appleton-Century-Crofts.

King, I. M. (1971). *Toward a theory for nursing: General concepts for human behavior.* New York: John Wiley & Sons.

King, I. M. (1981). *A theory of goal attainment: Systems, concepts, process.* New York: Wiley.

King, I. M. (1986). *Curriculum and instruction in nursing: Concepts and process.* Norwalk, CT: Appleton-Century-Crofts.

King, I. M. (2003). Assessment of functional abilities and goal attainment scales: A criterion referenced measure. In O. Strickland & C. Dilorio (Eds.), *Measurement of nursing outcomes* (2nd ed., pp. 3–20). New York: Springer.

Kravitz, M., & Frey, M. A. (1989). The Allen Nursing Model. In J. J. Fitzpatrick & A. W. Whall (Eds.), *Conceptual models of nursing: Analysis and application* (pp. 313–329). Norwalk, CT: Appleton & Lange.

Leininger, M. M. (1977). *Caring: The essence and central focus of nursing. The phenomenon of caring: Part V.* Kansas City, MO: American Nurses Foundation.

Leininger, M. M. (1985). Transcultural care diversity and universality: A theory of nursing. *Nursing & Health Care, 6,* 209–212.

Leininger, M. M. (1988). Leininger's theory of nursing: Culture care diversity and universality. *Nursing Science Quarterly, 1*(4), 152–160.

Leininger, M. M. (1991). *Culture care diversity and universality: A theory of nursing.* New York: National League for Nursing Press.

Levesque, L., Ricard, N., Ducharme, F., et al. (1998). Empirical verification of a theoretical model derived from the Roy adaptation model: Findings from five studies. *Nursing Science Quarterly, 11,* 31–39.

Levine, M. E. (1969). *Introduction to clinical nursing.* Philadelphia: F. A. Davis.

Levine, M. E. (1989). The four conservation principles: Twenty years later. In J. Riehl (Ed.), *Conceptual models for nursing practice* (pp. 325–337). New York: Appleton-Century-Crofts.

Majesky, S. J., Brester, M. H., & Nishio, K. T. (1978). Development of a research tool: Patient indicators of nursing care. *Nursing Research, 27*(6), 365–371.

Marchione, J. M. (1993). *Margaret Newman: Health as expanding consciousness.* Newbury Park, CA: Sage Publications.

Maynard, C. A. (1996). Relationship of critical thinking ability to professional nursing competence. *Journal of Nursing Education, 35*(1), 12–18.

McCaugherty, D. (1992). The Roper nursing model as an educational and research tool. *British Journal of Nursing, 1*(9), 455–459.

McEwen, M., & Wills, E. M. (2002). *Theoretical basis for nursing.* Philadelphia: Lippincott Williams & Wilkins.

McFarland, M. R. (1997). Use of culture care theory with Anglo- and African-American elders in a long-term care setting. *Nursing Science Quarterly, 10*(4), 186–192.

Meleis, A. I. (1997). *Theoretical nursing: Development and progress.* Philadelphia: Lippincott-Raven.

Mitchell, G. J. (1997). Theory and practice in long term care: The acorn doesn't fall far from the tree. *Long Term Care, 7*(4), 31–34.

Mosher, R. B., & Moore, J. B. (1998). The relationship of self-concept and self-care in children with cancer. *Nursing Science Quarterly, 11*(3), 116–122.

Munro, M., Gallant, M., MacKinnon, M., et al. (2000). The Prince Edward Island conceptual model for nursing: A nursing perspective of primary health care. *Canadian Journal of Nursing Research, 32*(1), 39–55.

Neuman, B. (1974). The Betty Neuman health-care systems model: A total person approach to patient problems. In J. P. Riehl & C. Roy (Eds.), *Conceptual models for nursing practice* (pp. 99–114). New York: Appleton-Century-Crofts.

Neuman, B. (1989). *The Neuman systems model.* Norwalk, CT: Appleton & Lange.

Neuman, B. (1995). *The Neuman systems model* (3rd ed.). Norwalk, CT: Appleton & Lange.

Neuman, B. M., & Young, R. J. (1972). A model for teaching total person approach to patient problems. *Nursing Research, 21,* 264–269.

Newman, M. A. (1979). *Theory development in nursing.* Philadelphia: F. A. Davis.

Newman, M. A. (1986). *Health as expanding consciousness.* St. Louis: Mosby.

Newman, M. A. (1990). Newman's theory of health as praxis. *Nursing Science Quarterly, 3*(1), 37–41.

Newman, M. A., Sime, A. M., & Corcoran-Perry, S. A. (1991). The focus of the discipline of nursing. *Advances in Nursing Science, 14*(1), 1–6.

Nightingale, F. (1859/1992). *Notes on nursing: What it is and what it is not* (Commemorative ed.). Philadelphia: J. B. Lippincott. [*Notes on nursing* was published originally by Harrison in London, England, in 1859. The above is an unabridged republication of the first American edition, from D. Appleton and Company in 1860.]

Nightingale, F. (1969). *Notes on nursing: What it is and what it is not.* New York: Dover.

Northrup, D. T., & Cody, W. K. (1998). Evaluation of the human becoming theory in practice in an acute care psychiatric setting. *Nursing Science Quarterly, 11*(1), 23–30.

Nursing Development Conference Group. (1973). *Concept formalization in nursing: Process and product.* Boston: Little, Brown & Co.

O'Conner-Francoeur, P. (1982). Children's concepts of health and their health behavior. Unpublished master's study. McGill University of School of Nursing, Montreal.

Orem, D. E. (1971). *Nursing: Concepts of practice.* New York: McGraw-Hill.

Orem, D. E. (1985). *Nursing: Concepts of practice* (3rd ed.). New York: McGraw-Hill.

Orem, D. E. (2001). *Nursing: Concepts of practice* (6th ed.). St. Louis: Mosby.

Orlando, I. (1961). *The dynamic nurse-patient relationship.* New York: G. P. Putnam's Sons.

Orlando, I. (1972). *The discipline and teaching of nursing process.* New York: G. P. Putnam's Sons.

Orlando, I. (1990). *The dynamic nurse-patient relationship.* New York: National League for Nursing.

Othaganont, P., Sinthuvorakan, C., & Jensupakarn, P. (2002). Daily living practice of the life-satisfied Thai elderly. *Journal of Transcultural Nursing, 13*(1), 24–29.

Palmer, I. S. (1977). Florence Nightingale: Reformer, reactionary, researcher. *Nursing Research, 26,* 84–89.

*Parker, M. E. (Ed.). (2001). *Nursing theories and nursing practice.* Philadelphia: F. A. Davis.

Parse, R. R. (1981). *Man–living–health: A theory of nursing.* New York: Wiley.

Parse, R. R. (1987). *Nursing science: Major paradigms, theories, and critiques.* Philadelphia: W. B. Saunders.

Parse, R. R. (1992). Human becoming: Parse's theory of nursing. *Nursing Science Quarterly, 5,* 35–42.

Peplau, H. (1952). *Interpersonal relations in nursing.* New York: G. P. Putnam's Sons.

Peplau, H. E. (1997). Peplau's theory of interpersonal relations. *Nursing Science Quarterly, 10*(4), 162–167.

Picot, S. J. F., Zauszniewski, J. A., Debanne, S. M., & Holston, E. G. (1999). Mood and blood pressure responses in Black female caregivers, and noncaregivers. *Nursing Research, 48,* 150–161.

Pope, D. S. (1995). Music, noise, and the human voice in the nurse-patient environment. *IMAGE: Journal of Nursing Scholarship, 27,* 291–295.

Reed, K. S. (1993). *Betty Neuman: The Neuman systems model.* Newbury Park, CA: Sage.

Reed, P. G., & Zurakowski, T. L. (1996). Nightingale: Foundations of nursing. In J. J. Fitzpatrick & A. L. Whall (Eds.), *Conceptual models of nursing: Analysis and application* (pp. 27–54). Stamford, CT: Appleton & Lange.

Rittman, M. R. (2001). Ida Jean Orlando: The dynamic nurse-patient relationship. In M. E. Parker (Ed.), *Nursing theories and nursing practice.* Philadelphia: F. A. Davis.

Rogers, M. E. (1961). *Educational revolution in nursing.* New York: Macmillan.

Rogers, M. E. (1964). *Reveille in nursing.* Philadelphia: F. A. Davis.

Rogers, M. E. (1970). *An introduction to the theoretical basis of nursing.* Philadelphia: F. A. Davis.

Roper, N., Logan, W., & Tierney, A. (1980). *The elements of nursing.* Edinburgh: Churchill Livingstone.

Roy, C. (1970). Adaptation: A conceptual framework for nursing. *Nursing Outlook, 18*(3), 42–45.

Roy, C. (1971). Adaptation: A basis for nursing practice. *Nursing Outlook, 19*(4), 254–257.

Roy, C. (1975). A diagnostic classification system for nursing. *Nursing Outlook, 23,* 90–94.

Roy, C. (1997). Future of the Roy Model: Challenge to Redefine Adaptation. *Nursing Science Quarterly, 10*(1), Spring.

Schaefer, K. M., & Potylycki, M. J. S. (1993). Fatigue associated with congestive heart failure: Use of Levine's conservation model. *Journal of Advanced Nursing, 18,* 260–268.

Schoenhofer, S., Bingham, V., & Hutchins, G. (1998). Giving of oneself on another's behalf: The phenomenology of everyday caring. *International Journal for Human Caring, 2*(2), 32–29.

Schorr, J. A. (1993). Music and pattern change in chronic pain. *Advances in Nursing Science, 15*(4), 27–36.

Sills, G. M. (1977). Research in the field of psychiatric nursing. *Nursing Research, 28*(3), 201–207.

Simmons, L. W. & Henderson, V. (1964). *Nursing research: A survey and assessment.* New York: Appleton-Century-Crofts.

Small, B. (1980). Nursing visually impaired children with Johnson's model as a conceptual framework. In J. P. Riehl & C. Roy (Eds.), *Conceptual models for nursing practice* (pp. 264–273). New York: Appleton-Century-Crofts.

Smith, M. C., & Edgil, A. E. (1995). Future directions for research with the Neuman systems model. In B. Neuman (Ed.), *The Neuman systems model* (3rd ed., pp. 509–517). Norwalk, CT: Appleton & Lange.

Soderhamn, O., & Cliffordson, C. (2001). The structure of self-care in a group of elderly people. *Nursing Science Quarterly, 14*(1), 55–58.

Stamler, C. (1971). Dependency and repetitive visits to nurses' office in elementary school children. *Nursing Research, 20*(3), 254–255.

Starr, J. (1984). The concept of health and health behaviors of physically disabled children. Unpublished master's study. McGill University, School of Nursing, Montreal, Canada.

Thompson, J. D. (1980). The passionate humanist: From Nightingale to the new nurse. *Nursing Outlook, 28,* 290–295.

Thorne, S., Jillings, C., Ellis, D., & Perry, J. A. (1993). *Journal of Advanced Nursing, 18,* 1259–1266.

*Tomey, A. M., & Alligood, M. R. (2002). *Nursing theorists and their works.* St. Louis: Mosby.

Wagner, P. (1976). Testing the adaptation model in practice. *Nursing Outlook, 24*(10), 682–685.

Watson, J. (1979). *Nursing: Human science and caring.* Boston: Little, Brown.

Watson, J. (1985). *Nursing: Human science and human care: A theory of nursing.* Norwalk, CT: Appleton-Century-Crofts.

Watson, J. (1988). *Nursing: Human science and human care. A theory of nursing.* New York: The National League of Nursing Press.

Watson, J. (1999). *Postmodern nursing and beyond.* Edinburgh, Scotland, UK: Churchill Livingstone.

Wilkie, D., Lovejoy, N., Dodd, M., & Tesler, M. (1988). Cancer pain control behaviors: Descriptions and correlation with pain intensity. *Oncology Nursing Forum, 15*(6), 723–731.

Woodham-Smith, C. (1951). *Florence Nightingale: 1820–1910.* New York: McGraw Hill.

Yamashita, M. (1999). Newman's theory of health applied to family caregiving in Canada. *Nursing Science Quarterly, 12,* 73–79.

Yamashita, M., & Tall, F.D. (1998). A commentary on Newman's theory of health as expanding consciousness. *Advances in Nursing Science, 21*(1), 65–75.

*The authors recognize the significant contribution of these texts in the completion of this chapter.

Critiquing Theory

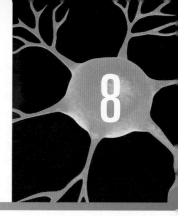

8

Intent: A criterion-based model for examining the intent, concepts, and propositions of theory is presented that results in making judgments about the usefulness of theory in nursing practice.

Key Words/Concepts

analyze	criterion based	judgment
application	criticism	model
assumptions	critique	proposition
boundaries	examine	variables
C-BaC	interpretation	
criterion; criteria	jargon	

Introduction

When students become involved in nursing theory, they tend to raise questions about relationships between theory and specific patient situations. This enables them to become familiar with how theory is used in nursing practice. At times it is retroactive. For example, a student might say: "I already knew that; I just didn't know it was part of a theory." In this chapter, we will explore the criterion-based critique model, called **C-BaC.** The model will help you to identify connections between your nursing practice and the various theories.

C-BaC is designed to help you make judgments about the value and use of theory. These judgments demonstrate how theoretical knowledge is incorporated into nursing practice and provides knowledge about theory and practice on which to build your practice. The C-BaC model helps you **examine** theories. When we examine something like theory, we inspect and explore, rather than **analyze**, which means appraise and evaluate. Exploring theory and its connections with practice will help you recognize the value of theoretical judgments.

In addition to being a useful tool for making judgments, C-BaC is also designed to focus on selected components related to nursing practice. Examples and illustrations from nursing and other disciplines illustrate the application of C-BaC. As your knowledge of theory increases, connections between nursing practice and theory become more evident. Exploring both nursing theories and theories that support nursing practice enables you to answer questions, solve problems, and describe and explain phenomena as well.

A Criterion-Based Critique Model

We begin by exploring the criterion-based critique model and how it is used. The title of the model contains two concepts: criterion based and critique. We will review the definition of a model and then define the two concepts.

Model

A **model** is a diagram or picture that helps explain or describe relationships between two or more objects, events, ideas, or components. The C-BaC model depicts some events expected to occur during an examination of components of nursing theory. The model provides specific criteria for you to use as you conduct your critique.

Criterion Based

A **criterion-based** model has definitive standards that guide the formation of judgments. These standards are called criteria. Although you could develop many more criteria related to theory, C-BaC limits the components to the following eight:

1. The meaning of the theory is clear and understandable.
2. Boundaries are consistent with nursing practice.
3. Language is understandable and includes minimal jargon.
4. Major concepts are identified and defined.
5. Concepts stimulate the formation of propositions.
6. Variables and assumptions help understand and interpret propositions.
7. Theoretical knowledge helps explain and predict phenomena.
8. Theory influences nursing practice.

Limiting the number of **criteria** in the critique simplifies the judgment process and assists in determining the usefulness of theory for nursing practice. Areas for assessment are selected for their importance to nursing practice. The simplicity of the tool allows you to expand the components as your knowledge about theory increases.

C-BaC criteria are designed to be broad to enable you to apply them to a variety of theories in nursing and other disciplines. As you use a criterion, try to narrow its application depending on the theory you are examining. For example, the second criterion for judging the intent of a theory states, "Boundaries are consistent with nursing practice." This criterion sets a standard for critiquing theory but allows you to stipulate what boundaries are consistent with specific areas of practice. You may select boundaries consistent with any setting where the nurse practices, such as a critical care unit or a patient's home, or you may select a specific nursing intervention, such as pain management of postsurgical patients or skin care of chronically ill patients.

Critique

Critique is a method used to judge the strengths and limitations of a research report or other scholarly activity. When you critique something, you make objective judgments about both positive and negative aspects of that report or theory. Although critique and criticism come from the same word stem, critique denotes a broad objective evaluation, whereas **criticism** tends to focus on weaknesses and limitations. C-BaC encourages you to focus on positive aspects of theory while taking limitations and weaknesses into consideration. Initially, the strengths of a theory will be easier to identify than its limitations. Your ability to make judgments about the usefulness of theory will expand as your knowledge and competence in nursing practice increase; as your competence and reasoning skills develop, your judgments about specific nursing situations will become more astute.

In summary, a criterion-based critique model is a representation of a set of standards that is used to examine designated components of nursing theory.

Using the Model

Now that you know what the C-BaC model is, we will explore how to use it. When you apply the C-BaC model, you rely on your knowledge about nursing theory and practice as well as your imaginative reasoning skills. You expand your knowledge base about nursing through reading, studying, listening, and discussing. As you examine relationships between theory and practice, you test your conclusions informally by focusing on specific aspects of practice. Your task becomes easier as you increase your ability to identify the knowledge you use for specific nursing actions. Nursing Story 8.1 will help clarify and simplify the process of developing a knowledgeable, theoretical approach to practice. Study the patient's story, but before you read the last section on theoretical application, think about the approach that Patricia Leegow, nurse practitioner, uses with Mr. Williams. You may think that theory is too abstract for practice, but you will soon recognize that many aspects of theory are very practical.

The implementation of C-BaC is carried out in three phases. The first phase critiques the intent of a theory as it is viewed from the meaning, boundaries, and language of the theory. The second phase focuses on its major concepts and propositions. Finally, judgments from the first two phases are incorporated into the third phase to examine the usefulness of theory in nursing practice. The model is illustrated in Figure 8.1.

Initially, you use C-BaC in a linear fashion; that is, you seek to understand the meaning, boundaries, and language of a theory before you explore its concepts and propositions and finally make judgments about its usefulness. When you learned to drive a car, you used a linear process. You inserted the key into the ignition, stepped on the gas pedal, turned the key, and so on. After

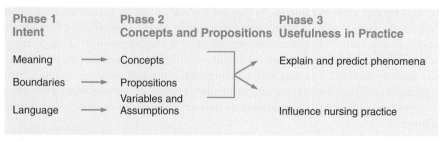

Figure 8.1 Criterion-based critique (C-BaC) model.

NURSING STORY 8.1

Developing a Knowledgeable, Theoretical Approach to Practice

The Patient's Story

Carl and Mary Williams have been married for 52 years. They raised six children and now are enjoying almost daily visits from one or more of their 10 grandchildren. They are both healthy, active, and looking forward to aging gracefully together.

Mr. Williams, however, has a growing, unspoken concern. Several months ago, he noticed that he had difficulty remembering some things. He had always prided himself on his good memory; now he had to work hard to recall dates and events, even some important ones. He almost missed playing golf last week with his foursome, when Mary reminded him. His forgetfulness didn't seem to bother her though. She just called it a "senior moment." At first Mr. Williams passed it off, too. "Everyone seems to forget when they get old," he thought. But it continued, and he was afraid to make an appointment with the doctor—and afraid not to as well. "What if I have Alzheimer's disease," he said to himself one day, "what will Mary and I do?" The church they attended had a new parish nurse. "I guess I'll just drop in and see her sometime," he thought, "and not bother Mary with it until I know more." Three days later, Mr. Williams dropped by the clinic to talk to the nurse.

Mr. Williams: Hello! I'm Carl Williams. I live over on Prospect Street with my wife Mary. We have been members of this church almost 50 years. If you have some time this morning, I wonder if I could chat with you about something?

Ms. Leegow: I am pleased to meet you, Mr. Williams, and I am very pleased you stopped by. My name is Patricia Leegow, the new parish nurse. I've seen you and your wife in church but haven't had a chance to meet you. I graduated from the university nurse practitioner program 3 years ago and worked with Dr. Roady, a family physician, until I started here last month. Do you know Dr. Roady?

Mr. Williams: I thought you looked familiar. Mary and I have been patients of Dr. Roady ever since he took over after Dr. Granster's retirement 10 years ago. We really like Dr. Roady. I hope he won't mind that I came to see you.

Ms. Leegow: I will tell Dr. Roady I saw you, and I know he won't mind; he encouraged me to take this position and we work on many cases together. Let's go into my office, and you can tell me about your concerns.

(continued)

NURSING STORY 8.1

Developing a Knowledgeable, Theoretical Approach to Practice (Continued)

Mr. Williams and Ms. Leegow talked for more than an hour. Initially, Ms. Leegow listened, speaking only to ask Mr. Williams to clarify his concerns. During this time, she focused on developing a relationship with Mr. Williams, obviously someone in need of support as well as information. They discussed possible causes of the changes he had noticed and set some short-term goals. Mr. Williams agreed to find a quiet time to talk about his concerns with his wife. In the meantime, Ms. Leegow would confer with Dr. Roady about some tests that might help in the diagnostic process.

Mr. Williams was still concerned as he walked back home from the church, but relieved that he had talked to Ms. Leegow. She had acknowledged that Mr. Williams might have something serious but also discussed many other possibilities and how they could be identified and treated. At least he didn't have to shoulder this entire burden by himself anymore.

Theoretical Application

One of the early nurse theorists, Hildegard Peplau, developed a theory dealing with interpersonal relations in nursing. Peplau viewed the nurse–patient relationship in four phases: orientation, or establishing a relationship; identification, or clarifying the problem; exploitation, or considering and selecting appropriate approaches to the problem; and resolution, or meeting the needs and evaluating the process. Obviously, Ms. Leegow has only begun to establish a relationship with Mr. Williams.

In addition to the four phases of the relationship, Peplau viewed nursing as an educational process. Although Ms. Leegow depends on her broad knowledge of health assessment, aging, diagnostic tests, medications, and treatments, her major focus is to educate Mr. Williams about his situation and answer his questions. Even in this early stage, Ms. Leegow recognized that his anxiety caused him to be confused about what was happening and the decisions he needed to make. Some of Peplau's work focuses on the concept of anxiety, which also helps explain why Mr. Williams was able to avoid discussing his concerns with his wife and rationalized the need to seek help. A researcher who studied Peplau's concept of anxiety has verified the conclusions Ms. Leegow made about the case (Reynolds, 1997).

you learned to drive, these actions become automatic; you no longer had to think about the steps. The same is true when you learn to use the nursing process; initially, you follow it step by step. Now you see the whole picture of starting a car and using the nursing process. In the future, you will be able to do the same with the C-BaC model.

By combining judgments about meaning, boundaries, and language from Phase I, you can focus your attention on the concepts and propositions in Phase II. If you experience difficulty understanding concepts and propositions, look again at the meaning, boundaries, and language. When you know the concepts and propositions of a theory, you will have the background you need to make judgments about a theory's usefulness in Phase III.

The following description focuses on separate phases—intent, concepts and propositions, and usefulness. Initially, questions associated with a criterion are posed to stimulate your thinking. In later sections, suggestions are made for your exploration. The questions and suggestions are not discussed here, although you may wish to do so in class. Three areas are discussed for each criterion: interpretation, application, and judgment. **Interpretation** describes the content of the criterion, **application** explains the process used to relate the content to the model, and finally, **judgment** speaks to how you arrive at decisions about the criterion. Measurement tools have been designed for most of the criteria. Keep in mind that each theory is different and will usually result in a different judgment.

Phase I: Intent of the Theory

Theorists have various intents or purposes for creating a nursing theory, such as to justify nursing knowledge and distinguish it from other disciplines, facilitate an understanding of nursing knowledge, contribute to nursing knowledge, and improve nursing practice. A primary purpose of theory is to establish the focus of disciplinary research or the phenomena of concern. Identifying areas of study in nursing is important for achieving the purposes of asking questions, solving problems, and explaining phenomena.

The intent of a theory is derived from its meaning, boundaries, and language. The following criteria will assist you in critiquing the intent of theory and help verify that your critique provides useful results:

1. The meaning is clear and understandable.

2. Boundaries are consistent with nursing practice.

3. Language is understandable and includes minimal jargon.

Criterion 1: The Meaning Is Clear and Understandable

The following questions will be helpful to you as you examine criterion 1:

- What was the reason for developing the theory?
- What is the theory about?
- How does the theory compare with other theories with similar meanings?
- What level of knowledge is needed to understand the language used in the theory?

Interpretation. Criterion 1, *the meaning is clear and understandable*, focuses on nursing knowledge and the area of nursing practice being considered. If a theorist does not clearly identify the area of practice in a theory, you may have to look for other elements in the theory or from research conducted about the theory. The following examples of the meaning and areas of inquiry of some nursing theories will increase your understanding of theory.

As indicated earlier, Margaret Newman's *theory of health as expanding consciousness* began to develop while she was caring for her mother during a lengthy illness, before she became a nurse (Newman, 1979, 1986, 1990). As a nurse enrolled in doctoral study, she observed the phenomenon that the state of health and physical mobility of individuals affected their perception of the passage of time. These observations were consistent with what she had observed while caring for her mother many years before. Knowing about the historical development of Newman's theory helps clarify its meaning, that is, assisting people to cope with the perception of time during lengthy illnesses. Nurse scientists who study this area may identify chronically ill patients, study how they spend their time, and explore diversions that could change their perception about the passage of time. In this instance, the theory title tells you little about its meaning, but examining its development makes it clear.

Another example comes from Madeleine Leininger's *theory of transcultural nursing* (Leininger, 1978, 1985, 1988). In 1950, Leininger practiced as a clinical nurse specialist in child mental health. She recognized that children from different cultures responded to health care in distinct ways. This discovery led her to the field of anthropology and ultimately to her theory of transcultural nursing. Initially, Leininger's attention focused on health care needs of children from various ethnic cultures, but later she expanded the focus to adults as well. Eventually, the theory encompassed the concept of cultural competence, that is, the nurse's ability to incorporate considerations of an individual's cultural background into nursing practice. Although inquiry in Leininger's theory remains focused on cultural needs, it crosses developmental stages, hospital and community-based health care settings, and a broad spectrum of cultural variations.

In some instances, clarifying the meaning of a theory is easier when similar theories are examined. For example, both Newman's *theory of health as expanding consciousness* and Rosemarie Parse's *theory of human becoming* draw from Martha Rogers' *theory of the science of unitary human beings* (Newman, 1979, 1986, 1990; Parse, 1981, 1992; Rogers, 1970, 1988). Looking at Newman's and Parse's theories will increase your understanding of the meaning of Rogers' theory. Although each theory is independent, all three use similar language, phenomena, concepts, and assumptions. When you critique a theory that is based on a related theory or shares concepts with it, it may be helpful to examine the meaning of the related theory as well as the one you are critiquing.

Communication theory provides another example of determining a clear and understandable meaning. Several models are mentioned in Chapter 5, with each focusing on a specific feature of communication. The health communication model speaks to relationships and transactions between a nurse and patient, and the context in which that communication takes place. It would be a simple matter to determine the meaning of this theory as well as its clarity.

Application. Before identifying the meaning of a theory, it is helpful to become acquainted with primary and secondary literature sources. Primary literary sources are the books, articles, and documents written by the theorist. Secondary literary sources, on the other hand, are written by individuals other than the theorist. Primary sources provide first-hand knowledge about the theory from the theorist. When you compare early and more recent sources, it will illustrate whether the theory's meaning has changed or not.

The ease with which you identify meaning varies from one theory to another. When you identify meaning, but before you make judgments about its clarity and understanding, you may try rewriting the meaning in your own words. The success with which you are able to do this will aid you in judging both clarity and understanding.

The title of a theory gives you clues about the theory's meaning but seldom provides sufficient information to document whether the clues are accurate. As theories develop, the titles may change. When Leininger developed her *theory of transcultural nursing*, many Americans viewed individuals from other countries as different, and nurses seldom learned the need to provide specialized care. As the demographics of America changed, Leininger's theory has as well. The theory is now known as the *culture care: diversity and universality theory*. The emphasis has expanded to include all individuals and their backgrounds, not just individuals from different countries and ethnic groups.

A new title for a theory may indicate several things: that the theory has changed, that the title has been brought into line with the original meaning of the theory, or that the theory is more consistent with current thought. Although Leininger's title may reflect some of each of these changes, it probably represents a change more consistent with current thought. Whenever a title changes, try to determine whether the meaning has also changed.

One other option for determining the meaning is to talk to or correspond with the author of a theory. Most contemporary nurse theorists are interested in talking with students and colleagues about their theories. You may also consult with faculty who know or have met some nurse theorists. The Internet is a source for pertinent information about nursing theorists and their theories (see Appendix A).

Judgments. A tentative judgment about the clarity and understanding of a theory's meaning should be made early in your critique. As you continue to study the theory, however, review and reconsider your initial decision. As indicated earlier, write the meaning of the theory in your words rather than adopting the theorist's language. Your ease or difficulty in doing this demonstrates your understanding of the meaning. The meaning of theory is seldom judged as completely clear or unclear. Figure 8.2, which provides a five-point scale, is more useful for ranking the criterion of meaning. As your knowledge about theory and nursing expands, you will begin to see some rays of light through the blurry images you saw early in your critique.

Criterion 2: Boundaries Are Consistent With Nursing Practice

Use the following questions to examine criterion 2:

- Does your definition of nursing fit with the definition in the theory?
- What aspects of nursing are studied and applied within the structure of the theory?
- How do you identify boundaries if they are not defined in the theory?
- Does the theory differentiate between nursing and other health disciplines?

Interpretation. Criterion 2 asks you to judge whether theory boundaries are consistent with nursing practice. These **boundaries** may include nursing care settings, recipients of nursing care, the role of the nurse in administrating that care, and legal and informal agreements that establish responsibilities of various health professionals. Where nursing takes place is important to know when we evaluate theory.

Criterion 1. The meaning of theory is clear and understandable.

The meaning of the theory of _____ is _____
(Name of theorist)   (Meaning in your words)

_____

_____

Circle the number closest to your perception of the clarity and understanding of the meaning of theory.

1	2	3	4	5
Fog too thick to see A blurry image		Starting to lift	Sun is breaking through	Clear as a bell

Figure 8.2 Clear and understandable meaning.

Nursing Care Settings. Settings where nursing care takes place are in a state of change. Until recently, more than 75% of nurses worked in hospitals; that figure has dropped to 65% (McBride, 1999). The length of time patients stay in hospitals is decreasing, and the emphasis on health and illness prevention is increasing. No longer are community-based health care settings limited to state health departments, nursing homes, traditional clinics, and homes; they are expanding to senior centers, churches, mobile units, and shopping malls. The shift to community-based care is expected to continue to increase, and the number of nurses working in the community will increase, as well.

Recipients of Care. There are five groups of recipients of care below, although others could be added:

- Development (infants, children, teenagers, adults, elderly, and the dying)
- Aggregates (individuals, families, groups, and communities)
- Illness, disease, surgery, and trauma entities
- Health–wellness continuum
- Acuity of care (acute, chronic, and preventive)

Many recipients fit into more than one group. For example, you may care for a 5-year-old child (development) recovering at home (family) after heart surgery (acute care), while the family provides the care under the daily supervision of a home health nurse. The boundaries for recipients of care are seldom geographic in nature but dictated by the particular needs of the individual, family, group, or community.

Role of the Nurse. Nursing is a multifaceted profession, and the nurse is responsible for fulfilling a variety of roles. The seven areas listed below are generally considered essential roles of the nurse:

- Caregiver
- Care manager
- Educator
- Leader
- Advocate
- Scientist
- Artist

In many instances, nurses fulfill two or more of these roles simultaneously. For example, when you administer hands-on care, you frequently serve as a health educator at the same time. In some cases, such as in an emergency room, you are the caregiver, although many nurses will continue to think of themselves as patient advocates.

Boundaries Between Professions. State and federal laws define formal boundaries between health professions. The state boards of nursing are responsible for enforcing laws about nursing enacted by their legislatures. In addition to these laws, there are informal agreements and institutional policies that help regulate the laws. At one time, physicians were the only health professionals with the authority to inject medications and only physicians could write prescriptions. Nurses have been giving injections for a long time, and initially, nurse practitioners (NPs) could only write prescriptions if physicians countersigned them. Laws now allow NPs to prescribe medications in every state, within specified classifications.

Boundaries exist between various groups of other health professionals, just as they do between nurses and physicians. Legal and informal agreements set important boundaries. Thinking about boundaries is consistent with what you learned about general systems theory earlier. Systems, subsystems, and environments lend themselves to examining boundaries between health professions.

For example, physicians, NPs, nurses, and pharmacists are involved in providing medications to patients. The physician and NP prescribe the medication, the pharmacist prepares the prescription, and the nurse administers the medication to the patient. Boundaries are dictated by laws and regulations, but all four health practitioners share responsibility to ensure that the patient receives the correct drug and dosage at the appropriate time and in the proper manner.

Application. To apply criterion 2, you need to collect information about recipients of care and the nurse's role in that care. While you search for clues to the boundaries, look at what the theorist and nurse researcher say about the theory. The emphasis of the theory will guide you to determine whether its boundaries are consistent with current or future nursing practice. When making such a determination, keep in mind that many nurse theorists are futuristic thinkers. Few nurses spoke or wrote about culture care before Leininger introduced the concept years before she published her theory. Now nurses recognize the importance of such care. Although nurses were aware of the need to encourage patients to care for themselves, when Dorothea Orem introduced the *theory of self-care deficit*, she changed the emphasis of nursing markedly (Orem, 1971, 1980, 1985, 1991). Nursing theories have boundaries consistent with both current and future nursing practice.

You may have difficulty accepting some theories that are very forward thinking. Try to imagine, for example, the difficulty that nurses in 1970 had accepting Rogers' *theory of the science of unitary human being*, when she wrote about nursing in space. When Leininger, Orem, and Rogers initially presented their theories to nurses, they set new boundaries for nursing practice.

Judgment. To decrease the complexity of making judgments about boundaries, the boundaries of the recipients of care (Fig. 8.3) and the roles of the nurse (Fig. 8.4) are illustrated. The wheels will help identify common nursing practice boundaries. As you identify the nursing practice boundaries consistent with a particular theory from the point of view of the recipient of care and the role of the nurse, examine the other options in each of the circles. Sometimes boundaries overlap. For example, a senior citizen visiting a clinic in a high-rise senior center is part of the developmental process, the health–wellness continuum, and the community (see Fig. 8.3). On the other hand, the nurse attending to that senior citizen in the clinic serves as educator, caregiver, and care manager, with the major emphasis on education (see Fig. 8.4). When numerous boundaries are to be considered, you might try to identify the one or two that are most relevant to the theory.

Criterion 3: Language Is Understandable and Includes Minimal Jargon

The following questions may be helpful in examining criterion 3:

- What words are new to you and how would you operationalize the meanings of these words?
- Are words in the theory defined the same as or different from your definitions?
- How many words did you look up in the dictionary in order to understand what the author was saying?
- What constitutes unnecessary jargon? What words could you substitute for jargon?

Interpretation. Understanding the language of theory is essential to making reasonable judgments about clarity, consistency, and usefulness to nursing practice. Expanding your vocabulary is also important as you critique theory. Theory that includes unfamiliar words, unusual word forms or definitions, or profuse jargon poses challenges to understanding and evaluation. You may wish to review the importance of using operational definitions in theories and related research as discussed in Chapter 4 to assist in your examination of this criterion.

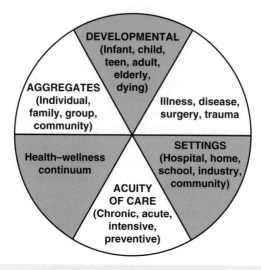

Theory evaluated: _____

List up to three recipients of care from the model and give a reason why each is relevant to the above theory.

1.

2.

3.

Indicate the level of consistency between the above theory and recipients of nursing care by circling one of the following:

high   **moderate**   **low**

Figure 8.3 Boundaries and the recipients of nursing care.

Disciplines and professions frequently develop a specialized language to name or label events and objects in their fields; we call this **jargon**. One use of jargon is to allow individuals in a discipline or profession to relay information to colleagues more quickly. As you examine a theory, you may need to differentiate between jargon and words that are unfamiliar to you.

Students of theory frequently question why nursing theories are so wordy and difficult to understand. The subject matter of theory is complex and can be difficult to interpret. Some theorists may assume that abstract language makes a theory more unique and distinguished. In an attempt to differentiate these words from common ideas, they seek unusual formulations of words. For example, Parse, in the *theory of human becoming,* uses participles to name concepts because she believes this emphasizes the process rather than a static orientation of the concept. Some examples of these concepts are *powering* instead of power, *valuing* instead of value, and *languaging* instead of language. The latter concepts may make the theory even more difficult to understand.

Application. Various strategies may be used to collect data for applying criterion 3, such as making lists of unfamiliar words, invented words, and jargon. If you have a copy of a document,

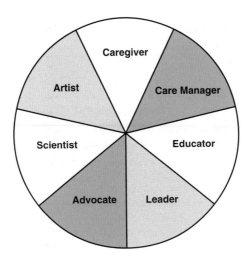

Theory evaluated: _____

List up to three roles of the nurse from the model and give a reason why each is relevant to the above theory.

1.

2.

3.

Indicate the level of consistency between the above theory and the role of the nurse by circling one of the following:

            high   moderate   low

Figure 8.4 Boundaries and the role of the nurse.

highlighting these words in different colors may be helpful. When you list them, you may wish to include the definition the theorist uses as well as a more common dictionary definition. Finally, note important words and concepts in a theory that you do understand. Comparing the list of concepts with the lists of unfamiliar and invented words may help determine your overall understanding of the language.

Judgment. The use of unusual language sometimes makes it difficult to do an accurate critique of the content of a theory. You may need to look up definitions and incorporate them into your understanding before you can achieve even a superficial acquaintance with some theories. Chapter 2 introduced you to some of the essential words in theory and their meanings. Think of words you currently use on a daily basis that you did not know when you entered nursing. Expanding your scientific and theoretical vocabulary is just one step in becoming an educated nurse who speaks the language of the discipline.

You can judge the language criterion using the five-point continuum illustrated in Figure 8.5. The scale uses arbitrary measuring levels of understanding of 30%, 50%, 70%, and 90%. Comparing your list of unusual words and jargon with abstract words and concepts that you do understand will help you make the appropriate judgment.

As you proceed with the second and third phases of the critique, refer back to your judgments about clarity and understanding of the theory's intent.

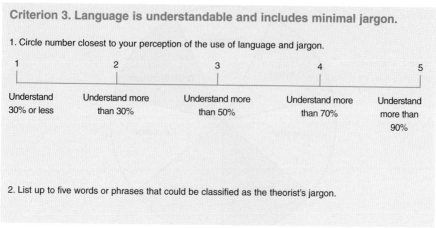

Figure 8.5 Use of language and jargon.

Phase II: Concepts and Propositions

When you complete your critique of the meaning, boundaries, and language of a theory, you are ready to proceed to Phase II, the critique of a theory's concepts, propositions, variables, and assumptions. C-BaC focuses on some theory building blocks because they lead you more quickly to the critique of the usefulness of theory in nursing practice.

The three criteria in Phase II are as follows:

4. Major concepts are identified and defined.

5. Concepts stimulate the formulation of propositions.

6. Propositions are related to the meaning of the theory.

Criterion 4: Major Concepts Are Identified and Defined

You may find the following questions useful in examining criterion 4:

- What are the major concepts used in the theory?
- How are these concepts related to nursing practice?
- Are definitions of major concepts consistent with what you know about nursing practice?
- Are definitions of major concepts consistent with those used in other theories?

Interpretation. In Chapter 2, you learned that concepts define objects, events, and ideas and provide them with boundaries and structure. When you use concepts that are generally accepted by the discipline, you can use shortcuts in written and verbal descriptions. You have learned and used many concepts, such as vital signs, surgical prep, history and physical, and charting, since entering nursing; you will learn many more concepts related to theory.

Theory includes two types of concepts: those that are commonly understood and generally accepted across the discipline and those that are unique to one or two theories. The concepts of health, nursing, person, and environment are found in many nursing theories. Most theories incorporate additional concepts as well, such as nursing process (Levine, 1967, 1969), pattern recognition (Newman, 1979, 1986, 1990), self-care (Orem, 1971, 1980, 1985, 1991), interpersonal process (Peplau, 1952), energy fields (Rogers, 1970, 1988), adaptation (Roy, 1970, 1975), and caring (Watson, 1979, 1985). When you identify a concept as being a major component of a theory, you will also need to examine how the theorist defines that concept.

Concepts that present clear, well-defined ideas are more useful than those that are defined in vague terms or are constantly changing. At one time, for example, nurses, physicians, and the health care community agreed on the meaning of the concept of *patient*. When nurses began to emphasize health and wellness, the concept of *client* was introduced, even though many nurses questioned whether client accurately represented the relationship with the nurse. More recently, the concept of *consumer* was introduced. We continue to see all three concepts used, but with varying definitions.

Application. Your initial task in applying the criterion will be to identify major concepts and their definitions. Primary sources may introduce concepts and their definitions, but some authors of secondary sources, who are attempting to interpret theory, will specify them more carefully. To apply this criterion, therefore, you will need to examine both primary and secondary sources, recognizing that secondary sources may be more helpful than primary. When you are able to identify major concepts and definitions, they may still be too complex to understand. In that case, you may benefit from rewriting the definition in more user-friendly language. Parse tends to define concepts that are difficult to understand. One of the definitions she uses is "health is a continuously changing process that man participates in co-creating" (Parse, 1981, p. 40). To help understand the meaning of health, we might rewrite Parse's definition to read: *health changes in response to the individual's relationships with his or her environment.* Someone else might rewrite the definition to read: *health is a constantly changing response to the choices an individual makes.*

You may wonder how to identify theoretical concepts that are major and how many you should select. Although there are many correct methods to determine major concepts, you might want to define the differences between a major and a minor concept before making selections. You might select concepts that are mentioned earliest or most frequently in the theory. You might select concepts that are relevant to a specific area of practice or about which the most is written. For example, if you locate several scientific publications about caring nurses based on Benner and Wrubel's theory, you may choose that as a major concept. The criterion says "concepts," so be sure you select at least two. Because this is a learning activity and not scientific research, you do have leeway in your choices.

Judgment. Although you have made judgments about selecting concepts, the critical judgment related to this criterion is the consistency of the concepts with nursing practice, both current and future. Figure 8.6 provides a scale that includes a midpoint that will yield to your perception about both current and future nursing practice.

Criterion 5: Concepts Stimulate the Formulation of Propositions

The following suggestions will help you explore criterion 5. You may think of other areas to explore as well. Determine who is responsible for defining concepts and the relationship between the concepts and propositions. Think about the importance of using concepts in propositions.

Interpretation. In criterion 4, you identified concepts and definitions. These concepts and their definitions are important in stimulating the formulation of propositions. Although the definition of concept is important to the theorist in the development of theory, it may not always serve the nurse scientist who attempts to measure the concept in actual practice. For example, Benner and Wrubel (1989) define caring as "persons, events, projects, and things [that] matter to people" (p. 1). The nurse scientist who studies the concept of caring may have difficulty identifying and measuring things that matter and therefore may try to operationalize caring in a way that yields more useful data. There are various ways to study caring by observing nurses' activities as they care for a patient. Scientists may study the amount of time the nurse spends with the patient, whether the nurse recognizes and fulfills the patient's needs, the

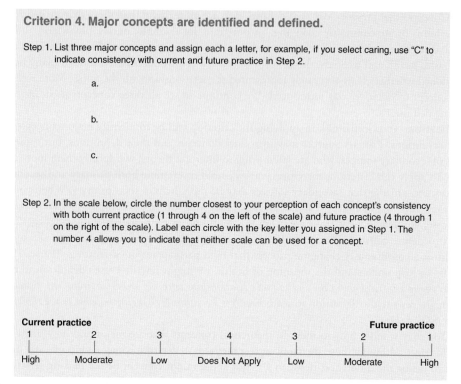

Criterion 4. Major concepts are identified and defined.

Step 1. List three major concepts and assign each a letter, for example, if you select caring, use "C" to indicate consistency with current and future practice in Step 2.

     a.

     b.

     c.

Step 2. In the scale below, circle the number closest to your perception of each concept's consistency with both current practice (1 through 4 on the left of the scale) and future practice (4 through 1 on the right of the scale). Label each circle with the key letter you assigned in Step 1. The number 4 allows you to indicate that neither scale can be used for a concept.

Current practice   **Future practice**

1   2   3   4   3   2   1

High   Moderate   Low   Does Not Apply   Low   Moderate   High

Figure 8.6 Definitions of major concepts and their consistency with current and future practice.

nurse's attention to family members, or actions of the nurse when nursing interventions are not successful.

Using these and other ideas, a nurse scientist may define the concept so it is measurable and able to be incorporated into hypotheses. An example of a proposition related to an earlier suggestion, the amount of time the nurse spends with the patient, might be: The caring nurse checks the patient at least four times during each 8-hour shift and talks with the patient for at least 20 minutes periodically during the day. Collecting quantitative data such as these requires monitoring the activities of the nurse.

Application. Theorists do not always identify propositions in their theories. In this exercise, you will find it helpful to write some propositions based on theoretical concepts. As you think about simple concepts, such as health, nursing, or caring, examine their definitions, how they relate to each other, and how they stimulate a proposition. Earlier, we mentioned Leininger's culture care theory and the importance of the concept of caring. An example of a proposition stimulated by the concept of caring might be: The nurse who learns about the culture of new immigrants from Southeast Asia will provide more effective teaching about therapeutic diets.

Judgment. Your judgment about whether concepts and their definitions stimulate propositions will require comparing concepts in a theory and related research findings. Attempt to find one or two propositions that you can trace back to a theoretical concept. You will also benefit from writing propositions. For example, return to Benner and Wrubel's definition of caring, "things that matter" (1989). If you are involved in an accident and are taken to the local emergency room, what would matter to you? If the nurse called your parents, would the same things matter to them that matter

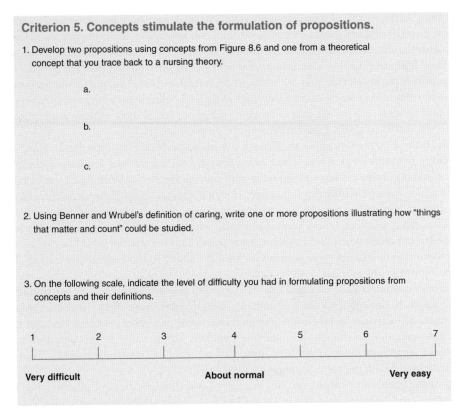

Criterion 5. Concepts stimulate the formulation of propositions.

1. Develop two propositions using concepts from Figure 8.6 and one from a theoretical concept that you trace back to a nursing theory.

   a.

   b.

   c.

2. Using Benner and Wrubel's definition of caring, write one or more propositions illustrating how "things that matter and count" could be studied.

3. On the following scale, indicate the level of difficulty you had in formulating propositions from concepts and their definitions.

1	2	3	4	5	6	7

Very difficult   About normal   Very easy

Figure 8.7 Concepts and propositions.

to you? When you hear individuals relate stories about being in an emergency room, they talk about how long they waited before being seen and how difficult it was to get information about what was happening. It is clear that "time" and "information" matter to them. Assume you are a nurse scientist and you decide to study this situation and base your study on Benner and Wrubel's work. Write one or more propositions using their definition of caring and what matters to you. Figure 8.7 provides an approach for using concepts in the development of propositions.

Criterion 6: Variables and Assumptions Help You Understand and Interpret Propositions

You have already explored concepts and propositions. Now you are ready to examine the role of variables and assumptions in propositions. Review the definitions of concepts, propositions, variables, and assumptions in Chapter 2, and think about how they relate to propositions.

Interpretation. A proposition is a statement that connects two or more concepts into a directional relationship, and is generally derived from experience or observation in the real world. Suppose a high school teacher notices that students who regularly attend class earn higher grades on final examinations. This proposition illustrates the direction and nature of the relationship between the concepts of class attendance and final exam grades. We call these concepts variables.

Variables are observable and measurable concepts with the ability to change. In the above proposition, the teacher can observe and measure attendance in class and final exam grades. Both attendance and grades can vary. The internal variables in the proposition are class attendance and grades. As the variable of class attendance varies, the final exam grade may also vary. In addition to these internal variables, there are external variables that may influence the internal variables. For example, if the classroom is too hot or too cold, the students fail to complete class assignments.

In addition to variables, assumptions also help you understand and interpret propositions. **Assumptions** are statements that are taken to be factual or true. Looking at the proposition above, you may make various assumptions, such as high school students want to go to college, are motivated to study, and attend class to learn. By accepting one or more of these assumptions as truths, you can focus on the basic concepts in the proposition.

Application. As you think about your contacts with home-bound or hospitalized patients, try to identify propositions pertinent to one or more of the nursing theories you have studied. The proposition may come from your familiarity with nursing practice or by studying the literature. You may also attempt to identify propositions from a theory and relate them to practice. In your contacts with hospitalized patients, for example, you may notice that individuals who are up and about frequently talk about going home. Individuals who are confined to bed, on the other hand, may be less apt to ask when they can leave the hospital. This observation would be easy to write as a proposition by making an association between the ability to move about and talking about the desire to leave the hospital.

Health care reform and managed care have changed how some decisions are made in regard to the length of time patients are hospitalized. These decisions may affect the relationship between patients' activities and their desire to go home. Some patients may express the need to remain hospitalized, even though they meet the standards for discharge. In this proposition, the variables change from measurements of individual recuperation to standards set by insurance companies and health maintenance organizations.

Judgment. Compose two propositions related to two different areas of practice. For each proposition, use the template in Figure 8.8 to identify the internal variables, and write one or two external variables. As you think about each proposition, identify two assumptions that help you understand and interpret the proposition.

Phase III: Usefulness in Nursing Practice

The third and final phase of C-BaC is the determination of the usefulness of theory in nursing practice. This is the most important consideration of the critique. Phase III criteria build on judgments that you made in Phases I and II. The two criteria in Phase III are as follows:

7. Theoretical knowledge helps explain and predict phenomena.

8. Theoretical knowledge influences nursing practice.

The basic functions of knowledge, as discussed in Chapter 3, include providing intellectual processes to the application of knowledge to stimulate new theory and knowledge. The first function, identifying concepts and relationships between concepts, relates directly to criteria 4 and 6 in Phase II. The second purpose, to provide intellectual processes for knowledge application, is relevant to Phase III. Phase III also focuses on the remaining processes: understanding propositions, explaining and predicting phenomena, and influencing and controlling phenomena.

Criterion 7: Theoretical Knowledge Helps Explain and Predict Phenomena

Think about the relationship between theory, theoretical knowledge, and nursing practice. Try to identify how your practice reflects theoretical knowledge and the explanations and predictions you are able to make about your practice.

Interpretation. As you study theory and the knowledge it generates, you will begin to make connections between theory, knowledge, and practice. These connections help you understand

Criterion 6. Variables and assumptions help you understand and interpret propositions.

Formulate two propositions related to two different areas in nursing. Identify two internal and two external variables for each proposition and two assumptions.

Proposition I.

A. Internal variables
1.

2.

B. External variables
1.

2.

C. Assumptions
1.

2.

Proposition II.

A. Internal variables
1.

2.

B. External variables
1.

2.

C. Assumptions
1.

2.

Figure 8.8 Variables and assumptions.

the application and outcomes of care. Nurses who are employed in long-term care facilities, for example, recognize that residents with hip fractures need considerable assistance with activities of daily living, such as dressing and basic hygiene. These individuals are unable to return to a state of independent living until they regain their everyday skills. The central theme of Orem's *theory of self-care deficit* is defining when the nurse must provide care and when adults are able to care for themselves. Nurses expect to spend more time assisting and educating these residents initially,

but as they regain skill, the self-care deficit decreases, and both resident and nurse assume different roles. Orem's theory illustrates connections between theoretical knowledge and nursing practice, as well as the practicality of theory that was mentioned earlier.

Evidence that knowledge helps explain and predict phenomena is found in Benner's exemplars about expert nurses. In one exemplar, a woman has difficulty making a fistula drainage bag
adhere to her skin for more than a couple of hours. This causes serious skin problems and is upsetting to the woman. An expert nurse convinces the woman that she has developed a successful
method and is confident it will work in the woman's case. With the nurse's insistence and teaching, the bag is applied and stays on for 3 days (Benner, 1984). The nurse had experimented with
various methods and procedures until she found one that would work. Although the nurse did
not conduct formal research, she tried various methods, collected data, and made decisions based
on her experience. In the woman's case, the expert nurse understood the problem, explained what
she would do, and then predicted the outcomes using the defined method. As an expert nurse,
she was able to incorporate the purposes of knowledge and science into her practice.

Application. Nurse scholars and scientists make judgments about the usefulness of theory by
identifying and studying phenomena that help explain and predict relationships between interventions and outcomes. Although you may be unable to test phenomena at this time, you can
benefit from the work of others by thinking about potential effects of the study on your practice.

Leininger's culture care focuses on relationships between the recipient's cultural background
and the nursing interventions and outcomes. One area of cultural concern is nutrition and diet.
In the United States, for example, many people view meat as an essential component of their
daily diet. In many developing or third-world countries, meat is too sparse and too expensive to
eat very often, so other foods, such as beans and rice, are substituted for meat. Unless a health
care professional understands the cultural background of an individual, a recommendation to eat
more meat may be ignored by the individual. You can use this theoretical knowledge to collect
information about a patient's diet and thereby influence your practice. When you are familiar
with an individual's cultural background, you are better able to understand and predict how he
or she will respond to the care and education you provide. Practicing nurses, as well as nurse scientists, are concerned about accuracy and adequacy of care, both of which contribute to the judgment of usefulness of knowledge and theory.

Generally, nurse scientists look for evidence that confirms, rather than contradicts, what
nurses know and are able to do. When it appears that changes are needed, research findings must
be replicated to verify the original findings. Both the scientific and practice communities in nursing must have confidence in the changes, not just the individuals who conduct the research.
When the nursing discipline adopts theoretical knowledge without adequate verification, the effect on practice could be neutral or negative. The same might be true if you allow knowledge to
influence your practice without collecting sufficient evidence. Searching for information that
confirms your decisions about care will have a positive effect on your practice.

Judgment. The most valuable result of criterion 7 is to identify phenomena from nursing practice
and determine whether theory helps explain and predict as well as understand the observation.
Figure 8.9 provides an approach that includes an example of a phenomenon and ideas about its relationship for the purposes of knowledge. It is your task to write your own statement of a phenomenon and give examples of explaining/predicting, understanding, and influencing/controlling.

Criterion 8: Theoretical Knowledge Influences Nursing Practice

To stimulate your thinking about the influence of theoretical knowledge on nursing practice,
think about its effects on your nursing practice. Identify concepts and their influence in a practice situation you have observed.

Criterion 7. Theory helps explain and predict phenomena.

1. State a phenomenon from your observation of nursing practice.
   EXAMPLE: Residents of a long-term care facility who eat in the dining room eat a more nutritious diet than those who eat in their rooms.
   PHENOMENON:

2. State one or two ideas that stem from the phenomenon that relate to the following purposes of knowledge; that is, explaining and predicting, influencing and controlling, and understanding.
   PURPOSES OF KNOWLEDGE:
   a. Example of Understanding: Individuals focus their attention on socializing with other individuals and less on the meal they are served and eating.
   RESPONSE:

   b. Example of Explaining/Predicting: In the United States, eating is viewed as a social activity.
   RESPONSE:

   c. Example of Influencing/Controlling: Individuals who do not eat a nutritious diet should be encouraged and assisted to the dining room and seated at a table with friends.
   RESPONSE:

3. When you have completed sections 1 and 2 above, evaluate your ability to carry out the exercise by circling the number below that best describes your feelings:

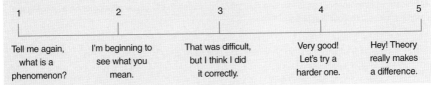

1	2	3	4	5
Tell me again, what is a phenomenon?	I'm beginning to see what you mean.	That was difficult, but I think I did it correctly.	Very good! Let's try a harder one.	Hey! Theory really makes a difference.

Figure 8.9 Explaining and predicting phenomena.

Interpretation. Throughout this book, we refer to relationships between theory and knowledge and between theory and practice. In Chapter 3, you became aware that research findings that support theory may be added to the body of nursing knowledge when nurse scientists have confidence in those findings. Criterion 8 focuses on your ability to identify research findings that can have an effect on practice, by locating research reports related to a particular practice matter. When you understand these connections, you will recognize the value of the influence of theory on nursing practice.

Learning about theory and the knowledge that it generates will not automatically influence your practice. You will benefit from using critical thinking and clinical reasoning skills to determine how ideas can be incorporated into your practice; whether you need to set guidelines about when they should be used; and, if adopted, how to evaluate the effect of the changes on patient care.

Application. Criterion 8 requires you to use observation and reasoning skills for the purpose of evaluating your practice and its relationship to theory. Most of your practice to this point has focused on tasks and procedures. Now you must think about what you do and why you do it and then identify how knowledge relates to your actions.

Locating the necessary information to critique whether criterion 8 can be met requires a search of the scientific literature. If you select a topic in which you have some knowledge and interest, you will have a better chance of success. Your search should explore the content of the topic as well as potential theoretical frameworks.

Judgment. Although you have probably evaluated your educational and clinical progress, it is unlikely you have been asked to do so at the level required by criterion 8. This is a good time to take an introspective view of your developing practice. Figure 8.10 assists you to make pertinent observations and to critique them. If you select an area of nursing in which you are interested and to which you have access, you will find it is easier to follow the exercise and collect the necessary information.

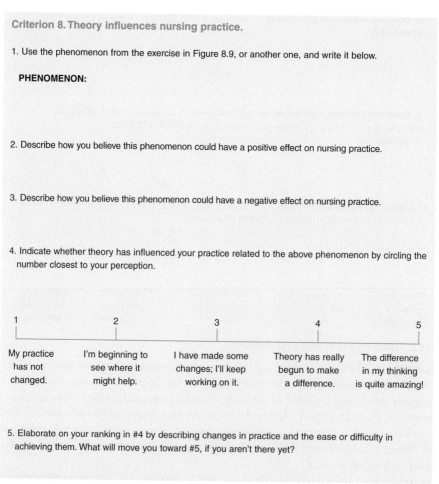

Criterion 8. Theory influences nursing practice.

1. Use the phenomenon from the exercise in Figure 8.9, or another one, and write it below.

   PHENOMENON:

2. Describe how you believe this phenomenon could have a positive effect on nursing practice.

3. Describe how you believe this phenomenon could have a negative effect on nursing practice.

4. Indicate whether theory has influenced your practice related to the above phenomenon by circling the number closest to your perception.

1	2	3	4	5
My practice has not changed.	I'm beginning to see where it might help.	I have made some changes; I'll keep working on it.	Theory has really begun to make a difference.	The difference in my thinking is quite amazing!

5. Elaborate on your ranking in #4 by describing changes in practice and the ease or difficulty in achieving them. What will move you toward #5, if you aren't there yet?

Figure 8.10 Influence of theory on practice.

Advanced Theory Analysis Models

C-BaC provides a fundamental approach to critiquing theory and knowledge that you can conduct with a growing practice background. Advanced students and practitioners who wish to generate questions for research, obtain funds for research, and ultimately add to the scientific body of nursing knowledge will require a more complex approach to analyzing theory and knowledge. The information below about a few advanced analytical models will help you to become acquainted with literature that you need in order to conduct your critique.

Several models for theory analysis, including Barnum (1998), Fawcett (1993), Walker and Avant (1995), and Meleis (1997), are briefly described. These four models require a level of scholarly reasoning beyond what most practicing nurses have. Both the basic and the advanced information you are learning will help you move to a higher level of knowledge and understanding in the future.

Barbara Barnum

Barnum's model of theory analysis divides criteria into internal and external criticisms. She uses the concept of criticism to include strengths and limitations, similar to the use of critique in C-BaC. Internal criticisms focus on how theory components fit together, whereas external criticisms examine the scope and complexity of theory.

Some examples of internal criticism include determining whether the pattern of the theory makes sense and whether propositions follow logically from assumptions and objective measures of clarity, consistency, adequacy, and logic. Because most people agree on how these internal judgments are made, Barnum assumes that the results are objective.

Examples of external criticism are the usefulness of theory, effects of theory on nursing practice, differentiation of nursing from other health fields, and the individual's definition of nursing. Barnum believes that these judgments are more subjective because they depend on the evaluator's educational background, the setting or specialty area of practice, and the individual's perception of the world of nursing, health, and recipients of care (Barnum, 1998).

Jacqueline Fawcett

Fawcett divides her model into analysis and evaluation. Analysis is a nonjudgmental, detailed examination of the scope, context, and content of a theory and concentrates on the theorist's writings. Evaluation requires the individual to make judgments about the testability of theory, the potential for practical and empirical research, and its significance to practice. Evaluation takes into consideration the results of the analysis but relies significantly on interpretations and critiques by others, research reports, and reports of practical application resulting from the knowledge. Fawcett provides separate lists of questions for analysis and evaluation (Fawcett, 1993).

The approaches used by Barnum and Fawcett are similar, although each uses different labels for some of the concepts. Of the four models discussed in this section, these are the easiest to understand and most similar to C-BaC.

Lorraine Walker and Kay Avant

Walker and Avant (1995) define theory analysis as a "systematic examination of a theory for meaning, logical adequacy, usefulness, generality (impact on other areas), parsimony (simplicity), and testability" (p. 133). They believe evaluation is part of analysis and that each step is important to a complete analysis. The purpose of Walker and Avant's analysis is to identify both strengths and weaknesses of theory. They believe that educators and practitioners usually focus on strengths because they rely on theory to improve nursing care and therefore need positive feedback. Researchers and scientists, on the other hand, focus on weaknesses in their search to identify unusual or unclear relationships that will justify studying the theory.

Afaf Meleis

Meleis' evaluation model is comprehensive, analytical, and evaluative. She uses tools such as description, analysis, critique, testing, and support. Although each component of theory can be evaluated separately, Meleis brings them together in a large complex model featuring "nursing theory" and "theoretical nursing" (Meleis, 1997). Evaluation for each component can be conducted separately, but all components must be included in the final result. Meleis believes that criterion-based critiques are essential to the development of knowledge but that scientists benefit from applying healthy skepticism as well. Although you may feel that the language Meleis uses is more familiar, she takes more liberty in her definitions in implementing her model. For example, Meleis talks about using a criterion-based evaluation but leaves the formulation of criteria to the evaluator.

Walker and Avant's model is more intricate than those of Barnum and Fawcett; of the four models, Meleis' model is the most comprehensive. When you choose to extend your exploration of theory evaluation, starting with Barnum and Fawcett will be most helpful.

Summary

Chapter 8 has described a criterion-based critique (C-BaC) model limited to eight areas of concern. The model provides a foundation for beginning exploration of theory and theoretical knowledge. C-BaC includes components of more advanced models but limits the examination to the intent of the theory, concepts and propositions, and usefulness in practice. The knowledge acquired from this beginning approach to the evaluation of theory will form a foundation for further education.

A brief discussion of four advanced models illustrates relationships between them and C-BaC and provides ideas about the importance of continuing exploration of scientific knowledge and its use in practice.

Learning Activities

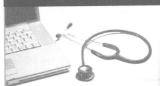

1. The story writers: Divide into small groups to compose stories about incidents from your nursing experience. Identify relevant concepts from these stories and link them to one or more specific nursing theories using the critique model presented in the text. For example, is the concept of caring as viewed from the perspective of Leininger or Watson more useful to explain what happened in the story? Which concept of self-care explains a situation most effectively: Henderson's definition of nursing or Orem's self-care deficit theory? (See Chapter 7.)

2. Editor for a day: Divide into groups of three to four. Identify a section from a nursing theory that is particularly difficult to understand. Rewrite that section using as little jargon and as few words as possible. Ask other student groups to analyze the edited version and verify that they understand it.

References

Barnum, B. S. (1998). *Nursing theory: Analysis, application, evaluation.* Philadelphia: Lippincott Williams & Wilkins.

Benner, P. (1984). *From novice to expert: Excellence and power in clinical nursing practice.* Menlo Park, CA: Addison-Wesley.

Benner, P., & Wrubel, J. (1989). *The primacy of care: Stress and coping in health and illness.* Menlo Park, CA: Addison-Wesley.

Fawcett, J. (1993). *Analysis and evaluation of nursing theories.* Philadelphia: F.A. Davis.

Leininger, M. (1978). *Transcultural nursing concepts, theories and practice.* New York: John Wiley & Sons.

Leininger, M. M. (1985). Transcultural care diversity and universality: A theory of nursing. *Nursing & Health Care, 6*(4), 209–212.

Leininger, M. M. (1988). Leininger's theory of nursing: Cultural care diversity and universality. *Nursing Science Quarterly, 1*(4), 152–160.

Levine, M. E. (1967). The four conservation principles of nursing. *Nursing Forum, 6*(1), 45–59.

Levine, M. E. (1969). *Introduction to clinical nursing.* Philadelphia: F.A. Davis.

McBride, A. B. (1999). Breakthroughs in nursing education: Looking back and looking forward. *Nursing Outlook, 47*(3), 114–119.

Meleis, A. I. (1997). *Theoretical nursing: Development and progress.* Philadelphia: Lippincott-Raven.

Newman, M. A. (1979). *Theory development in nursing.* Philadelphia: F.A. Davis.

Newman, M. A. (1986). *Health as expanding consciousness.* St. Louis: C.V. Mosby.

Newman, M. A. (1990). Newman's theory of health as praxis. *Nursing Science Quarterly, 3*(1), 37–41.

Orem, D. E. (1971). *Nursing: Concepts of practice.* New York: McGraw-Hill.

Orem, D. E. (1980). *Nursing: Concepts of practice* (2nd ed.). New York: McGraw-Hill.

Orem, D. E. (1985). *Nursing: Concepts of practice* (3rd ed.). New York: McGraw-Hill.

Orem, D. E. (1991). *Nursing: Concepts of practice* (4th ed.). St. Louis: Mosby–Year Book.

Parse, R. R. (1981). *Man–living–health: A theory of nursing.* New York: John Wiley & Sons.

Parse, R. R. (1992). Human becoming: Parse's theory of nursing. *Nursing Science Quarterly, 5*(1), 35–42.

Peplau, H. E. (1952). *Interpersonal relations in nursing.* New York: G.P. Putnam.

Reynolds, W. J. (1997). Peplau's theory in practice. *Nursing Science Quarterly, 10*(4), 168–170.

Rogers, M. E. (1970). *An introduction to the theoretical basis of nursing.* Philadelphia: F.A. Davis.

Rogers, M. E. (1988). Nursing science and art: A prospective. *Nursing Science Quarterly, 1,* 99–102.

Roy, C. (1970). Adaptation: A conceptual framework for nursing. *Nursing Outlook, 18*(3), 42–45.

Roy, C. (1975). A diagnostic classification system for nursing. *Nursing Outlook, 23,* 90–94.

Walker, L. O., & Avant, K. C. (1995). *Strategies for theory construction in nursing.* Norwalk, CT: Appleton & Lange.

Watson, J. (1979). *Nursing: The philosophy and science of caring.* Boston: Little, Brown.

Watson, J. (1985). *Nursing: Human science and human caring—a theory for nursing.* Norwalk, CT: Appleton-Century-Crofts.

Introduction to Research

Sean Clarke, RN, PhD, CRNP

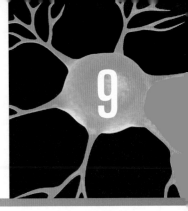

9

Intent: This chapter provides an overview of the philosophical foundation of research and its relationship to theory, knowledge, reasoning, and practice. It discusses specific steps associated with the research process, as well as criteria used to critique completed research. The chapter also introduces you to some of the specific issues associated with conducting and utilizing research in nursing and other health professions.

Key Words/Concepts

confounding variable	methodology	reliability
dependent variable	modernism	replication
descriptive statistics	neomodernism	research critique
empirical	observational	research design
evaluation	operational definition	research discourse
evidence-based practice	peer review	research questions
experiment	population	sampling
generalizability	postmodernism	theoretical framework
independent variable	primary research	triangulation
inferential statistics	protection of human subjects	validity
informed consent	qualitative research	
literature review	quantitative research	
measurement tool	randomized clinical trial	

Introduction

Albert Einstein (1927) wrote, "If what is seen and experienced is portrayed in the language of logic, we are engaged in science. If it is communicated through forms whose connections are not accessible to the conscious mind but are recognized intuitively as meaningful, then we are engaged in art" (p. 30). This quote captures some of the philosophical underpinnings of nursing theory, knowledge, research, and practice. Understanding the dichotomy between art and science also helps to bring essential differences between major types of research into focus and provides you with some insight into the ongoing debate about philosophies and methods of knowing and understanding in nursing. Keep this dichotomy in mind as you explore this introduction to nursing research.

Philosophies Influencing the Development of Nursing Research

As nursing researchers, past and present, worked to develop a scholarly knowledge base for the profession, they were, and continue to be, influenced by two specific philosophies. These philosophies are modernism and postmodernism.

Modernism

Modernism is a philosophy of thinking and knowledge development that emphasizes logic, objectivity, the discovery of facts, linear cause and effect, and a belief in universal principles and laws. Embedded in modernism is the concept of logical positivism, which is the belief that questions or problems can be resolved through the application of logic. Working in concert with logical positivism is the concept of logical empiricism, which is the belief that logical assertions can be scientifically verified through experimentation or through the gathering and analysis of statistical data. Logical empiricism has had a significant impact on modern nursing because of its focus on verification or testing of principles and the implication that phenomena are only scientifically meaningful if they are empirically verifiable through the senses, logical proof, or mathematics (Reed & Shearer, 2009). Modernism and research are linked through methodologies that are designed to keep research objective and untainted by values and influences of everyday life (Reed, 2009).

Modernism has been and continues to be extremely influential in the world of academia. When nursing education moved from 3-year, hospital-based programs into university settings in the mid-20th century, nurse researchers and theorists began to emerge, and the primary philosophy guiding their work was a modernistic one. Modernism was not without critics, inside and outside of nursing. It is a philosophy that is optimistic about the ability of scientific endeavors to solve problems. It places a great deal of faith in science's ability to explain, predict, influence, and control knowledge in a responsible manner. Interestingly, wars and atrocities, along with rapid societal changes throughout the world in the 20th century caused scholars in many disciplines to question whether modernism could answer all questions, solve all problems, and explain all phenomena (Lister, 1997). As a result, they began searching for alternative methods of knowledge development. As nursing's science evolved over the second half of the 20th century, by the 1980s, a considerable number of nurse scholars came to adopt this skepticism and share this quest.

Postmodernism

As valuable as modernism was and is to theory development in nursing, researchers in a number of disciplines, including nursing and the social sciences, found that it fell short in some respects. Its focus on facts and objectivity failed to adequately address many phenomena observed in nursing practice. For example, how does one empirically prove the effect of a person's faith on his or her health, measure the benefit of a hospice nurse to the dying, or research the complexity and multiplicity of human feelings and emotions in empirical terms? How could the experiences of patients, families, and their communities coping with dizzying social change be explored and explained (Lister, 1997)?

Modernism could not address these types of phenomena. As a result, many nurse scholars embraced a second philosophy in knowledge development, called **postmodernism.** According to Reed and Shearer (2009), postmodernism, which began as a philosophical and social movement among literary theorists in France during the 1960s, began influencing nursing around the end of the 20th century. Simply speaking, whereas the focus in modernism was on proving theory, the focus of postmodernism was on the development of new theory through the discovery of meaning without empirical evidence.

Today, postmodernists value nonlinear thinking, which is a very different approach from the more linear sequencing of the research process that much of this chapter deals with. They recognize that phenomena can be observed from the outside or experienced from the inside and accept the possibility that multiple empirical and nonempirical truths may surround the same phenomenon (Reed & Shearer, 2009; Watson, 1999). They are open to participative theory discovery, where researchers and participants in research interact with each other to allow the researcher to discover the practical reality of people's life experiences. Postmodernists draw meaning from stories and narratives and acknowledge the existence of a practical reality that cannot be confirmed with physical senses. Instead of answering questions or solving problems in the traditional sense, postmodernists deconstruct phenomena, which means they take them apart and critique them. Using the deconstructed concepts, they then build new patterns, identify new relationships, and discover new meanings and values associated with the original phenomena. Exciting new perspectives that challenge prevailing wisdom can result from this approach. It is sometimes said that modernists look upon the meaning of the world and their place in it, and that postmodernists re-make the world as their science demands it (Britt, 1989).

Of particular significance to nursing, the postmodern view represents an epistemological shift in nursing theory development to include not only the modernistic search for truth and validity of empirical findings, but also the exploration of phenomenological findings unique to human beings and their experiences.

Neomodernism

Has another philosophy of knowledge discovery emerged that moves past postmodernism? According to many scholars, there is (Best & Keller, 1991; Cheek, 2000; Reed & Shearer, 2009; Watson, 1999; Whall & Hicks, 2002). This third philosophy, called **neomodernism,** draws tenets from both modernism and postmodernism, and proposes breaking down boundaries and meanings that currently shape nurses' perspectives on themselves as human beings and as professionals, as well as citizens within society. Neomodernism breaks from the idea that human experience can be adequately described by "grand" theories that establish a set of pre-established truths, emphasize cause-and-effect relationships, and attempt to explain all major phenomena across an entire field of study. Neomodernism proposes a multidimensional reality and multiple positions from which reality can be viewed (Cheek, 2000), including the careful use of some positivist ideas and research traditions when appropriate.

Neomodernism questions the traditional idea of advances and progress in health care, "both in terms of what actually constitutes progress and advances, and concomitantly, whether developments and change in the health care system are necessarily progressive" (Cheek, 2000, p. 19). Reed and Shearer (2009) assert that postmodernistic and neomodernistic attitudes are dislodging beliefs about dichotomies, such as research and practice, inductive and deductive reasoning, qualitative and quantitative data, and so on. They indicate that 21st-century approaches to developing knowledge will move past these dichotomies. Watson (1999), in her discussion of neomodernism, indicates that even the name "nursing" should be done away with because it is too embedded in modernistic practices. Throughout her career, Watson has challenged established thought in many areas, including the nature of human beings and their experiences. She does so again in her views of neomodernism:

> *Perhaps this postmodern Era . . . and beyond can best be captured metaphorically as the age of light, which takes us into a new relationship with our being-in-the-world as embodied forms of light intersecting and coming into our light, metaphorically and evolutionary. We are becoming more god like and divine as we move towards the light of our divinity, a level of connectedness, the oneness of all, attending to the implicate spiritual unfolding and evolving (Watson, 1999, p. 271).*

It is thought that revolutions in knowledge development occur periodically because existing paradigms are found to be inadequate or incomplete, which may be why neomodernism has emerged. Many postmodernists are pessimistic that research and theory testing in their conventional senses are meaningful activities. In contrast, neomodernists are optimistic about the ability of scholars and scientists to help improve society, but keep the skeptical attitudes inherent in postmodernism. Whall and Hicks (2002) note that there seems to be a lack of interest in the United States in neomodernism compared to other countries. "The reasons for this difference are not clear but may represent a view in the US that the paradigm shift does not exist or is unimportant" (p. 72). Nonetheless, a number of writers have seen neomodernism as offering nurses important tools for dealing with the uncertainties and challenges in applying evidence-based practice (an idea you will return to later in this chapter) in their work (Whall, Sinclair, & Parahoo, 2006).

Modernism and postmodernism have had and continue to have a tremendous impact on nursing research, and the potential impact of neomodernism remains to be seen. Table 9.1 provides an overview of these philosophies and their associated research methods.

Introduction to Research

Perhaps your first contact with the word research was in elementary school when you went to the library to "research" a topic for a school project by consulting books and encyclopedias; however, the word research also means discovering new information that may not have been written about.

Table 9.1	Relationship Between Major Knowledge Development Philosophies and Major Research Methodologies	
Philosophy	**Focus**	**Research Methodology**
Modernism	Logical positivism/Empiricism	Quantitative
Postmodernism	Examination of phenomena as they occur in the world	Qualitative and other non-quantitative methodologies
Neomodernism	Futuristic existentialism	Undiscovered methods

This type of research is referred to as **primary research** and is highly valued worldwide because of its potential benefits to society. In conducting primary research, important variables and relationships are discovered that may help you answer questions, solve problems, or explore newly observed phenomena. For example, while observing interactions between patients recently diagnosed with myocardial infarction (MI) and their families, a researcher may arrive at the following question: Do MI patients who have familial support recover more quickly than those who do not? The researcher could take this question and develop a research study to determine the relationship between supportive family relationships and speed of recovery from MI. Once the research was completed, the findings might influence how nurses identify, relate, understand, explain, influence, and control concepts associated with caring for patients experiencing an MI.

A single research study never completely resolves a research question or results in the formation of established theory. Nursing practice is guided by theory that has developed from multiple original and/or replicated research studies. Refer to Figure 9.1.

There is an interesting difference in the way clinicians and researchers look at the world. Clinicians make decisions about one patient at a time and use a combination of their knowledge, skills, values, meanings, and experiences, whether supported by scientific evidence or not, to decide what is best for each patient at any given moment in time. If a patient has a good outcome and recovers, the soundness of decisions is not usually questioned. Researchers, on the other hand, generally look at patient situations differently. They look at groups of patients with the same or similar health-related conditions and try to draw conclusions about their collective experiences.

Unlike clinical decisions about a single patient, research results, especially in health care, are intended to be shared with other professionals who may interact with similar groups of patients. What also sets research apart is that it is presented using a structured process that is designed to ensure the integrity of its conclusions for outside audiences.

Although research is an essential approach for building theory, it is important to recognize that conducting research is only one way of knowing and understanding nursing and the world.

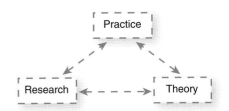

Figure 9.1 Major relationships between practice research and theory.

Experiencing the clinical world firsthand and reflecting on one's experiences in terms of what is right and good for patients and the profession are other valid ways of knowing about the world (Carper, 1978). Nurses who apply scholarly and systematic attention to phenomena of interest without using a formal research process are also making important contributions and may choose to publish their conclusions for others to consider and discuss.

The Western tradition of health care has come to emphasize scientific proof that treatments are effective for patients. In the United States and many other countries, governments and foundations provide money for researchers to develop usable clinical theory. For a variety of reasons, today, research is emphasized as an essential way health-related disciplines can justify their place in academic settings. Nursing is considered scholarly in that there is research support for what is taught in educational programs preparing its members for practice and because many faculty in schools of nursing are involved in generating new knowledge. As you continue your education, you will note that researchers are well respected in education and service. You may even choose to become a researcher who will contribute to ongoing knowledge development in nursing.

Types of Research

After deciding to conduct a study, a researcher must make many choices. One of the first choices relates to the type of research design to use. Selecting a **research design** involves determining the "best" way of exploring a particular phenomenon. As you read about research, you will note that the term **methodology** is sometimes used in place of "research design," as in the question, "What will the methodology for your study be?" Methodology is usually labeled as qualitative, quantitative, or triangulated. Triangulation research is usually a combination of quantitative and qualitative methodologies. Methodological strengths and weaknesses refer to the degree to which a particular research design or methodology helps or hinders the drawing of conclusions about a phenomenon of interest. Major research methodologies and their guidelines are discussed below.

Quantitative Research Designs

The simplest way to describe what all **quantitative research** has in common is that it measures or assigns numbers to concepts or variables and their relationships within a particular phenomenon. The goal of quantitative researchers is to identify and describe concepts or variables and their relationships within a particular phenomenon in an objective manner using **empirical** or statistical measurements. This empirical description may then lead to a better understanding of the phenomenon and how it may be influenced or controlled.

A very important idea in quantitative research is the notion of variables. As explained in Chapter 2, variables are concepts that have the ability to take on different values and either influence or be influenced by other concepts or variables. In addition, you learned about independent and dependent variables. In any research study, the **dependent variable** is the one you believe is being influenced, and the **independent variable** is the one you believe is doing the influencing. Whether a variable is dependent or independent can change from study to study. For example, a nurse researcher may study breastfeeding as a dependent variable, such as in the question: "What predicts whether a mother breastfeeds her infant or not?" It could also be an independent variable, as in the question: "Does breastfeeding predict the nature of a mother's relationship with her child?" It is important to keep the distinction between dependent and independent variables and the ability of the same concept to change position in research questions in mind as you read about the different types of research methodologies.

Experimental Designs. The most basic quantitative methodology is the **experiment.** The primary characteristic of experimental methodology is that it is tightly controlled by the researcher.

It usually involves one or more groups of subjects that receive a "test" treatment as well as a control group that does not receive a treatment. Subjects are assigned to these groups at random. Random assignment means that each subject has an equal chance of ending up in either the experimental group or the control group.

In experimental research, consistent measurements of the dependent variable are taken before and after the introduction of the independent variable(s), which helps isolate the effect or influence the independent variable(s) has on the dependent variable.

In health care, experiments where most, but not all, conditions are controlled are referred to as quasi-experimental. This methodology is most commonly used when human beings are the subjects of study because there are many aspects of humans and human behavior that cannot be controlled. Some studies using the quasi-experimental methodology are referred to as **randomized clinical trials** (RCTs). In RCTs, patients with a similar health care problem (dependent variable) are selected and randomly assigned to receive a new treatment or new medication (independent variable). Measurements of the dependent variable(s) are taken before patients are exposed to the independent variable and then are taken again after the exposure. The influence or effects of the independent variable are assigned a numerical value and analyzed statistically. Conclusions about the effectiveness of the treatment or medication are then drawn based on this analysis. For example, researchers may want to investigate the effectiveness of a new antihypertensive medication. They would solicit subjects with hypertension (dependent variable) and divide them into an experimental group and a control group. The experimental group would receive the medication (independent variable) and the control group would receive a placebo. The researcher would measure each subject's blood pressure at the beginning the study, administer the medication or placebo for a predetermined period of time, measure the blood pressure during the time the medication or placebo was being administered, and measure it again at the end of the study to see if there was a difference in the readings that could be attributed to the medication (independent variable). The researcher would then determine if this difference was statistically significant. Or, two or more antihypertensive medications could be administered at random to different groups of patients and the results compared. This is actually a more likely scenario in actual practice once at least one effective clinical approach or treatment for a condition exists. Examples of significant treatments tested in past RCTs include the use of citrus fruit to prevent scurvy in British soldiers at sea and the use of streptomycin for patients with tuberculosis (Berwick, 2003; Hart, 1999), and RCTs have become a very popular method for testing a variety of nursing interventions for patients, families and communities.

Nonexperimental/Observational Designs. Sometimes new treatments, medications, or interventions cannot be tested in RCTs without risking patient safety. Ethical concerns restrict the ability to intentionally manipulate many independent variables that influence the health and well-being of patients. Imagine, for example, the negative consequences of intentionally manipulating or causing a patient's fluid and electrolyte balance to go out of normal physiological range for the purpose of observing the effects. Because of these ethical considerations, there are limitations on how extensively experimental and quasi-experimental designs can be used in the study of human beings. Fortunately, there are nonexperimental (or observational) research designs, where the measurement of different variables can be accomplished without conditions needing to be controlled by the researcher or putting the research subjects at risk from the manipulation of conditions. Relationships between variables found when using nonexperimental designs must be interpreted differently than the results of an experimental or quasi-experimental study, and nonexperimental results are considered weaker evidence of an association between independent and dependent variables. A great deal of knowledge regarding human science has been generated using observational research studies.

Qualitative Research Design

Qualitative research involves a very different approach to collecting, analyzing, and interpreting data. Qualitative researchers believe that not all of the variables and relationships within a particular phenomenon can be measured objectively and that in order to fully understand a phenomenon they need to draw on the richness of the language, both verbal and nonverbal, and behavior people use to describe their health-related experiences. In support of this intent, people participating in qualitative research are often called participants instead of subjects. Qualitative methodologies involve using techniques such as analyzing transcripts from interviews with participants and notes made during observation of or interactions with participants to draw conclusions about a particular phenomenon. Indeed, if one had to draw a cartoon of qualitative and quantitative research, the qualitative researcher immersed in data would be surrounded by words and the quantitative researcher by numbers. Qualitative research involves setting aside many of the assumptions used in quantitative research, such as the ability to use numbers to describe relationships among concepts or variables.

There are many types of methodologies for qualitative research. Some of the most common include:

- Phenomenology: description and inductive analysis of phenomena associated with experiences
- Grounded theory: using data from experiences to formulate, test, and redevelop hypotheses until a theory emerges
- Ethnographic research: using methods from anthropology to systematically gather information about a particular culture
- Historical research: using interviews and descriptive analysis of documents to establish the details regarding events in the past
- Philosophical inquiry: systematic reflection and analytic writing on concepts, their value, and meanings in society

What all of these methods have in common is a setting aside of traditional numerical measurement in favor of a concentrated and systematic analysis of communication, ideas, and behavior to discover and interpret patterns.

Qualitative researchers have a different point of view than quantitative researchers about the role of research in constructing theory and about the use of data and data analysis techniques to establish relationships between concepts. In nursing and many other disciplines, there is professional tension between qualitative and quantitative researchers. Many observers would consider quantitative research methods to have the "home" advantage, so to speak, because of its long tradition as the primary research method in the sciences and in nursing. At one time, there were clear sides in the so-called "methods debate," with qualitative and quantitative researchers showing little interest in or respect for each other's work. Today, there is much less polarization of opinions than even a decade ago, suggesting that nurses have broadened their outlook on ways of knowing and understanding. Qualitative research methods have generated incredible enthusiasm and have unquestionably enriched nurses' understanding of patients' and families' health and health care experiences. At the heart of this renewed enthusiasm is the idea that not all phenomena are equally well suited to study using one method (Silva, 1999) and that every discipline dealing with human experience, including nursing, has **research questions** that can benefit from qualitative exploration. Furthermore, qualitative research appeals to many nurses because it offers an alternative to quantitative research approaches and creates opportunities for those lacking interest in quantitative research methods to contribute to the scientific basis of the discipline.

While qualitative researchers consider the subjectivity of human experience and of the research process as fundamental and unavoidable, qualitative research is far from a free-for-all.

Just as there are many subjective decisions in quantitative research design and analysis, there are many activities that are recognized as "best practices" in conducting and reporting qualitative research. Qualitative research studies must be undertaken with a diligent and systematic approach to yield credible results.

Critiquing qualitative research requires a slightly different set of questions than are presented in this chapter. However, good quantitative studies contain clear research questions, clear explanations of methodology, concisely presented findings, and suggestions of how the findings fit into the broader literature and relate to nursing practice.

A recurring theme in this book is that theory and research are important because they contribute to improved nursing care for patients. Interestingly, several authors (Packard & Polifroni, 1999; Polit & Beck, 2008) have pointed out that much of the ongoing debate about the preferability of qualitative or quantitative methods has resulted from nursing's continued focus on the means of doing the research instead of the results of research efforts. It has become clear that nursing must employ qualitative and other nonlinear research methods to study some of the phenomena that affect patients and practice, with some scholars even calling for nursing as a science to develop its own methodologies to deal with areas that cannot be adequately addressed within existing qualitative or quantitative approaches (Barrett, 2009; Dekeyser & Medoff-Cooper, 2009; Moccia, 1988; Phillips, 1988). Retaining an open but reflective stance to research conducted using different methods and examining the merits of each study individually is important, rather than prejudging research findings based on their qualitative or quantitative methodology.

Triangulation

Triangulation means using multiple methodologies, commonly a mix of qualitative and quantitative designs, to study the same phenomenon, with the goal of arriving at a richer, more complete picture of a phenomenon. The term triangulation is taken from a navigation technique used to locate a fixed point by knowing the distances of two related points from it and the angles involved. The idea that qualitative and quantitative methodology and the strengths of each can somehow be combined in the same study (a technique often referred to as "mixed methods") is a provocative and exciting one (Sale, Lohfeld, & Brazil, 2002). The potential advantages to blending or mixing methods involve the precision possible in quantitative work and the richness of experiences that can be captured in qualitative analyses. Many researchers find the idea of triangulation appealing, at least up to the point where they are challenged to carry out both methodologies equally well and weave the findings together into a coherent report. Some scholars believe that methodological triangulation is not advisable because qualitative and quantitative methods involve such fundamentally different assumptions about the nature of knowledge (Moccia, 1988). They suggest that triangulation of approaches across different studies, rather than within single studies, may be a more realistic approach in trying to better understand phenomena in nursing. Now that you have a clearer sense of how quantitative and qualitative researchers work and what some of the issues in research are, a closer look at the research process for quantitative studies is in order.

The Research Process

The research process is best described as the step-by-step process for designing, implementing, and disseminating findings from a research study. The process involves the identification of a research question and is followed by studying relevant literature; selecting a supporting theoretical framework; identifying variables, assumptions, and their relationships; selecting a methodology; securing funding to support the study; carrying out the study; collecting and analyzing data; and disseminating findings. Dissemination of findings allows for professional discourse or discussion about the epistemological contribution of the research and directs future studies. Future studies often examine something more specific about the relationships identified in the conclusion of the first study or may simply replicate the original study to confirm findings. The following are essential steps of the research process.

Phase I. Initiating a Research Study
Step 1. Identifying the Research Question

Identifying and articulating a research question is the most important part of the research process. Research questions, sometimes stated as propositions or hypotheses, indicate the focus of a research study and propose a relationship between independent and dependent variables. Yogi Berra has been quoted as saying, "If you don't know where you are going, you'll wind up somewhere else." So it is in research. A well-framed research question or series of questions is at the core of every sound, useful, and influential research study. Researchers who rush through this essential step often find they are left with useless data that do not assist them in producing an epistemologically significant study. The development of a research question is influenced by reading related research studies and other literature on the topic, thinking about what types of data best address the question, and reflecting on how feasible it is to collect those data. It is during this process that external variables and/or assumptions related to the research question may be identified. External variables may also be referred to as **confounding variables** because of their potential to confound, confuse, or influence the internal variables and relationships under investigation in the study. If external or confounding variables and assumptions and their potential influence on the research question are not identified early in the research process, they may cause difficulties in measuring variables, analyzing data, and drawing conclusions. While a preliminary version of a research question, external variables, and assumptions must be in place at the outset of a study, all of these elements may undergo modifications at subsequent stages in the process.

Research questions come from many sources. They may emerge from phenomena observed in nursing practice or be stimulated by other research studies or theoretical writings. They may even emerge from the observation of unique phenomena that occur without warning. For example, nurse researchers in Hong Kong and Canada sought to examine how hospital nurses addressed outbreaks of severe adult respiratory syndrome (SARS) and on very short notice developed research studies using data collected during the SARS epidemic. These researchers had selected research questions before proceeding and, therefore, were indeed following the traditional research process; however, when a research study of this type is initiated, the researchers must be very careful to ensure that their questions are carefully framed. If not, then their studies yield data that cannot be analyzed in a meaningful way or produce results that are of little interest to anyone, and the researchers' efforts are apt to be labeled "research done for its own sake."

It is important that researchers narrow their research questions, because questions that are too broad can be difficult, if not impossible, to research effectively. For example, broad questions relating to personal or professional values, such as "Are baccalaureate programs the preferred form of education for all nurses?" and "Are services provided by nurse practitioners sound and an acceptable way to provide health services?" are so complex and multilayered that they cannot be answered by one or two specific research studies. However, questions that are extrapolated from these broader issues can be addressed by individual research projects. For example, consider the recent study, "Are patient outcomes different in hospitals with different proportions of staff nurses prepared at the baccalaureate level?" (Aiken, Clarke, Cheung, Sloane, & Silber, 2003; Estabrooks, Midodzi, Cummings, Ricker, & Giovannetti, 2005; Tourangeau et al., 2007). This more narrow type of question is valuable in beginning to address a broader issue because it is focused in such a way that methods of measurement can be identified, and data can be collected and analyzed. Research questions need to be deconstructed in the postmodernistic sense, and their smaller parts identified and studied through research in order to obtain meaningful and usable results that can collectively address broader issues.

Step 2. Reviewing the Literature

The second step in phase I of the research process is the conduction of a comprehensive literature review. A **literature review** reveals what previous research studies and theoretical writings have established as reliable information about a particular phenomenon. Reviewing previously published work helps clarify relationships between concepts or variables of interest and also can give important clues about how to design a new study in terms of whom to study, what research tools to use in data collection, and which analytic methods to use. In addition, a comprehensive review of the literature may reveal gaps in understanding a particular phenomenon, which helps with selection of a research question.

You will undoubtedly conduct at least one literature review before completing your nursing education, and this is an excellent, often eye-opening way to discover the challenges of locating relevant literature and weighing evidence about the state of the science in a particular area. You will discover why, in terms of time and expertise, it is impossible for anyone to review systematically all of the research that relates to the questions within his or her practice. Fortunately, researchers and clinical scholars often conduct and publish systematic reviews of all research studies available in very specific areas, carefully and critically review them, and develop summaries of the results, highlighting what is known, the degree of certainty by which it is known, and what remains to be studied. Such reviews can be found in a variety of general or specialty peer-reviewed or refereed professional journals, or in reports prepared by or for various government agencies, such as the Agency for Healthcare Research and Quality (www.ahrq.gov), or various private foundations. They may also be found in special databases available through libraries and the World Wide Web, such as the Cochrane Collaboration (www.cochrane.org). It is rare that researchers start "from scratch" to review existing literature unless a topic is very new. However, researchers always need to seek out relevant work that authors of reviews may have failed to include for one reason or another or that was published after the review was written.

Step 3. Selecting a Theoretical Framework

Once the research question is decided and the literature review completed, it is time to move to the third step in phase I of the research process, which is to select a supporting **theoretical framework.** During this step, the researcher draws upon previously established theory and knowledge to provide structural support and beginning validity for the research study. Theoretical frameworks provide the foundation for the research process and are extremely valuable roadmaps for connecting what is known to what is hoped to be learned.

An effective framework not only guides the researcher in relating the study to what is known and has been demonstrated in the past, but also provides some insight into possible relationships among concepts or variables that can be or need to be examined in the research. As a result, frameworks help polish and refine research questions, external variables, assumptions, and methods of measurement.

Frameworks are often found in books, research articles, or theoretical writings and are frequently discovered during a comprehensive review of the literature. If an established, supporting framework is not found, then the researcher may have to develop a map or model that demonstrates the relationships. It is important to note that while many creative models and theoretical frameworks began this way, new frameworks do not have the same initial credibility as established, validated frameworks. Whether drawn from existing literature or newly generated, theoretical frameworks are essential to conducting research.

In summary, before designing a research study, there are sequential steps that must be taken, which include the identification of a research question, proposition, or hypothesis; a comprehensive review of the literature; and the selection of a supporting theoretical framework. One way of looking at this process is to view it as a journey. Research questions provide the intended destination; the review of literature serves as a travel guide—a useful, and in many ways, vital guide—to what others have experienced in similar journeys; and the theoretical framework provides the roadmap that details how to get to the destination.

Phase II. Designing the Study

After phase I of the research process is completed, the researcher must decide how to examine the relationships stated in the research question. This is referred to as designing the study or selecting the methodology for the study. It is at this point that the researcher will make decisions about the following:

- Which methodology best fits the research question
- Who or what will be studied
- What tools will be used to collect data
- When, where, and under what circumstances the data will be collected

Step 1. Selecting the Methodology

As discussed previously, the selection of the research design or methodology is dependent upon the nature of the phenomena of interest, the intent of the research question, and the characteristics of the concepts or variables and relationships involved. The methodology may be quantitative or qualitative in nature or a combination of the two.

The decision about methodology is also influenced by how similar research questions are addressed in the review of the literature, as well as the direction provided by the theoretical framework. Selection of the most appropriate methodology is essential to the conduction of a meaningful and valuable study. Regardless of which methodology is used, rigor in implementing it is essential if the study is to be useful.

Step 2. Selecting a Research Sample

The second step in phase II of the research process is to decide who the subjects or population of a particular study will be. The notion of **population** is an important one. The phrase *population of interest* or *target population* refers to the entire group of individuals to whom a researcher would like to apply research findings. For example, researchers may study a group of adolescents with anorexia nervosa in New York City and want to apply the research findings to the same population across the United States, or they may want to study the occurrence of pressure ulcers in residents of nonaccredited skilled nursing homes in one particular state and have the findings generalized across all nonaccredited skilled nursing homes in the country. In a perfect world, you could study all of the individuals in the target population that is of interest to you; however, you have no way of finding all such people, nor do you have the resources in terms of time and money to do this. Instead, you must find a representative sample of the target population with whom to work.

To increase the likelihood that research findings can be applied across an entire target population, the sample should be selected at random. This would mean selecting subjects from a target population in a manner such that any person in that population has an equal chance of being selected for the study. The researcher would then collect and analyze data and develop conclusions that would presumably apply across the entire target population. The likelihood that a sample population reflects a larger target population in the real world is called **generalizability.** You can see why selecting random samples could get extraordinarily time consuming and expensive. Nevertheless, random samples of nurses and patients in health care facilities, schools, and other settings are selected for nursing and health care research studies every day.

In many research studies, a target group easily accessed by the researcher—for instance, the patients on a particular hospital unit during a specific week or month (not selected at random from a larger population)—is chosen as the research sample. This sample is referred to as a *convenience sample*, regardless of how difficult it is to find the subjects, get their consent, or gather data on them. A major drawback in using a nonrandom or convenience sample is that its characteristics and responses may not represent the larger target population, which would decrease the generalizability of the findings.

Despite their disadvantages, convenience samples are commonly used in research because drawing random or representative samples of patients or subjects from an entire target population is often not possible for practical or financial reasons. However, when convenience samples are used, the reader must be convinced that conclusions are really generalizable to the broader population of interest.

Step 3. Selecting Measurement Tools

The third step in phase II relates to the selection of measurement tools. As discussed previously, one of the distinguishing features of quantitative research is reliance upon measurement, that is, assigning numbers as indicators of relationships among concepts or variables. Researchers use **measurement tools** to do this. The most common measurement tool with which you were familiar before studying nursing was most likely a ruler or tape measure, marked off in inches or centimeters and used for measuring length. As a nursing student, you are familiar with temperature and blood pressure measurements, intake and output measurements, oxygenation measurements, and so on. Some of the most common measurement tools in nursing research include paper-and-pencil questionnaires that measure knowledge, perceptions, and feelings about phenomena related to nursing and health. The researcher must select a method for measuring every concept and variable whose relationship is specified in a research question. This can be very challenging at times.

Researchers must ensure that each measurement tool they select possesses good **reliability** and **validity.** Reliability and validity are also called *psychometric properties* or simply psychometrics. Simply stated, a measurement tool is reliable when the results are the same or are very close to the same each time it is used to measure something. For example, using a ruler to measure a piece of wood over and over again should give you the same measurement each time.

Validity is a somewhat more complicated idea than reliability and refers to evidence indicating that a particular measurement tool is really measuring what it is intended to measure. In the case of the ruler, you might determine its validity by determining how closely the markings on the ruler correspond to measurements available from the National Institute of Standards and Technology. With regard to the validity of measurement tools used in nursing research, the researcher would determine the amount of evidence indicating that a tool actually measures the concept or variable of interest. For example, using the previous example of familial support influencing the recovery of MI patients, the researcher would need to ensure that the measurement tools actually measured familial support and not a different but related concept, such as friendship, guilt, or obligation.

Researchers often invest many years in developing reliable and valid measurement tools, because without them, it is almost impossible to support the conclusions of quantitative studies. Reliable and valid measurements are the very foundation of quantitative research. For this reason, using brand new, homemade instruments with untested reliability and validity greatly weakens the credibility of a study. Often measurement tools have been used in the past under specific circumstances, lending confidence in their reliability and validity when used in similar circumstances. For example, there may be sufficient evidence that a particular thermometer works well with outpatients in an ambulatory care setting but insufficient evidence about its effectiveness when used with hypothermic critically ill patients. There may also be sufficient evidence supporting the reliability and validity of a particular questionnaire when it is answered in a pencil-and-paper format but insufficient evidence regarding the tool when the items are read out loud to subjects.

Step 4. Location, Timing, and Circumstances of Data Collection

The fourth step in phase II begins with the question of when, where, and under what conditions subjects will be studied. Will they be approached where they normally seek health care or will they be asked to come to a different place? Will they be seen one time or will they be seen at several times over the course of the study? A closely related question involves whether or not the study exposes subjects to treatments or manipulations (independent variables) and subsequent measurements, such as in an experimental study; or whether subjects will be observed and their characteristics measured without any treatments or manipulations, such as in an **observational** study. If the subjects in the study are to undergo a new treatment or manipulation, decisions must be made about the exact nature of this manipulation, how it will be done, how the researcher will make sure it is done correctly and consistently, and what the control or comparison conditions are for the subjects.

There are other aspects of research design not discussed in this introductory chapter; however, the topics introduced here are among the most important. Once phase II has been completed, attention needs to turn toward resources needed to conduct the study, such as time, money, and access to potential sample subjects. These issues will need to be addressed before the researcher begins collecting data. Indeed, in many cases, the research team may need to outline their plan for data collection and justify their expenses before initiating the study in order to obtain financial support.

Phase III. Collecting Data

Data collection is part science, part art, and mostly hard work. When a research study enters the data collection phase or "goes into the field," subjects must be recruited and the sequence of procedures, called the study protocol, followed precisely. Unless all data needed from subjects can be gathered in one encounter, arrangements must be made to gather data on subsequent occasions, particularly if manipulations are involved and change in the subjects over time is of interest. Researchers must ensure two things about the information gathered during the data collection phase: consistency—all data must be collected from all subjects in exactly the same way or as close to the same way as possible—and completeness of the data. The number of subjects for which data are missing must be kept to an absolute minimum.

Phase IV. Data Analysis

At the heart of all quantitative studies is a desire to identify measurable relationships among concepts. In phase IV of the research process, data are analyzed to determine the existence and significance of these relationships. Data collected during this phase are assembled into what is referred to as a dataset. The techniques used to uncover patterns and relationships in a dataset are referred to as data analysis or statistics. All health professionals study statistics for at least one semester. Future researchers study statistics considerably longer. They do this for two reasons. The first is to gain a sense of how to find and express patterns in numerical data. The second is to get a sense of how statistics are used within the language and thinking of researchers to support persuasive conclusions.

Data analysis is sometimes referred to as data crunching, which is an apt metaphor in many ways for what researchers and their readers expect statistics to do. Statistics bridge the distance between research data and the questions that are of real interest to the researchers and consumers of the research. Researchers often start by reducing or distilling many individual pieces of data into smaller, and usually more meaningful, statistics in the form of graphs and tables. As their name suggests, **descriptive statistics** help paint a simplified, easily understood picture of the research data. The main forms that you will see are summary statistics, such as the mean or average, and graphs of various types. The challenges in descriptive statistical work are to present an accurate picture of data trends without misleading readers about the true patterns.

The second type of data analysis is called *statistical hypothesis testing* or **inferential statistics,** which assists researchers in answering two basic types of questions. The first is whether there is a difference between two or more groups of subjects on a certain measure or set of measures, and the second is whether there is a relationship between two or more variables among the subjects in a sample. Selecting and interpreting statistical tests can be very complex. However, simply put, statistical tests involve comparing research data against the values in mathematical models to determine whether differences or relationships among variables are larger or greater than would be expected by chance alone. The correct statistical methods for any specific study's data depend on whether or not data meet certain criteria called statistical assumptions. Some statistical assumptions relate to the study's sample, measurement tools, and measurement conditions and are predictable, while others cannot be clarified until the study is undertaken and the data actually in hand.

Because there is much to know and learn about statistical analysis, there is a certain mystery to it, especially among newcomers to research. Remember that data analysis is done to help answer research questions and is only one part of the research process. However, which research questions can be answered in a quantitative research study depends on having the right types of data and being able to apply appropriate statistical tests to them. So thinking about data analysis from the beginning of the research process is essential. While statistical analysis cannot and should not be the primary focus for the beginning researcher or research consumer, sound statistical analysis, along with reliable and valid measurement tools, are major elements that allow quantitative researchers to draw credible conclusions from their studies.

Phase V. Interpreting Research Findings

The final phase in the research process involves reporting, interpreting, and explaining results obtained in phase IV. During this phase, the researcher will often begin by summarizing the results of the data analysis. The researcher then relates the results to the research questions(s) identified in phase I as simply and directly as possible. For example, did data collected from the MI patients really support the contention that familial support was associated with recovery? The researchers then list ways their results are similar and different from those of other researchers and offer some explanations as to why results turned out the way they did. Strictly speaking, researchers do not intend to prove relationships among variables. They may believe certain relationships exist and may even hope that certain results will emerge, but ultimately, they let the data speak for themselves. When researchers do not obtain expected results or results are inconsistent with what other researchers found, there are two possibilities they must confront: Either their study design was flawed in some way, or the theoretical framework guiding the research was incorrect. After outlining and explaining the expected and unexpected findings, researchers usually end the research report with conclusions for practice and offer insights about what the next logical steps are in studying the phenomenon in future studies.

Once research findings are summarized and conclusions drawn, findings are ready to be disseminated, which is the intentional sharing of research results to other interested professionals and is the last step in the research process. How research findings enter the literature will be discussed later in the chapter, but suffice it to say the researcher attempts to convince relevant audiences that the research reveals something of meaning or use for their practice.

Phase VI. Reporting and Reading Research

Prior to reporting and disseminating their studies and conclusions, researchers revisit all of the decisions made during the research process in an attempt to ensure the integrity of the study. When researchers produce posters, paper presentations, articles, or books, they are essentially establishing a trail of information that is similar to an electrical circuit that runs from an electrical outlet to a light bulb, with the research question serving as the energy source, the steps in the research process serving as the connecting points, the researchers' writing being the wiring, and the authors' conclusions being the bulb. If there are problems with the bulb, the power source, the wiring, or the connection points within the circuit, the bulb will not light up. As mentioned before, a well-formulated research question is an essential ingredient of any study. Furthermore, if there are problems with any of the components of a study at any point in its development, its conclusions will be suspect and its contribution weak, if there is a contribution at all. Design flaws in a study are sometimes referred to as fatal flaws because they ruin any chance of drawing valid conclusions from the data. Less dramatically, just as the light from the bulb may go off and on unsteadily if there is a small problem with the wiring, if there are smaller nonfatal flaws in a study, the researchers may be able to make the connections clearer and more defensible by rewriting one or more of the sections.

Each time researchers report results, their readers must decide whether or not the researchers have conducted a sound study capable of supporting its conclusions and whether the points about connections between research questions, design, and conclusions are sufficiently answered. When there are problems, and there often are, the reader has to decide whether the flaws are fatal or not and which conclusions are actually supported by the data.

Research Discourse

Research studies begin to influence others when researchers report and disseminate the study and its conclusions. The report must be read and interpreted by peers and viewed within the context of what has been believed and written about the topic in the past. It is during this process that a research study is said to have entered into the **research discourse.** Discourse is the dialogue that goes on between the researcher and the consumers of the research, including other researchers in the field and related disciplines, practitioners, and the public over an extended period of time.

Discourse begins when researchers, following the rules of evidence, publish new studies in peer-reviewed literature. Rules of evidence include presenting sections in the report that parallel the research process. These sections include:

- Introduction: what the study is about and what the phenomenon of interest is; a review of specific research studies that have either established or raised questions about the major linkages between the concepts of interest, followed by an explicit description of relationships between them that will be tested
- Methods: how the phenomenon was explored, and, if applicable, how any tests of relationships between variables were conducted
- Results: what was observed and the statistical analyses that summarize or support findings
- Discussion: what the research findings mean in the context of previously published research and theories about the phenomenon, how the findings should be used in practice, and where research in this area should go next

This consistency of format serves a useful purpose in that it gives readers a logical, predictable, and organized outline of the researchers' thoughts and data. In particular, a detailed methods section helps the reader judge how logical the testing of the relationships among variables was.

Researchers frequently write research reports in the third person, present only the most relevant details of their studies, and lay out information about the phases and components of their studies in a consistent order in each paper. The editors of scientific journals insist authors write their studies for publication this way. They also ask other researchers and experts in a particular discipline to read and critique the research article before deciding to publish it, which is a process called **peer review**. Peer review of a research study assists editors in determining how significant and interesting the phenomenon and variables of interest are, how meaningful the testing of relationships among variables was, and whether the conclusions reached by the researchers were reasonable. In other words, journals have experts review all aspects of the research study.

One of the most important jobs of the journal editor and peer reviewers is to make sure the researchers write about the results they actually show in the article and do not go any further in drawing conclusions than the study design supports. The journal editors must also ensure that unsupported ideas or assertions be kept to an absolute minimum and, when included, are clearly identified as untested.

Whether or not conclusions of a study are reasonable is the judgment a reader must make after considering the research design, analysis, presentation and flow of findings, and conclusions the researcher has presented. As mentioned before, if any of the connections in this electrical circuit are thin or missing, the light bulb will not light up. If any of the major elements in the study are not clearly and accurately described, the conclusions the researcher hoped to make will be questioned. For example, consider the previous discussion about a relationship between familial support and recovery in MI patients (Mookadam & Arthur, 2004). Links in the chain or connection points in this particular circuit include the following:

- Which patients were studied and whether they adequately represent the target population, which influences the generalizability of the results **(sampling)**
- How familial support and patient recovery were operationally defined and measured and whether these measures made sense (key measures)
- Identification and measurement of external or confounding variables that relate to recovery, familial support, or both that could interfere with interpreting the relationships among variables, such as how serious the patient's heart attack was

- Consistency and objectivity of data collection
- Determination of the accuracy of the statistical analysis
- Results discussed in relation to strengths and limitations in sampling, measurement, completeness of controls, and overall design

Because everyone, from researchers to journal editors to readers, wants to see interesting and even dramatic research results, consumers of research must be very careful that conclusions are not based on overstating or misinterpreting the data presented. Researchers need to confine their conclusions to those based on actual data and should take care to mention any known flaws in the research design, particularly any external or confounding variables they could not or chose not to consider.

Discourse as Debate

As the term discourse might suggest, more than one researcher or group of research collaborators are usually involved in the discussion about a particular phenomenon. What happens when two or more groups reach different conclusions about a set of relationships between variables of interest? Essentially, they debate their points of disagreement, but not usually face to face, except at scientific meetings where findings are presented and discussed "live." Debate is conducted through published articles in peer-reviewed literature, relying on research data whenever possible.

One of the more dramatic and contentious discourses in nursing science involves therapeutic touch, a noninvasive healing method involving the transfer of energy from the hands of the healer to and from the patient without physical contact (Krieger, 1979). Supporters of therapeutic touch have a speculative theory about why and how therapeutic touch works and cite a body of literature suggesting that it has beneficial effects for patients (Gordon, Merenstein, D'Amico, & Hudgens, 1998; Heidt, 1981; Quinn, 1993; Turner, Clark, Gauthier, & Williams, 1998). Detractors claim that the theory behind therapeutic touch is false and that it has no real benefits (Rosa, Rosa, Sarner, & Barrett, 1998; Satel, 2000). Researchers on both sides of the debate criticize the work of the other on exactly the same elements of research design that have been discussed thus far in this chapter, including sampling of patients and nurses, measurement tools, circumstances of measurement, and connections between methods and conclusions. While both sides in this debate have claimed some degree of victory, as the literature stands, nurses and health care agencies must weigh the evidence themselves before deciding whether or not to use this technique with their patients (Tall, 2003). You might find it interesting to examine this particular body of literature.

One factor that influences the use of research in building theory is the fact that random luck or conscious or unconscious decisions on the part of researchers can push research findings in a specific direction. However, when different researchers investigate the same question by applying the same or different research designs with different groups of subjects at different times and places and find the same patterns, it is considerably more difficult to attribute the original findings to accidents, guesswork, or wishful thinking. The idea that mistaken conclusions will, over time, be fixed by other researchers conducting subsequent studies, including repeating or replicating the study as closely as possible, is referred to as the self-correcting nature of science and is very important in the ongoing development of a body of theoretical knowledge. The phrase "over time" is an important qualifier, however, because it can take many years for sound scientific data to provide authoritative answers in an ongoing scientific debate.

When reviewing the state of research literature on a specific topic, you are trying to uncover the essence of the discourse in a particular area of research and determine what the areas of agreement and disagreement between researchers are. Researchers may disagree about the conceptual definition of a phenomenon of interest and its related concepts or variables, or they may disagree about how to measure the concepts and variables. They may also have different points of view about how the phenomenon operates in the real world. Reviewing research studies can clearly be a very demanding process, but when it is done well, it reveals changes in our understanding of the phenomena over time. More importantly, it guides practice in terms of what is known with certainty, what is still under debate, and what treatments are and are not helpful to patients. When sufficient research studies have been conducted on a particular phenomenon to the point that consistent patterns in their conclusions can be identified, these conclusions form established theory. The use of established theory to improve patient care has received a great deal of attention since 1997 and is commonly referred to as **evidence-based practice.**

Replication of Research

One principle of quantitative research is that a single study may appear to find a relationship or fail to find a relationship between variables of interest not because of flaws in the methodology, but rather because the population sample was unusual or skewed. Because of this and because there are many conscious and unconscious decisions that researchers make, the results of a single study are not, strictly speaking, considered sufficient grounds for drawing final conclusions about a particular research question. Researchers and consumers of research need to see the same or similar findings in several different studies before ruling out the possibility that the findings are due to chance or the result of a specific methodological decision. In everyday life and in clinical practice, you use similar thinking. For example, you need to get to know an individual for some time and under different circumstances before feeling comfortable guessing how he or she will respond in a new situation. Similarly, you usually need to see the same or a similar phenomenon in several different patients before concluding that you have an idea worth sharing with colleagues or researchers. Subsequent research studies that use the same or closely related methodologies to verify conclusions of a previous study are called replication studies or simply, **replications.** In Western countries, much attention is given to original research that presents fresh findings that have never been shown in the literature before. Unfortunately, replication research, even if it manages to disconfirm some or all of the results of an original study, commonly receives less attention than it should.

Ethical Considerations in Nursing Research

Responsibilities of Researchers

From your first class in nursing, professional conduct has been emphasized in your education. Clinicians are guided by principles that protect patient safety and privacy, as well as patients' rights to make informed decisions about their health care. In research, as in clinical practice, there are concerns about professional ethics that relate to researchers doing the right thing for their subjects and society. Because nurses are already familiar with the need to protect patients and understand that the intent of nursing research is to improve patient care, it may not be clear why so much attention is paid to ethics in research and why so often research is delayed or derailed due to ethical concerns.

In the nurse–patient relationship, everything the nurse does is specifically intended to benefit the patient, and the patient's best interest always comes first. In research, this is not necessarily the case. Research subjects contribute time and effort and commonly agree to somewhat different health care treatments than they would normally receive. In nearly all situations, research benefits nursing's body of knowledge, future patients, and society at large, but not necessarily the subjects of the studies. Researchers benefit as well, because they are valued and respected in our society and often receive special credit for completing and reporting their work. The possibility that subjects might not benefit or might even be harmed by research they are volunteering for creates responsibilities on the part of researchers to protect subjects in clinical research and ensure that they are not inconvenienced or endangered any more than is absolutely necessary.

Some would argue that there is always a power imbalance in the subject–researcher relationship and that there is an important element of trust involved whenever research is conducted with human subjects. Even if subjects appear able to make a choice about participating in a study, researchers will often be in a real or perceived position of authority. Researchers, by virtue of their education and experience, understand more about the complexities of the study and the real benefits and risks to which subjects will be exposed. Many subjects in nursing research are also patients in the health care system and are recruited for the study during treatment, so there is an additional obligation for researchers to protect them, because they are especially vulnerable. Twentieth-century history contains many examples of how trust has been abused by researchers. Two particularly appalling incidents included Nazi experimentation on prisoners and concentration camp internees in the Second World War, and what was called the Tuskegee Study, where African Americans were purposely denied access to medical treatment for syphilis so that researchers could observe the progression of the disease (Wolinsky, 1997). Every researcher in nursing or any other discipline who works with human subjects is taught about these egregious violations of the most basic principles of research ethics so that they understand why close regulation of research is necessary.

Risks Versus Benefits

Deciding whether risks outweigh benefits is not always easy. Some feel that research is essentially harmless if it does not expose patients to medications or treatments and involves only questionnaires and measures that are not physically invasive. However, harmlessness is in the eye of the beholder. All subjects participating in studies give of their time and effort. That time can never be recovered, and therefore adequate justification should be provided for why the subjects' investments of time will be rewarded with scientific advances. Indeed, the time of subjects who are seriously ill, especially those with terminal diseases, is particularly precious and should only be taken by studies of considerable scientific merit. Furthermore, merely asking questions about private thoughts, feelings, and behaviors, especially regarding sensitive topics, may prove to be upsetting. Lastly, even if every precaution imaginable is followed, such as locked offices and filing cabinets, code numbers for participants, and so forth, there is always a risk that someone other than the researchers could access subjects' personal data or health information and then link that information back to that person. Because of the potential for such breaches of confidentiality, researchers must be very diligent in protecting the privacy of their research subjects by collecting and storing data securely.

Oversight

To protect subjects, a basic ground rule in research ethics is that all research studies need to be reviewed and overseen by qualified individuals outside the research team. Important areas reviewed by oversight personnel include who the subjects are, how they are recruited, the kinds of treatments or other conditions the subjects are exposed to, and what researchers hope to understand from the study. The basic structure and goals of the studies are also examined. Researchers must clearly show how they intend to protect subjects' rights to choose whether or not to participate and their rights to withdraw from the study at any time. In addition, researchers must be explicit about their plan to maintain confidentiality of subjects' personal data.

Researchers always have the ethical groundwork of their proposed research reviewed by others through an ethical review panel or human subjects institutional review board (HSIRB). Before a study is allowed to proceed, the HSIRB, which consists of researchers, ethicists, nurses, physicians, clergy, patients and families living with specific illnesses, and other members of the general public, come together to review formal research applications. The panel looks for evidence that whatever risks or demands subjects are exposed to are justified by the possible contributions of the research. In making their decisions, the HSIRBs debate the worthiness of studies under review, and how researchers can best reduce risk to the subjects. Without prior HSIRB approval, researchers cannot normally implement their studies. As an assurance that researchers follow through on the obligation to seek and obtain HSIRB approval, research conducted without this clearance is considered "fruit from a poisoned tree" and, if conducted, is usually not accepted for publication in scientific journals.

Informed Consent

There are many practical issues in conducting research studies that you will learn about during your coursework and through experience. One of these issues is the necessity of obtaining **informed consent,** which is the voluntary agreement of a competent individual to be a subject in a study, after he or she has reviewed all relevant information about the study. In effect, after the study has passed an HSIRB, every prospective subject is asked to evaluate the risks and benefits of participating for himself or herself. In fact, HSIRBs will usually examine all materials and informed consent forms used by the researchers.

Researchers must find a way to explain to prospective subjects in clear and concise language all of the aspects where participation will involve activities that are not usual and customary clinical treatment. The need to keep research and clinical practice separate is essential so that neither patients nor researchers become confused about the distinct purposes of the two activities. Responsible researchers actively refer patients who are their subjects to other health professionals when needs, especially potential emergencies, are identified during the course of conducting research. There are also special considerations about informed consent for those who may not be able to decide independently about participating, such as critically ill and mentally ill individuals, infants and children, prisoners, members of isolated communities, and so on.

Privacy

For many years, researchers have recognized the need to maintain anonymity of subjects. This includes taking measures to ensure that only appropriate research staff have access to subjects' personal information collected during the course of a study. With implementation in 2003 of the privacy provisions in the federal Health Insurance Portability and Accountability Act (HIPAA), there has been renewed attention to confidentiality issues in health care and in research, especially in relation to the potential harming of subjects if personal health information falls into the hands of those who have no need to know. Regulations associated with HIPAA impose heavy fines on health care professionals and institutions if confidential health information is shared inappropriately. It is not surprising that HIPAA has dramatically changed the way subjects are recruited for clinical research and how research data are handled when studies are implemented (Annas,

2003). Some researchers fear that overly rigid privacy rules or extremely literal interpretations of them may be holding up scientific progress (Ness, 2007).

Research, Reasoning, and Evidence-Based Practice

Evidence-based practice (EBP) involves putting the most reliable and valid research-based information possible into the hands of health care professionals. The process is relatively simple: Clinical decisions are made based on relevant, peer-reviewed research that has been intentionally sought out and critiqued for soundness of design, usefulness of findings, and replication (Sackett, Straus, Richardson, Rosenberg, & Haynes, 2000).

It is generally agreed that patients are entitled to nursing care that reflects the best scientific knowledge available. Yet there is significant variation in nursing and health care services across the United States and around the world. It has become clear that these variations are not always in patients' best interests. It can be very revealing to think through rationale for decisions nurses make in practice on a daily basis, especially when considering how many decisions are based on the following:

- Replicated research evidence
- Established theory that may or may not have current research support
- Speculative theory that has yet to be tested and proven reliable and valid
- Tradition that follows the idea that "it has always been done this way"

It is generally accepted that very few treatments used in health care have received rigorous research scrutiny in the form of randomized trials. While most of what is taught and practiced is based on the best theory available, sometimes established theory can be useless or harmful. Experience has shown, more often than you might think, that some long-accepted treatment approaches used with patients are ineffective or even dangerous. For example, until recently, hormone replacement therapy was thought to offer important health benefits, including protection against cardiovascular disease, for women during and after menopause; now hormone therapy is believed to increase risk of cardiovascular disease (Heiss et al., 2008; Manson et al., 2003).

Nurses should make patient care decisions based on the best evidence available. Hopefully, this is represented in established theory; however, the only way to know for sure is to delve into the research literature. Researchers try to keep up with the needs of the public and the nurses and other health care professionals who care for them. Unfortunately, the needs are great and there are insufficient numbers of researchers; this should serve as a stimulus for education and service settings to focus attention on the need for more researchers and usable research.

Nurses and others must accept that there will always be clinical decisions that are made without compelling research evidence. However, it is apparent that health professionals are not making use of the research evidence that is available. Even after researchers have conclusively established effective and noneffective ways of caring for patients, many professionals and institutions still do not utilize these research results. They rely instead on traditional yet out-of-date approaches to care (Berwick, 2003; Committee on Quality in Health Care, 2001). Given that the lives and well-being of patients are at stake and considering all of the time, money, and energy being invested in health care research, this needs to change.

The biggest challenge in evidence-based practice is deciding which research findings are reliable, valid, and useful for application in clinical practice. As previously discussed, there are differing levels of confidence in conclusions of different research studies depending on the strengths and limitations of the study. The identification of sound, relevant research occurs as researchers and consumers of research discuss papers in the surrounding discourse. Each study must stand or fall on the merits of its research design and the accuracy of its conclusions when subjected to scrutiny. Drawing accurate conclusions about what research does or does not support in terms of clinical practices requires that those involved in the discourse analyze and reflect on the entire body of literature available. The stakes are simply too high to expose patients to risks involved in applying unsound or speculative research findings. The challenge here is that to do this takes a significant amount of time, which may be part of the reason research findings are not integrated into practice in a more expeditious manner.

Systematic reviews of published findings are indispensable to practicing clinicians. A perusal of the Internet in the area of systematic reviews in health care or a visit to any health sciences library will acquaint you with the growing range of resources that now exist to help you access the most reliable and valid clinical evidence available. This distilled information is much easier and more helpful for busy practicing nurses to absorb than having to read, analyze, and critique each study individually. Staying up to date in terms of new research findings can and will be a challenge, particularly in rapidly moving areas of research, but consulting evidence-based databases that are updated on a regular basis can be an excellent strategy for offering your patients the best of what science has to offer.

Even when there is a critical mass of evidence supporting or discouraging use of a treatment, it bears mentioning that EBP is not intended to provide recipes for "one size fits all" or "cookie cutter" health care—it allows for, and even demands, health professionals consider their professional judgment, special patient circumstances, and patient and family preferences in making clinical decisions. It requires clinicians to use treatments demonstrated to be effective more often than not, and that they steer away from treatments found to be ineffective or harmful by research studies. It is also important to remember that EBP doesn't only address treatment or intervention decisions. Clinicians using the EBP framework also shape their assessments and care planning for particular patient populations to reflect what is known about the evolution of health problems and the experiences patients typically have when dealing with them.

Criterion-Based Critique for Research (C-BaCR)

While systematic reviews of literature are the best source of reviewing comprehensive summaries of research, the building block of a systematic review is the critique of individual research reports. A modified version of the C-BaC, the criterion-based critique model presented in Chapter 8, is presented here that can be used to critique individual research studies and examine factors influencing the validity of a study. Below is a summary of C-BaCR for research:

Phase I. Intent

Criterion 1: The purpose of the study is clear and understandable.

Criterion 2: Boundaries are consistent with nursing practice.

Criterion 3: Language is understandable and includes minimal jargon.

Criterion 4: Major concepts/variables are identified and operationally defined.

Criterion 5: Protection of human subjects is evident.

Phase II. Relationships

Criterion 6: Operationally defined concepts/variables form the research question.

Criterion 7: Assumptions are identifiable.

Criterion 8: Research question reflects the purpose of the study.

Criterion 9: Research design is sound and follows the Rules of Evidence.

Criterion 10: Findings and conclusions are clear and understandable.

Phase III. Usefulness

Criterion 11: Findings have the potential to help nurses understand, explain, predict, influence, or control nursing phenomena.

Phase I. Intent

Criterion 1: The Intent of the Study Is Clear and Understandable

The report of a research study, by means of its title and introduction, should rapidly and clearly inform the reader about the study's purpose. Use the following questions to evaluate criterion 1:

- What is the phenomenon being investigated?
- Is it a replication study?
- Is there sufficient evidence that this phenomenon warrants investigation?
- What was the target population and sample the researchers examined?

Criterion 2: Boundaries Are Consistent With Nursing Practice

The intent of the study should address an area of need within nursing practice as described in the discussion of boundaries of nursing practice under criterion 2 in Chapter 8. If efforts are going to be made to integrate study findings into nursing practice, it should be possible to identify the nursing care settings, recipients of care, and nursing roles for which the phenomenon being addressed has relevance. Boundaries may also be influenced by the degree to which nurses independently exercise influence or control over selected aspects of the phenomenon being addressed or the degree to which they collaborate with other health professionals. The issue of disciplinary boundaries may be viewed from a different perspective by reviewing articles published in research journals in other scientific fields. Use the following questions to evaluate criterion 2.

To which recipients of care is the study relevant? Possible ways to classify groupings include the following:

- Developmental stage (infants, children, teenagers, adults, elderly, and the dying)
- Aggregates (individuals, families, groups, and communities)
- Illness, disease, surgery, and trauma entities
- Health–wellness continuum
- Acuity of care (acute, chronic, and preventive)
- Relevant role of the nurse:
  - Care manager
  - Educator
  - Leader
  - Advocate

- Scientist
- Artist

Criterion 3: Language Is Understandable and Includes Minimal Jargon

Research studies are rarely light, entertaining reading. A certain amount of jargon is to be expected, because correct scientific or clinical terminology enables researchers to write shorter and cleaner sentences. However, operationally defining new or unusual concepts or variables and clarifying new terms is a courtesy to the reader and very important for dissemination of findings. A certain amount of research terminology to explain the type of research designs, measurement tools, and specific data analysis techniques is common, so it is important that you assimilate this language into your working vocabulary over time as you learn to read the research literature. Overall, you need to determine if the researcher's use of terminology and operational definitions helps or interferes with making sense of the research report. Additional questions to consider include the following:

- Does the researcher use terms that have a common meaning?
- Does the researcher adequately operationally define new terms, concepts, and variables?
- Does the researcher invent new terms when common terms might work as well? Does the researcher appear to invent new meanings for words?
- Does the researcher use different terms for the same concept or variable or is language throughout the study report internally consistent?
- Are abbreviations or acronyms explained the first time they are used? Do abbreviations used by the researcher make the text more difficult to read?

Criterion 4: Major Concepts/Variables Are Identified and Operationally Defined

The internal concepts or variables being investigated in a particular study will most likely be identified in the title and introduction of a study. They may be explicitly stated in the form of a research question or hypothesis or implicitly implied. It is essential that you identify the independent and dependent variables to interpret the study and its significance.

External or confounding variables and assumptions associated with the study may also be explicitly expressed or implicitly implied in the introduction as well, or they may be scattered throughout the remainder of the report. Regardless of where, how, and if external variables and assumptions are identified or implied, it is important that you try to identify them in order to determine the significance of the findings and conclusions of the study.

Each concept or variable in the study must be operationally defined in an explicitly clear manner so other researchers can select subjects, circumstances, and measurement variables in an identical or similar manner if they wanted to replicate the study. **Operational definitions** may be identified together in a separate section of the report, or they may be named alongside the conceptual framework explaining the variables and their relationships. They could also be introduced in the list of measurement tools in the methods section. The names and descriptions of measurement tools and evidence regarding their reliability and validity are helpful in determining how variables are defined and then measured using that definition. For example, consider the study about the influence of familial support on a patient's recovery from an MI. The variable of familial support could be operationally defined and measured according to criteria in the Norbeck Social Support Questionnaire (Norbeck, Lindsey, & Carrieri, 1981).

The following will help you evaluate a research study using criterion 4:

- Identify the internal variables and the relationship being explored in the study. Mark the independent variables with the letters "IV" and the dependent variables with "DV," and see if you can identify the relationship being addressed in the study.
- Identify the external variables and assumptions. Mark the external variables with an "EV" and assumptions with an "A."
- Identify the operational definition of each concept and variable.
- Determine if the operational definitions accurately define the concepts and variables being investigated.

Criterion 5: Protection of Human Subjects Is Evident

As previously discussed, protecting human subjects in research is essential. Institutions and journal editors nearly always demand proof that appropriate procedures have been followed to ensure protection of the rights of human subjects. As a result, you may be reasonably assured that research studies appearing in refereed, peer-reviewed journals meet this criterion. However, you may wish to ask these supplemental questions:

- Was a formal statement in the report made about approval of a study by an institutional review board (or similar body) and procedures that were followed for obtaining informed consent?
- Are there any aspects of the study population or the information collected that suggest that extra caution should have been exercised in protecting subjects (e.g., vulnerable populations such as minors, confused or mentally impaired patients, or prisoners)?
- Did any aspect of the procedures create possible threats to the physical or emotional well-being of the participants?
- If any of these potentially problematic ethical issues are identified, did the authors indicate how they reduced risks for subjects?

Phase II. Relationships

Criterion 6: Operationally Defined Concepts/Variables Form the Research Question

The need to be clear connections throughout research papers regarding the concepts and variables, their operational definitions, the research questions, and measurement methods. Identifying internal consistency is very important when critiquing a study. Research questions are usually located near the end of the introduction of a study, prior to the methods section, and most of the time, the independent and dependent variables are easily identifiable within the question. Operational definitions for the concepts and variables may be specifically identified in the introduction or subsumed within the general discussion about the research question. The operational definitions then must be reflected in the measurement tools used for the study. For example, in the research question "Do MI patients who have supportive families recover more quickly than those who do not?" the four variables of patient, MI, familial support, and recovery are identified, operationally defined, and then measured with tools that are based on the operational definition, such as the Norbeck Social Support Questionnaire (Norbeck et al., 1981).

Sometimes research questions or hypotheses and their concepts and variables are not specifically identified in the title or introduction of the study. These are called implicitly stated research questions and you must figure them out as you read the study. When working with implicitly stated questions, the title of the study, the introduction, and the measurement method may be used to identify the question, concepts, and variables. The following will help you evaluate a research study using criterion 6:

- Determine if the study has an explicit or implicit research question in which concepts and variables can be identified.
- Determine if each concept or variable has been operationally defined in an accurate and measurable format.
- Determine if the concepts and variables being investigated are accurately reflected in the title of the study, the research question, and the measurement tools.

Criterion 7: Assumptions Are Identifiable

Assumptions are relationships among concepts or variables that are assumed to be true, and it is these assumed truths that serve as ground rules for a research study. Quantitative researchers use several assumptions about the nature of the world, about the phenomenon they are researching, and of research itself. Specifically, they believe it is possible to measure various concepts or variables and to set up situations in research studies whereby the truth or falseness of research questions or hypotheses can be tested. The operational definitions of essential variables within specific studies are assumed to be accurate and reasonable indicators of the concepts or variables involved, and the sample of subjects chosen to participate is assumed to be representative of the larger target population. These assumptions are so basic to the research process that they are not usually mentioned in research reports.

In some studies, researchers will explicitly describe other major assumptions on which their studies are built. In other words, they will explain linkages between concepts or variables that have already been established and may be taken for granted. In the example of the hypothetical study about the influence of familial support on the recovery of MI patients, the researchers would probably make an assumption that support is a positive phenomenon that patients want to experience. Identification of assumptions is more common in longer studies, such as theses and dissertations. You may also see assumptions mentioned in the discussion section of the research report where limitations of the study are presented. It is relatively uncommon to see assumptions in most research journal articles, probably because of space limitations.

This may be the most challenging of the 11 critique criteria, because assumptions may be difficult to identify unless the researcher introduces them. However, the following will help you to evaluate a research study using criterion 7:

- Determine if the researcher identifies assumptions within the body of the study. If so, identify how these assumptions are related to the research question and research methodology. If not, look for relationships among concepts and variables on which the research question is built.
- Ask yourself, "What must be true about the concepts or variables and their relationships for this data collection to be reasonable and informative?"

Criterion 8: Research Question Reflects the Purpose of the Study

The research question and variables identified in criteria 4 and 6 should logically connect to the intent or purpose of the study as described under criterion 1. Therefore, you can address whether this criterion has been satisfied by explaining in your own words how testing the researchers' question (from criterion 6) would lead to a better understanding of the phenomenon the study aimed to investigate (in criterion 1). If a logical connection is not demonstrated, one of two things may have happened: Either the study did not measure what it was intended to measure, or in an attempt to summarize a study for publication, the authors or editors changed some aspect of the title, operational definitions, or conclusions that would have linked them together more explicitly. The following will help you evaluate a research study using criterion 8:

- Clearly identify the intent of the study.
- Identify how the research question reflects the intent of the study.

Criterion 9: Research Design Was Sound and Followed Rules of Evidence
While entire books have been written about evaluating research methodologies or designs, the focus here is on critiquing the appropriateness of the methodology selected for a reported study and how well that methodology was implemented. Use the following questions to evaluate criterion 9:

- Was the sample reasonably chosen in light of the target population?
- Do the measurement tools appear to be a reasonable way to measure the concepts or variables of interest?
- Do the authors provide references to other publications that have used the tool, which helps to establish reliability and validity of the tools? If the measurement tools appear to have been created by the researchers for use in this particular study, is there any evidence that they examined the reliability and validity, such as implementing a pilot study?
- Was the independent variable in the study an intervention or manipulation? If so, was it explicitly identified and described, along with the subjects who received it?
- Were subjects randomized?
- Was the data collection process described in sufficient detail that it could be replicated?
- Do you think the measurement(s) used were reasonable and appropriate for the design?

Until you have taken additional courses in research methods, this may also be a challenging criterion to evaluate without consulting references or obtaining assistance from a teacher or colleague who has specific education or experience in reading research; however, keep studying and critiquing, and over time, your skill will increase.

Phase III. Usefulness
Criterion 10: Findings and Conclusions Are Clear and Understandable
Research findings and conclusions in terms of differences across groups, or relationships between or among variables of interest, should be relatively easy to identify. However, unless you complete coursework in research methods or statistics, it may not be easy for you to understand exactly what the researchers present as the results of their study unless they are summarized in some way. Many, but not all, research articles will outline statistical findings both in detailed numerical and technical terms and in interpreted form. Interpreted statistics are the conclusions of the statistical analysis regarding which concepts or variables are similar, different, related, or unrelated within a study. If researchers have satisfied criterion 10, you should be able to state in your own words what the most important findings of the study were, particularly in terms of the characteristics of the subjects and the variables of interest, and in terms of differences or relationships involving the independent and dependent variable(s). The following will help you to evaluate a research study using criterion 10:

- Determine if findings are presented in technical or interpreted form. If presented in technical form, use your statistics references to help you to begin to understand what they are saying. If in interpreted form, use the interpretation to go back to the statistical data and see if you can understand how the interpretation was derived.
- Determine to what extent the findings are supporting the conclusions being drawn.

Criterion 11: Findings Have the Potential to Help Nurses Understand, Explain, Predict, Influence, or Control Nursing Phenomena

As stated at the outset of this chapter, research is useful only if it helps develop theory that assists nurses in understanding, explaining, predicting, influencing, and in some cases, controlling nursing phenomena. Here are some questions that may help you determine to what extent a study's findings and conclusions may be useful in advancing nursing practice, particularly with regard to nursing phenomena, recipients of care, and nursing roles outlined in your evaluation of criteria 1 and 2:

- Do the researchers explain ways their results are similar and different from those of previous studies?
- Do the researchers state clearly how this research contributes to an understanding of the phenomenon under investigation?
- Do the persuasive arguments made by the researcher hold up under scrutiny? Have the researchers convinced you that their findings are relevant to patients in the real world?
- To which patients could you apply the findings of this study and how would you do it?
- Do the reported results need confirmation or replication before being applied in practice?
- Assuming that the findings and conclusions are correct and confirmed in other studies, what would you do differently with patients? How do conclusions from the study differ from common practice or popular understandings of the phenomenon of interest?

Becoming a Sophisticated Consumer of Research

Reading and critiquing research studies can be a useful exercise, even if the results have not been replicated or do not lead to firm conclusions about changing interventions. Research studies raise awareness of issues and questions in practice. They help nurses broaden their thinking regarding factors influencing patients and their families. They also stimulate thinking about which traditional approaches to care might be discarded, what new uses might exist for traditional approaches, and what new approaches might be considered.

It is important to remember that clinical background and familiarity with the population under study is fundamental to being able to read and critique research intelligently. If you are well informed about patients, how their care is expected to proceed, and what their usual experiences are, you often have at least half of the knowledge required to evaluate the applicability of research findings and conclusions to your practice. Furthermore, even if the findings of a research study are difficult to apply directly in practice, it is nearly always possible to learn something either about the phenomenon of interest or how research is conducted and reported.

It is also important to maintain a healthy skepticism about research findings. Just because a research paper is published by researchers from a prestigious university or appears in a peer-reviewed or refereed journal is no guarantee that errors of various kinds have not been made, albeit inadvertently in most cases. Keep in mind that science does indeed correct itself over time. This means that in the long run, conclusions that are incorrect today are discovered and corrected by other researchers tomorrow.

One of the most important phrases to remember when reading research is "correlation is not causation." What this means is that just because two concepts or variables are associated with each other does not necessarily mean that one variable actually caused something to happen to the other. A good example of the need to heed this caution that also illustrates how research corrects itself over time appeared several years ago. A research group published a scientific paper in 1999 suggesting that keeping night-lights in the rooms of infants might cause nearsightedness (myopia) later in childhood (Quinn, Shin, Maguire, & Stone, 1999). However, a later study involved a more representative sample of children not skewed toward those referred for workup of vision problems and also examined a possible confounding variable—whether the children's parents were nearsighted. Myopic parents, the second group reasoned, might have wanted or needed a night-light to check on their children in the night. In fact, the second group's work suggested that the higher rate of nearsightedness in the children with night-lights in their rooms was due to the inherited nature of myopia, not the presence of a night-light. The use of night-lights was linked to parental nearsightedness (Zadnik et al., 2000) and researchers found no support for a causal relationship between a night-light and the development of myopia in children. Always remember the importance of considering the best interests of patients and not endangering their welfare by implementing inadequately verified research results in practice.

While a healthy skepticism is definitely advisable, it is important not to be totally dismissive or cynical about research findings either. When beginning to read research studies, many students and nurses tend to be very impressed with nearly any research article. However, once they learn the mechanics of research and all of the possible pitfalls in research design, they often become very critical and negative about every research study they read. This is not surprising, because very few studies are methodologically perfect. For reasons of time, money, and often both, researchers must often make compromises and do not recruit as many subjects or carry out as many measures or use measurement techniques of the caliber one might like to see. Researchers can also have "blind spots" about problems in their research designs that do not occur to them or others until the study is published and discourse has begun.

The dilemma for the novice research reader becomes being able to "see the forest for the trees" once she or he has learned how to critique research thoroughly. It is challenging, but essential, to learn to weigh data and identify contributions of any study that is less than ideal in one way or another. This takes time and experience, and as in the case of clinical practice, practice really does make perfect. The more research studies you read, the more comfortable it will feel and the faster you will be able to zero in on strengths, weaknesses, and valid critiques with an eye toward potentially applying their findings.

While being able to read and critique individual articles is a very valuable and rewarding skill, as discussed in the section on evidence-based practice, well-conducted literature reviews can summarize and distill "good" research and save a great deal of time. The explosion of literature in the health sciences has made it virtually impossible for nursing students and practicing nurses to keep up to date with every research article that is of potential value to their practice. More importantly, individual research studies are of less use in changing clinical practice than are trends across multiple research articles. Nurses and nursing students who are sophisticated consumers of research know that it is important to check existing databases for systematic, comprehensive reviews of similar literature to avoid reinventing the wheel when they need rapid answers about state-of-the-science research findings to drive their practice.

Summary

This chapter reviewed philosophies of theory development and how these philosophies influence the research process. Components of the research process, as they apply to quantitative research designs, were discussed in some depth. "Big picture" issues, including why participants in research need to be explicitly protected and implications for replication research, were discussed, as was the process by which individual articles become part of scholarly discourse in the community of professionals. In addition, how research "fits" with reasoning in clinical practice was analyzed, as were strategies for critiquing research for its clinical significance. The chapter also provided essential information on how students and practicing nurses can begin to critique research. Themes about the role of research in building theory in nursing were explored, as was the need for nursing practice to be based on the best evidence available at the time. Becoming a researcher or expert reader of research will take further investments of your time and energy, but hopefully your appetite to seek out opportunities to learn more about conducting, critiquing, and applying research has been stimulated.

Learning Activities

1. Using the C-BaCR worksheet located in Appendix B, critique several quantitative research studies and compare your findings with those of other students.

2. Investigate one or more resources that summarize large, yet related, research studies. When in the clinical setting, identify how research findings and conclusions are being implemented.

References

Aiken, L. H., Clarke, S. P., & Cheung, R. B., et al. (2003). Education levels of hospital nurses and surgical patient mortality. *Journal of the American Medical Association, 290*, 1617–1623.

Annas, G. J. (2003). HIPAA regulations—a new era of medical-record privacy? *New England Journal of Medicine, 348*(15), 1486–1490.

Barrett, E. A. M. (2009). What is nursing science. In P.G. Reed & N. B. C. Shearer (Eds.), *Perspectives on nursing theory* (5th ed., pp. 644–657). Philadelphia: Wolters Kluwer/Lippincott Williams & Wilkins.

Berwick, D. M. (2003). Disseminating innovations in health care. *Journal of the American Medical Association, 289*, 1969–1975.

Best, S. & Keller, D. (1991). *Postmodern theory: Critical interrogations.* New York: Guilford Press.

Britt D. (1989). *Modern Art: Impressionism to postmodernism.* London: Dhames & Hudson.

Carper, B. (1978). Fundamental patterns of knowing in nursing. *Advances in Nursing Science 1*, 13–23.

Cheek, J. (2000). *Postmodern and post structural approaches to nursing research.* Thousand Oaks, CA: Sage Publications.

Committee on Quality in Health Care, Institute of Medicine. (2001). *Crossing the quality chasm: A new health system for the 21st century.* Washington, DC: National Academy Press.

Dekeyser, F. G. & Medoff-Cooper, B. (2009). A nontheorist's perspective on nursing theory: Issues on the 1990s. In P. G. Reed & N. B. C. Shearer (Eds.), *Perspectives on nursing theory* (5th ed., pp. 59–67). Philadelphia: Wolters Kluwer/Lippincott Williams & Wilkins.

Einstein, A. (1995 [1927]). Letter to the editor of a German magazine. In A. Eddington (Ed.), *Essential Einstein* (p. 30). Rohnert Park, CA: Pomegranate Art Books.

Estabrooks, C. A., Midodzi, W. K., & Cummings, G. G., Ricker, K. L., & Giovannetti, P. (2005). The impact of hospital nursing characteristics on 30-day mortality. *Nursing Research, 54*(2), 74–84.

Gordon, A., Merenstein, J. H., D'Amico, F., & Hudgens, D. (1998). The effects of therapeutic touch on patients with osteoarthritis of the knee. *Journal of Family Practice, 47*(4), 271–277.

Hart, P. D. (1999). A change in scientific approach: From alternation to randomized allocation in clinical trials in the 1940s. *British Medical Journal, 319*, 572–573.

Heidt, P. (1981). Effect of therapeutic touch on the anxiety level of hospitalized patients. *Nursing Research, 30*(1), 32–37.

Heiss, G., Wallace, R., & Anderson, G. L., et al., for the WHI Investigators. (2008). Health risks and benefits 3 years after stopping randomized treatment with estrogen and progestin. *Journal of the American Medical Association, 299*(9), 1036–1045.

Krieger, D. (1979). *The therapeutic touch: How to use your hands to help or to heal.* New York: Prentice-Hall.

Lister, P. (1997). The art of nursing in a 'postmodern' context. *Journal of Advanced Nursing, 25*, 38–44.

Manson, J. E., Hsia, J., Johnson, K. C., Rossouw, J. E., Assaf, A. R., Lasser, N.L., et al., for the Women's Health Initiative Investigators. (2003). Estrogen plus progestin and the risk of coronary heart disease. *New England Journal of Medicine, 349*, 523–534.

Moccia, P. (1988). A critique of compromise: Beyond the methods debate. *Advances in Nursing Science, 10*, 1–9.

Mookadam, F., & Arthur, H. M. (2004). Social support and its relationship to morbidity and mortality after acute myocardial infarction. *Archives of Internal Medicine, 164*, 1514–1518.

Ness, R. B., for the Joint Policy Committee, Societies of Epidemiology. (2007). Influence of the HIPAA Privacy Rule on Health Research. *Journal of the American Medical Association, 298*(18), 2164–2170.

Norbeck, J. S., Lindsey, A. M., & Carrieri, V. L. (1981). The development of an instrument to measure social support. *Nursing Research, 30,* 264–269.

Packard, S. A., & Polifroni, E. C. (1999). *The dilemma of nursing science: Current quandaries and lack of direction.* In E. C. Polifroni & M. Welch (Eds.), *Perspectives on the philosophy of science in nursing* (pp. 498–506). Philadelphia: Lippincott Williams & Wilkins.

Phillips, J. R. (1988). Research issues: Research blenders. *Nursing Science Quarterly, 1*(1), 4–5.

Polifroni, E. C., & Welch, M. (1999). *Perspectives on Philosophy of Science in Nursing: An Historical and Contemporary Anthology.* Philadelphia: Lippincott Williams & Wilkins, p. 482.

Quinn, J. F. (1993). Psychoimmunologic effects of therapeutic touch on practitioners and recently bereaved recipients: A pilot study. *Advances in Nursing Science, 15*(4), 13–26.

Quinn, G. E., Shin, C. H., Maguire, M. G., & Stone, R. A. et al. (1999). Myopia and ambient lighting at night. *Nature, 399*, 113–114.

Reed, P. G. (2009). A treatise on nursing knowledge development for the 21st century: Beyond postmodernism. In P. G. Reed & N. B. Shearer (Eds.), *Perspectives on the nursing theory* (5th ed.). Philadelphia: Wolters Kluwer/Lippincott Williams & Wilkins.

Reed, P., & Shearer, N. B. C. (2009). *Perspectives on the nursing theory* (5th ed.). Philadelphia: Wolters Kluwer/Lippincott Williams & Wilkins.

Rosa, L., Rosa, E., Sarner, L., & Barrett, S. (1998). A close look at therapeutic touch. *Journal of the American Medical Association, 279*(13), 1005–1111.

Sackett, D. L., Straus, S. E., Richardson, W. S., Rosenberg, W., & Haynes, R. B. et al. (2000). *Evidence-based medicine: How to practice and teach EBM.* New York: Churchill Livingstone.

Sale, J. E. M., Lohfeld, L. H., & Brazil, K. (2002). Revisiting the quantitative debate: Implications for mixed-methods research. *Quality and Quantity, 36*(1), 43–53.

Satel, S. (2000). Nursing grudges. In S. Satel (Ed.), *How political correctness is corrupting medicine* (pp. 77–101). New York: Basic Books.

Silva, M. (1999). The state of nursing science: Reconceptualizing for the 21st century? *Nursing Science Quarterly, 12*(3), 221–226.

Tall, F. D. (2003). A close look at therapeutic touch. *Nursing Outlook, 51*(3), 126–129.

Tourangeau, A. E., Doran, D. M., & McGillis-Hall, L., et al. (2007). Impact of hospital nursing care on 30-day mortality for acute medical patients. *Journal of Advanced Nursing, 57*(1), 32–44.

Turner, J. G., Clark, A. J., Gauthier, D. K., & Williams, M. (1998). The effect of therapeutic touch on pain and anxiety in burn patients. *Journal of Advanced Nursing. 28*(1), 10–20.

Watson, J. (1999). *Postmodern nursing and beyond.* New York: Churchill Livingstone.

Whall, A. L., & Hicks, F. D. (2002). The unrecognized paradigm shift in nursing: Implications, problems, and possibilities. *Nursing Outlook, 50*(2), 72–75.

Whall, A. L., Sinclair, M., & Parahoo, K. (2006). A philosophic analysis of evidence-based nursing: Recurrent themes, metanarratives, and exemplar cases. *Nursing Outlook, 54,* 30–35.

Wolinsky, H. (1997). Steps still being taken to undo damage of "America's Nuremberg." *Annals of Internal Medicine, 127*(4), 143–144.

Zadnik, K., Jones, L. A., & Irvin, B. C., et al. (2000). Myopia and ambient nighttime lighting. *Nature, 404*(674), 143–144.

Internet Sites

www.ahrq.gov

www.cochrane.org

Theory and Practice

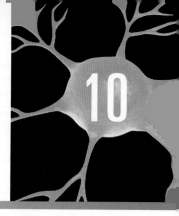

10

Intent: Observation, intuition, questioning, and comparing and contrasting are intellectual skills that help build a theory-based practice. Examples and stories illustrate how these skills are developed and used.

Key Words/Concepts		
comparing	evidence-based nursing (EBN)	purposeful observation
comparison	intuition	questioning
contrasting	intuitive observation	theory-based practice

Introduction

By now you are acquainted with theory, reasoning, knowledge, and research and have an appreciation for the role that theory has in nursing practice. You are able to implement a plan of care based on the assessment of patient needs and to evaluate the outcomes of that care. Your primary focus, the care of the patient, requires you to incorporate scholarly activities into your practice. This chapter focuses on developing purposeful and intuitive observation, questioning, and comparing and contrasting skills and sharpening decision-making skills to enable you to build a theory-based practice.

Many nurses attribute their level of practice to education and experience but are unable to justify why practice differs among nurses with similar backgrounds. They provide few answers to why some nurses advance more quickly than others. Benner, in her book *From Novice to Expert: Excellence and Power in Clinical Nursing Practice* (1984), describes five levels of nursing expertise based on a study of skill acquisition using the Dreyfus model (Dreyfus & Dreyfus, 1980). She named these levels novice, advanced beginner, competent, proficient, and expert and documented the division of practice into these levels by collecting information from practicing nurses. Currently, you are a novice, but when you become licensed, you will probably function as an advanced beginner and quickly move on to a competent level. By reading the exemplars that Benner collected from nurses practicing at these levels, you begin to see the significance of theory for nursing. Benner (2000) helped increase the understanding of how nurses achieve higher levels of practice and how education and experience guide improvement.

As you care for patients who require higher levels of care, you will depend on your intellectual skills to a greater extent. For example, nurses who care for dying patients are as concerned and passionate for their patients as nurses who care for patients who are returning to full health. You may raise questions, such as: Doesn't the patient who has the best chance of getting well deserve more care than the dying patient? If the goal of nursing is to improve someone's life, isn't caring for the dying patient acknowledging failure? You may decide to state these observations in the form of a proposition. For example, the level of care and concern the nurse demonstrates for a patient is not affected by the individual's prognosis. If you review Henderson's (1966) definition of nursing, you find that she assumes that death is a part of a person's life, not a separate entity. You then begin to understand why nurses view the dying person worthy of their attention. By comparing and contrasting the reactions of various nurses to patient situations, you can extend your knowledge about nursing practice. In another situation, you may identify the importance of goal setting in nursing practice, but not understand why goal setting is valuable. When you review King's (1981) theory of goal attainment, you begin to understand this phenomenon. In both instances, theory plays a significant part in identifying, understanding, and explaining nursing practice on a daily basis.

Skills for Building a Theory-Based Nursing Practice

As you build a practice based on theory and clinical knowledge, you benefit from developing intellectual skills, such as observation, intuition, questioning, comparing, and contrasting. Using these skills in nursing helps you make positive changes in your practice. These skills are not new to you; however, in the future you may use them in expanded ways that differ from how you used them in the past.

Observation: Purposeful and Intuitive

Early in your nursing studies, you learned the importance of observation. Now you must learn how to make critical observations for nursing practice. Initially you developed observational skills to assist in assessing patient needs and patient care responses. Using the nursing process and health assessment guidelines, you are able to develop an organized approach for observing and recording data. When you gain the ability to observe and provide care simultaneously, you are able to resolve problems that you initially found difficult. Observation skills will always be important in your practice, but you need to expand them as you build a theory-based practice. There are two types of observation: purposeful and intuitive.

Purposeful Observation

Purposeful observation is the intent to collect information about patients and their symptoms, nursing care, and nursing outcomes. Your observations about a patient are useful in your plan of care, and they add to your knowledge and understanding of nursing more broadly. Purposeful observation requires you to adopt strategies that enable you to collect and organize data about patient needs, nursing interventions, patient responses, and outcomes of care.

Developing Purposeful Observation Skills. Think about when you learned to play tennis, golf, or a similar sport. The first time you held a racket or club in your hands, you were probably concerned about holding it correctly, swinging it properly, and connecting with the tennis or golf ball. As you practiced, you may have observed the relationship between how you struck the ball and the direction, height, and distance the ball traveled. You purposefully observed your position, movement, and aim with a goal of improving your game.

Now think about your first patient assignment. You had little or no professional experience on which to base your observations, questions, or actions. When a patient asked about a medication or diet, you had to rely on your instructor or another nurse for the answer. By discussing questions with your instructor and thinking about various incidents, you built a framework of knowledge on which to care for future patients. Nursing Story 10.1 describes an experience of a nursing student's first encounter with a patient.

NURSING STORY 10.1

A Student's First Patient

Melissa Brown, a new nursing student, is assigned to Harriet Gibson, a 70-year-old woman with a serious burn on her right arm. This is the first clinical contact Ms. Brown has had with a patient. As soon as preconference is over, Ms. Brown enters the patient's room and notices Mrs. Gibson's breakfast tray on the over-bed table.

Ms. Brown: Good morning, Mrs. Gibson. I am Ms. Brown, your . . . ah . . . nurse today. I'll let you eat first and come back later.

Mrs. Gibson: If you have a minute, Ms. Brown, I could use some help. The doctor just changed this bandage and my arm is pretty sore right now.

Ms. Brown: Oh, I didn't know. Of course I'll help you. You probably need the head of your bed elevated.

Mrs. Gibson: That would be good, and I need that pillow over there under my arm. [Ms. Brown elevates the bed, positions the pillow under Mrs. Gibson's right arm, moves the tray table in front of Mrs. Gibson, and uncovers the food.]

Ms. Brown: Let's see what you have to eat this morning—orange juice, a poached egg, toast, and some coffee. Where would you like to begin?

Mrs. Gibson: Could you please help me brush my teeth and wash my hands and face before I eat?

Ms. Brown remembered a discussion about feeding patients in preconference and now she wished she had listened more carefully. She did not realize how important the discussion was at the time and, besides, she was nervous. She did not know what to say to Mrs. Gibson, and she wanted to do the right thing. Because Ms. Brown is a novice with no prior experience on which to base her actions, she will need assistance. As she thinks back on the experience, however, Ms. Brown, a bright, enthusiastic student, decides she learned a great deal more from Mrs. Gibson than just helping her to eat.

What are three things Ms. Brown might have learned from this episode? First, she learned to ask patients about their pain, not just assume they would tell her if they were uncomfortable. Second, she learned that eating in bed with one arm immobilized is difficult and that assistance in getting prepared to eat may be essential. Third, she learned to focus on the patient's needs rather than her own needs. These three things constitute a significant learning opportunity for Ms. Brown in her first patient encounter and provide a simple example of how much you can learn from one patient when you purposely use your observation skills.

Purposeful observation is important, but how you use the observations when you revisit situations not only improves your observation skills, but also focuses on improving your responses to patient needs. Although the skills required for nursing, tennis, and golf are very different, mentally reviewing your experience in each will aid in improving them.

Using Purposeful Observation. Using basic assessment theory and skills, Ms. Brown realized that Mrs. Gibson would need assistance in carrying out activities of daily living, such as bathing, eating, and moving into a comfortable position. In this, her first patient exposure, Ms. Brown, with help from her instructor, became aware that Mrs. Gibson wanted to become independent. To achieve this goal, Mrs. Gibson needed to care for herself as much as possible. Remember, in Orem's theory of self-care deficit, the nurse's role is to assist the individual to achieve self-care, but to also provide care until the patient is able and willing to do so. When Mrs. Gibson requested assistance, Ms. Brown was able to provide the care. She focused on immediate tasks, not on Mrs. Gibson's ability to improve. If Ms. Brown discusses her experiences in postconference, the instructor may point out theoretical elements between the nurse's provision for Mrs. Gibson's needs as well as designing a plan for self-care. Ms. Brown was able to make these observations with assistance from her instructor.

Intuition

Not all observation is purposeful or directed by what you see, hear, or feel. At times, you know something without consciously being aware of what or how it was observed. We call this **intuition.** Silva (1977) cautioned nurses "to value intuition and introspection as much as those [observations] arrived at by scientific experimentation" (p. 62).

A mother may check on her toddlers who are playing in another room, for example, even though the children have not called her attention to their activities. When she goes to check on them she finds them removing books from a bookshelf or emptying a desk drawer. The mother reports, "I just had a feeling they were up to something." She might add, "Maybe they were just too quiet, or maybe it was a mother's intuition."

Similar circumstances occur in nursing. Expert and proficient nurses report that they return to check a patient at times, not because they observed a change in the person's condition, but because they felt it was important to do so. Benner (1984) discusses these situations at length using labels such as *early detection, early warning systems, specialized knowledge, subtle changes, anticipation of deterioration,* and *future think.* These labels confirm that nurses, using their knowledge and experience, are programmed to be alert to what is different from what is expected.

More recently, Ruth-Sahd (2003) included intuition as one of the critical ways of knowing. She sees intuition as having a place at all levels of nursing education, starting with initial assessment courses. According to Moch (1990), intuition, one of the components of personal knowledge, is essential to the development of nursing knowledge. In 1978, Carper identified patterns of knowing within nursing knowledge that are unique to the discipline of nursing. While it is likely that intuitive knowing is an advanced form of patterning, at this time, scientific investigation has not revealed how it occurs.

Highly proficient and expert nurses experience clues and feelings they are unable to explain or attribute to observable patient behavior. From past experiences, they know it is important to act on these clues. Nursing Story 10.2 describes such an instance. Expert nurses say that when things do not look or feel right or when a patient's response does not fit the pattern they usually see, they take another look, literally and figuratively. After several years of practice, expert maternity nurses are aware when patients are about to deliver, even before verifying those feelings with an examination. Expert critical care and emergency room nurses respond to specific situations before diagnoses are made or confirmed, even before they know the patient. Experienced nurse

---

NURSING STORY 10.2

Using Intuitive Skills

Anne Collins, MSN, RN, an expert nurse on the surgical unit in an academic health center, describes a time when she acted on intuition:

"As soon as report is over, I visit every postsurgical patient on my unit. Then I return to the workstation to organize my evening schedule. Last Thursday, about 5 minutes after returning to the station, I had this feeling that I needed to check Dolores Hector again. She had undergone radical breast surgery early in the day and had progressed so well that she returned to the unit from the recovery room early. When I visited Ms. Hector shortly after 4:00 PM, everything seemed normal. Her vital signs, the surgical dressing, everything about her was just fine, or so I thought. I finished my rounds and started my evening planning. Now I knew I had to return to her bedside and look again.

When I returned to Ms. Hector's room, she still seemed okay, but I decided to check her dressing. I saw blood just starting to break through the surface of the dressing. Of course, I applied additional dressings and pressure to the site and called the surgical resident. Ms. Hector is doing fine now.

Later that evening when things quieted down, I thought about the episode. I wondered why I had this feeling something was wrong when nothing seemed out of the ordinary during my first visit. Maybe I noticed a restless movement, maybe her color wasn't just right, maybe she talked a little more than usual. I have worked on this unit for so long, I seem to have a second sense about patients. I have learned to rely on my feelings, like I did with Ms. Hector, not just my overt observations of dressings, skin color, and vital signs.

I don't recall experiencing such feelings when I first was assigned here. And I don't remember the first time I returned to check a patient without objective data. Now I know how important it is to act on these early warnings. I hate to think what might have happened to Ms. Hector if I had not checked her again last Thursday."

practitioners are able to focus quickly on the most relevant symptoms of an ill child brought to the community health clinic before conducting a complete history and physical examination.

Developing Intuitive Skills. As you observe how patients react to symptoms, illness, surgery, and medication, you build patterns of recognition that help you care for other, similar patients. Developing intuition, or advanced patterns of recognition, cannot be rushed, although there are actions you can use to sharpen your intuitive skills (Correnti, 1992). As you increase your direct contact and experience with patients and listen to their descriptions of illnesses, health problems, and goals, you will enhance your ability to make **intuitive observations.** Developing caring relationships with patients, keeping journals about your practice, and reviewing those journals periodically are strategies that also enhance your skills.

Describing your experiences with patients in the form of stories rather than clinical reports or cases allows you to identify caring relationships between the patient and nurse. When you tell a story, you select information that provides insight into the lived experiences of the patient and nurse. When you present a clinical report, you depend on objective documentation. When you have a particularly exceptional patient experience and you want to share it with your colleagues, write a story and read it to them. The discussion that follows your storytelling will focus on relationships between you and your patient, as well as the diagnosis, treatment, and prognosis of the patient.

Telling a story is more difficult than reporting a clinical episode. Stories about your patients are really stories about your nursing practice. You learn different things from clinical reports than you do from stories. Health care tends to emphasize objectivity, but being aware of relationships, feelings, and caring allows you to recognize the benefits of your subjectivity as well. There are many stories in this book. Some include clinical or objective information, but all focus on building a theory-based practice.

Using Intuitive Skills. After reviewing several stories in the nursing literature, a group of students wrote a clinical-based report about a patient of one of the students. The students discussed the differences between clinical reports and stories and revised the report as seen in Nursing Story 10.3.

How does this short story help you as a student? What would you and other nurses learn by hearing and discussing the story? Although knowing about chemotherapy and its side effects is very important for both the nurse and the patient, the story illustrates the control Ms. Smith can exert over her response to chemotherapy. The nurse also becomes aware of the role that family members play in the patient's progress. This is powerful information that is important for you as a nurse to know. If Jane Dickson had not commented about Ms. Smith's attitude and offered her a chance to talk about it, she would have lost an opportunity to build on her prior experience with patients in chemotherapy. She may change her approach to patients as they begin their therapy. Suppose Ms. Dickson had never talked to a patient with a similar experience. She is now encouraged to elicit information from future patients. She may determine the frequency of such coping mechanisms and begin to differentiate characteristics of patients who cope from those who do not. Ms. Dickson may note that some patients have close family ties and supportive friends and others do not. Some individuals thrive on challenges; others turn toward the basics.

When nurses hear a story, they may change their focus from a rigid clinical view of patients in chemotherapy to the role the patient plays. A number of nursing theories and research studies speak to nurse–patient relationships (Peplau, 1952), the role of the family (Orem, 1991), caring (Benner & Wrubel, 1989; Leininger, 1988; Watson, 1985), and research (Baumann, 1996; Ducharme, Ricard, Duquette, Lavesque, & Lachance, 1998; Hagerty & Patusky, 2003). It is helpful for Ms. Dickson and for you to relate these experiences to theoretical concepts and propositions.

NURSING STORY 10.3

Ms. Smith's Attitude

Sally Smith, the mother of three adult children, has been married for 28 years. When she was diagnosed with breast cancer and scheduled for chemotherapy, she tried to remain strong. Family and friends told her that chemotherapy was devastating and that she would be very ill after each and every treatment. Ms. Smith decided to go ahead with the treatments despite what she had heard. Jane Dickson, BSN, RN, was the outpatient nurse the day Ms. Smith received her final chemotherapy treatment.

> *Ms. Dickson:* You have such a great attitude, Ms. Smith. I am sure it has been helpful to you and your family during your chemotherapy.
>
> *Ms. Smith:* Thank you, Ms. Dickson, but when I started my treatments, my attitude wasn't very good. After the first treatment, I just fell apart.
>
> *Ms. Dickson:* Fell apart?
>
> *Ms. Smith:* At first, I did not want to believe that chemotherapy would make me sick. But so many people told me how sick I would be, I must have believed them anyway. Within hours after my first treatment, I was so dehydrated, I had to be admitted to the hospital. I was devastated. I didn't know how I would ever make it through the next 6 months. During those 2 days in the hospital, I decided I would not allow myself to become that sick again despite what others told me. I needed to be strong for my family, and I needed to get my life back. I didn't tell anyone about my decision, but I promised myself I would stay well.
>
> *Ms. Dickson:* That must have been very difficult keeping that promise without telling your family.
>
> *Ms. Smith:* I finally did tell my husband about my decision, and he helped by being very positive and supportive. But, after that first treatment, I never did get sick again. Oh, I felt a little tired the day after the chemotherapy, but I was back to my routine by evening. I am thankful it is over, but now I know I can make it. And, I am going to beat the cancer, too.

Being aware of patterns of recognition or intuition in your experience may seem too far in the future at this time. However, the tools discussed above allow even novice and advanced beginner nurses to make more effective use of their experience than viewing each patient as a completely new entity. Focus on the opportunities each experience provides to strengthen your intellectual skills, such as reasoning, decision making, judgment, negotiation, and assessment.

During the past several decades, the nursing process, nursing care maps, nursing diagnoses, critical pathways, and other standardized learning tools have been used to organize nursing practice. Although these tools assist you to learn basic practice techniques, they may interfere with developing an openness to learn from experiences with patients and your ability to reason critically and independently. As you move to competent, proficient, and expert levels of nursing practice, you will depend less on the prescribed, linear tools you use as a student and focus more on the intellectual skills discussed here. These skills will help you to interpret both concrete and abstract information and make better use of both purposeful and intuitive observational skills.

Questioning

In Chapter 4, you read that Socrates taught his students by asking questions focusing on who, what, where, why, how, and what if. Now it is your turn to ask questions and to respond to questions that others ask you.

As the complexity of patient care increases, you will ask and respond to more questions. Even when you ask appropriate questions, you may be at a disadvantage if you do not trust your judgment to use the knowledge effectively. Suppose you have a power outage at your home. Your neighbors still have power, and all the circuits in your house are functioning properly. At this point, you have reached the limits of your knowledge about electricity and call the power company or an electrician. When the electrician arrives, you may lack the knowledge to discuss the situation. You simply ask him or her to fix the problem. You may discuss the problem later, so you will be able to identify the problem if it happens again.

When you study nursing, you might encounter a similar situation. You know how to identify the patient's room and something about the patient's health problems, and you are probably acquainted with some equipment in the room. If the patient asks you questions, you may have difficulty answering without consulting the instructor or another nurse. Whether you are learning about electricity or nursing, adding to your knowledge or focusing on new problems in light of prior experience will increase your ability to ask and answer questions.

Developing Questioning Skills

You probably are proficient in basic **questioning** but interested in expanding the scope of the questions you ask. When you study, think about questions related to the content. In class, listen to questions that your professors ask. While you are thinking about an answer, try to classify the type of information being requested. As indicated above, the first word in a question is your clue. For example, *What* is the pancreas? *Where* is it located? *What* substance does it secrete? When you hear questions that ask "what" and "where," think of related ones starting with "how," "why," and "what if." Beginning questions with how, why, and what if indicates that you are moving to a higher level. *Why* do people get diabetes? *How* does insulin control diabetes? *What happens if* a patient forgets to take insulin? You may not be able to answer every one of these questions, but you are preparing yourself to expand your scope of questioning.

When you are in the hospital, clinic, health department, or other clinical site, listen to conversations among nurses and between nurses, physicians, and other health professionals about patient care. At first the conversations may be confusing, but try to differentiate between *what* and *when* questions and the *why, how,* and *what if* questions. Discuss some of these questions in preconference and postconference, especially when they relate to patients you have cared for. When you have questions, your professor may suggest that you look for answers, while at other times, you may decide to investigate the questions before bringing them to class or conference. These are strategies that you need in practice.

If every health care question had one answer, computers and robots could make diagnoses and dispense medicines. Because that is not the case, health care professionals are expected to be able to explain how and why individuals respond in different ways to illness, treatments, and medications. Patients depend on nurses to discuss options that are available for dealing with specific situations. That does not mean that there is a definitive answer for every question the patient asks. For example, if parents ask you what the physician will do if their child is unable to retain food, it is helpful to know some of the options, even if you are not aware which one the physician might use. Over time, you will build a knowledge base for responding to such questions.

Participating in a debate about health care issues is helpful in developing questioning skills. Debates focus on unresolved issues when there are two or more viewpoints. Many ethical issues in health care are debated, such as abortion, assisted suicide, selecting recipients for organ transplant, and using embryonic tissue in research. Approaches to patient care can also be the basis for a debate. In Nursing Story 10.2, Anne Collins, an expert surgical nurse, attributes her return to check the postoperative condition of Ms. Hector to a "second sense" or intuition. Some nurses view intuition as mystical or unscientific and do not believe it should play a part in nursing. A nurse who debates the pro side of the issue—*Intuition plays an essential role in the level of practice of the expert nurse*—has an opportunity to formulate and explore many questions, such as: What scientific evidence validates intuition as a tool of the expert nurse? How do nurses develop intuition? What happens if a nurse misses a clue? How can intuition and scientific assessment be used together? The debater will find support from Benner (1984), whereas the opposition might look to Roy (1970) or Orem (1991).

As you prepare for a debate, examine both sides, not just the one you are arguing. Your position will be stronger if you can identify potential positions of your opponent. You can do this by posing questions that are logical and illogical, as well as viewpoints that are sensible and absurd. Even when there is no formal debate, speak up and be able to support your views, especially when they differ from those of others in the group. You can prepare yourself more effectively by posing questions about both sides and then seeking alternative responses. Nurses as a group tend to think along similar lines. As a student in a college or university, you have opportunities to enroll in a variety of courses and seek out students from other majors who hold opinions in opposition to yours. When you find individuals with different opinions, initiating discussions with them will stimulate you to broaden your questioning skills.

Using Questioning Skills

As you develop your questioning ability, you may wonder how this relates to building a theory-based practice. When you face routines, procedures, and structured plans, you are forced to think by habit. To overcome this passive approach to patient care, you need to make different choices by thinking about how theory, research outcomes, and scientific knowledge are related to practice. You may seek information about new interventions to improve your practice. When you are dissatisfied with the status quo, you may capitalize on it by striving for a higher level of practice. You may also purposely focus on theoretical concepts and propositions and relate them to your practice. As your theoretical knowledge base increases, your practice will provide better illustrations of the concepts and propositions you have learned.

Novices and advanced beginners strive to provide safe, error-free nursing care that meets basic needs. As your knowledge expands and your skills improve, you begin to question some of the things you encounter. For example, you may ask yourself: Why didn't Mr. Wilson have better results from his surgery? What can I do to comfort 3-year-old Mitzi when her parents leave in the evening? How can I develop a better relationship with Mr. Gardner, who is so depressed about physical therapy? What would experienced nurses do in these situations? In the process of considering these questions, ideas about theoretical sources that were not available to you before you studied theory will arise. For example, how would Benner and Wrubel's *primacy of caring* help you understand Mr. Wilson's delayed recuperation? Does the stress he is experiencing interfere with his coping? What clues can you get from Watson's *theory of human caring* that might help you comfort Mitzi? Would Peplau's *theory of interpersonal relationships* help you relate to Mr. Gardner during his depression?

Typically, nursing students are unhappy when they earn a course grade of B or C after they have studied hard to achieve at a higher level. Most practicing nurses are also unhappy when patients do not respond to the care they give when they believe they have given the best care possible. You may need to study and think differently to achieve a higher grade, and the practicing nurse may need to seek new intellectual tools to achieve a higher level of care. Although theoretical ideas are somewhat obscure and abstract for use with daily problems, they may help guide your search for ideas from clinical laboratories, research reports, and conferences with more experienced nurses.

Proficient and expert nurses not only know what questions to ask and symptoms to check, but are also confident in their decisions. Their knowledge and confidence developed over time, along with their experience and their ability to integrate new ideas and theoretical concepts into nursing practice. Responding to difficult questions and being confident of your knowledge increase your ability to deal with new situations and your efforts to improve.

Comparing and Contrasting

You were familiar with observation and questioning before entering the nursing major. Comparing and contrasting are intellectual skills that may be new to you. **Comparing** is the identification of common features of two or more entities, while **contrasting** is the identification of differences between these entities. The concept of **comparison** includes both comparing and contrasting. You have probably heard people say, "You cannot compare apples and oranges." Apples and oranges have many common features; for example, they are both fruits, have an outer covering and seeds, and grow on trees. They also have significant differences, including the type of covering, the location of the seeds, the texture of the fruit, and the taste. An orange is a citrus fruit from the rue family, whereas an apple is from the rose family. Both are sources of vitamin C, although the orange has a richer supply. Therefore, you can compare apples and oranges, and you can also contrast them.

How do you use compare and contrast in nursing practice? You use observation skills to compare or contrast two or more patients, their symptoms, and their responses to care. You use your reasoning skills to compare and contrast experiences with different theoretical options.

Developing Comparing and Contrasting Skills

Thinking about apples and oranges and how they are similar and different has already given you an opportunity to develop some new skills. You use observation skills to make comparisons and examine both common and uncommon features. Just as you developed a mechanism or plan to make purposeful observations, you need to plan to make purposeful comparisons. Initially, your attention to these comparisons will be during postconference discussions, when you think about your experiences at the end of the day, and when you recognize the similarity between current patients and those you have cared for in the past.

The development of comparing and contrasting skills will be more difficult than developing the skills of observation and questioning. As you build observation and questioning skills, you will recognize improvements in making comparisons. Finding time to study and think about comparisons is critical in developing these skills. Formulate personal exercises and questions that focus on comparing and contrasting two patient experiences or a patient experience and a specific theory. When you arrive at conclusions concerning these exercises, you may want to discuss them in class or conference.

Using Comparing and Contrasting Skills

You can become quite adept at identifying and using theory in clinical situations. For example, a student who was concerned that patients and families had difficulty coping with the news of eminent death contrasted the views of Henderson and Johnson. The student described Henderson's nurse as one who encourages the patient to be as independent as possible and invites the patient to communicate emotions, fears, and concerns. Johnson's nurse stays with the patient during this time and teaches the patient and family members about the psychology and physiology of death and dying (Henderson, 1966). On the other hand, Johnson takes a more impersonal stance and divides care into psychological care, physiological care, and care after death. The nurse is still a listener but is not responsible for teaching about death and dying (Johnson, 1980). The student concluded that Henderson's nurse supplements the patient's need for independence and knowledge but recognizes the need for continual attention. In Johnson's theory of behavioral systems, the nurse regulates the patient's behavior, providing comfort and support, but without the personal attention Henderson's nurse gives. Although these conclusions may seem simple, they illustrate that the student gave considerable thought to the phenomenon and how it might affect her practice in the future. The student's view is more consistent with Henderson's definition. As the student expands her knowledge about the definition and the care of a dying patient, she will be preparing for future theory-based practice.

Another student explored the phenomenon that patients in intensive care units are less likely to develop complications or die when nurses are assigned to only one or two patients. The student compared Orem's *theory of self-care deficit* with Neuman's *systems model* and arrived at some interesting observations. Orem's theory is appropriate for a patient in the intensive care unit who is unable to exercise self-care or meet few, if any, basic needs. The student recognized this and based the argument on that issue. The nurse who has to meet the demands of the dependent patient will need adequate time to do so and, therefore, should care for only one or two patients at a time. When a patient's demands are not met, his or her health status may suffer (Orem, 1991).

In Neuman's *systems model* (1995), the nurse's role is to assist the patient to adapt to and reduce stressors. On Neuman's wellness–illness continuum, the patient in intensive care would be at the illness extreme and is likely to need time-consuming nursing interventions. The patient who continues to experience stress is unable to move toward wellness and is more apt to face complications. Contrasting the theories of Orem and Neuman illustrates that the difference is in goal achievement, not necessarily outcomes. Hindsight like this helps you recognize the value of theory. Looking closely at your practice helps you modify your intellectual approach to resolving nursing care problems and dilemmas. As you gain experience, comparing your practice to what you know about theory sharpens your interest and ability to move beyond traditional policies, procedures, and routines.

These two examples of identifying phenomena and comparing and contrasting theoretical positions illustrate how to use theory in nursing practice. By comparing and contrasting theories related to phenomena you observe in your clinical experience, you also gain insights about practice.

Integrating Research Outcomes Into Nursing Practice

The goal of developing skills of purposeful and intuitive observation, questioning, and comparing and contrasting is to change your practice from one of routine procedures to one that emphasizes the best that we know about nursing and that is theory based. You may wish to review what you learned about reasoning in Chapter 4 as you study these strategies.

As a student, you expect to build knowledge, skills, values, meanings, and experiences related to nursing practice. This is accomplished in class and through clinical knowledge, from reading textbooks and journals, and by listening to and observing your professors and other nurses. You depend on these sources and expect the information to be accurate and relevant. At times, you hear or read about research breakthroughs in the mass media. When you hear about these discoveries in nursing and health care, you need to verify and judge the usefulness of the information and determine whether they can be incorporated into your practice. We will explore each of these areas as well as evidence-based nursing in this section.

Verification of Information

Whether you can verify health information you hear or read about in the media depends, in part, on the source. Frequently, radio and television commentators announce breakthroughs in health care and attribute their information to a scientific journal, such as the *Journal of the American Medical Association* (JAMA) or the *New England Journal of Medicine* (NEJM). Peer-reviewed journals such as these are highly regarded by health care professionals as well as by the public; therefore, you assume that the research outcomes being reported have high degrees of reliability and validity. When you hear a report that is of special interest to you, however, you may wish to note the name of the journal and the date of publication. By obtaining a copy of the journal, you can assess whether the information the media provided is consistent with the scientific information provided to the medical community. Television news commentators and newspaper columnists frequently focus on details of a study that capture the attention of the audience, not necessarily what is most pertinent to health care professionals. As a professional, you are responsible for verifying the information before adopting it. Remember that reliability and validity of research depend on replication of the study and demonstrating the same or similar outcomes over time. When the outcomes of subsequent research do not support the initial tests, action must be taken. For example, when the weight reduction drug fenfluramine hydrochloride (Fen Phen) was introduced, millions of people used the drug. Within several months of being released, however, the Food and Drug Administration pulled it from the market, because new data showed it was harmful to cardiac muscle (www.rec-law.com/fen-phen/legalinfo.htm, 2002).

One way to verify research outcomes reported in an article is to determine whether it was published in a peer-reviewed journal. Peer-reviewed journals only publish articles that have been reviewed and recommended for publication by two or more anonymous peers of the author who are experts in the field. Although peer review does not guarantee the results of the study, it does validate the methodology, conduct, and background of the author. Some nursing journals are peer reviewed, but many are not. You will usually be able to determine whether a journal is peer reviewed by information provided in the journal. Articles in peer-reviewed journals are generally research based, whereas articles in journals that are not peer reviewed may present the authors' opinions. All the journals mentioned in Chapter 6 are peer reviewed. Journals such as the *American Journal of Nursing, RN*, and *Nursing [Year]* are not in this category. In these journals, the editor selects articles for publication and, while these articles may include useful information, they do not meet the standard for research articles.

Reviewing the primary sources of information is also important. Rather than relying on a news commentator's interpretation of research findings, you should locate the journal and read the original article. If you are concerned about the findings in the article, examine the references listed at the end of the article. Most journals provide information about where authors can be reached. If you have questions that the article does not answer, you may wish to call or e-mail the author or write a letter to the editor of the journal. Many sources can be used to determine whether information is reliable and valid, and you need to make use of as many of these as necessary.

Scope of Information

You hear and read about numerous changes in nursing and medical practice. Some of these changes are interesting, and a few may even be useful in your practice, depending on the scope of the research. When results from a research study can be used with populations other than the ones studied, they are generalized to the new group of patients. In some research studies, it is obvious which conclusions can be used with other groups. In others, you need to compare the demographics and characteristics of the subjects in the study with your patients for similarities and differences. For example, in a report of a study of low–birth-weight, premature infants, you would need to ascertain the exact definition of low birth weight as well as prematurity to determine whether the characteristics of infants under your care are consistent with those in the study (Gennaro, Brooten, Raucoli, & Kumar, 1993). There may be other attributes to take into consideration before accepting the results as useful in your practice as well, such as birth order, the infant's gender, and age of the mother.

Gender and age limit the application of some research findings. You would not apply conclusions from a study about cardiac problems in adult males to adult females until you explored the implications of doing so. For many years, studies of cardiac problems limited participation to white males, although some reports inferred that the results could be applied universally. In 1976, a study was initiated to investigate the long-term consequences of the use of oral contraceptives. Nurses were selected for the study because they would be able to respond to technically worded questionnaires.

Approximately 122,000 nurses received questionnaires related to the use of oral contraceptives and similar health topics every 2 years. An additional 123,000 nurses were added to the study group in 1989. Two- and four-year questionnaires continue to be used, with response rates at 90% (Nurses' Health Study History, 2002). The study has stimulated the increased diversity of females and other less represented populations in research studies.

When you face problems in your practice, you cannot always wait until you hear about discoveries of new practices. Sometimes you must actively seek ideas to solve problems. Experienced nurses constantly accumulate information to help solve current and future problems. They are aware of the literature and other sources of information and assistance and are ready to determine whether a new intervention will be useful in their practice and to apply it as needed. In Nursing Story 10.4, Mavis Jones, BSN, RN, discusses a scenario in which she actively seeks new information and ideas to solve a clinical problem.

Implementation of Outcomes

The experience you gain as a student and later as a registered nurse will provide more evidence to use in your practice. Observation is a helpful tool for building a theory-based practice.

When Melissa Brown, the student discussed earlier, faced her first patient, she was so concerned about what to say and do that she was unable to observe the physical and mental state of Mrs. Gibson. Think how Melissa Brown, RN, would act in the same situation, as shown in Nursing Story 10.5.

Melissa Brown, BSN, RN, is now a graduate student and demonstrates purposeful observations from the nurse's report and patient's chart and applies them to the experiences she encounters

Actively Seeking New Information and Ideas

Mavis Jones, BSN, RN, a home health nurse with 5 years' experience, tells a story about Selma Nelson, an elderly woman who is temporarily living with one of her daughters following hip surgery:

"I've been a home health nurse for more than 5 years now, and I know how hard it is for elderly patients to exercise and learn to walk after surgery. I've always been able to convince patients and their families how important exercise is, but not the Nelsons. Let me tell you about Selma Nelson, who is 85 years old, and her two daughters, Mabel and Nancy, who live about a block from each other.

Mrs. Nelson fractured her right hip about 2 months ago. The surgery went very well, and she made excellent progress at the Uptown Rehab Center. Two weeks ago, the center held a conference with Mrs. Nelson and her daughters. The next day, Mrs. Nelson was discharged to Mabel's home. The discharge plan that was discussed at the conference included the following:

Get up and dress with minimal help every morning.

Eat all meals with the family.

Nap after lunch for an hour.

Exercise three times a day for 30 minutes.

Encourage independence.

The therapist suggested that Mrs. Nelson would be able to accomplish most of her personal needs, except for meal preparation. The therapist was scheduled to come to the house twice a week, and as soon as Mrs. Nelson met the exercise regimen, he would cut that back to once a week. Mrs. Nelson's goal was to return to her apartment as soon as possible. It just didn't work that way.

Mabel and Nancy are afraid their mother will fall again. They gave her a bell and instructed her to ring it whenever she needed anything. They feed her breakfast in bed and let her stay there most of the morning. It was unusual for her to exercise for more than 5 minutes a couple times a day. When the therapist visited yesterday, he said Mrs. Nelson had regressed at least 30% in the past 2 weeks.

I have cared for 40 or more patients with fractured hips in the past couple of years. Between her daughters and I, we should be able to solve this problem. Then I saw two former patients, Ms. Estes and Mrs. Walters, several weeks ago at the shopping center. They are doing so well. I remember them saying, if they can ever help someone, to call them. Mrs. Nelson might just be the patient who needs their encouragement to get moving—I need to arrange for them to meet with Mabel and Nancy and their mother."

NURSING STORY 10.5

Melissa Brown Revisited

From the shift report and patient's chart, Ms. Brown knew what care Mrs. Gibson would need and also that she would be discharged the following day.

While preparing Mrs. Gibson for breakfast and setting up the tray, Ms. Brown determines that the pain medication Mrs. Gibson received 2 hours earlier is still effective. Mrs. Gibson is already moving around on her own, although she needs assistance with eating and bathing.

Ms. Brown has been working on the surgical floor for 2 years and is beginning to notice that patients request pain medication more frequently when they are sitting up than they do in the reclining position. When she mentioned this to Dr. Elton, he suggested using a sling on his patients when they are up, so that the arm is more relaxed, and then removing it when the patient returns to bed. Although Mrs. Gibson was not a patient of Dr. Elton's, Ms. Brown observed and made notes about her pain complaints as well as those of other patient's with similar problems. She plans to use these data in a paper she is writing for the nursing research class she is taking at the university. Dr. Elton asked to have a copy of her paper when she completes it.

---

in nursing practice. She not only contributes to better health care, but also recognizes the benefits of thinking about patients in relation to their common problems and relating her observations to what she is learning in her graduate research class.

When you feel competent in observing patients' conditions and responses to care, you benefit from analyzing your purposeful observations and your practice. You need to examine some situations as if you have not seen them before. Sometimes, "new eyes" use other senses as well, such as hearing and feeling. Many times, people respond to the emotions and moods of the people with whom they talk. Listen to how you speak to patients. Are you monotonous, abrupt, and hurried? Are you sad, depressed, and remote? Are you concerned, interested, and pleasant? Watch your facial expression as you talk with patients. Are you serious, distracted, and bored? Or are you involved, attentive, and listening? When you teach a new diabetic patient how to inject insulin, think how you would respond to the instructions if you were the patient. Would you understand everything the nurse said and did? How would you change the lesson? Finally, try to incorporate these ideas with the nursing stories discussed earlier.

You can increase your knowledge and skill as you care for patients when you consider what you have learned from prior experiences in similar situations. When you find yourself on a plateau, you may be caring for patients as if each is a new and separate experience, rather than using past experiences to plan and give improved care. You need to individualize and improve care for patients by being alert to your observations of patient problems and responses. When you incorporate new ideas into your knowledge base, both you and your patients benefit. Many clinical nursing research projects, such as the one Melissa Brown is doing for her research class, result from purposeful observations about a phenomenon and proposing new strategies for future situations.

What Is Evidence-Based Nursing and How Does It Affect Nursing Practice?

In the 1970s, a British physician/epidemiologist introduced the concept of evidence-based medicine (EBM) (Cochrane, 1979). The purpose of EBM was to provide better care at lower cost to more individuals. The definition of EBM stressed the use of evidence from random clinical trials (RCTs) and de-emphasized intuition, unsystematic clinical experiences, and pathophysiological rationale. The primary emphasis of medical evidence was on techniques and procedures rather than on the broader concept of patient care. EBM was expanded to evidence-based practice and evidence-based health care (Jennings & Loan, 2001).

In 1997, more than 20 years later, **evidence-based nursing (EBN)** was cited in the nursing literature for the first time (Simpson, 1997). The EBN movement started in Canada and the United Kingdom, and the major publications and organizations remain there. EBN has also been labeled evidence-based practice and evidence-based nursing practice. For consistency, we use EBN to represent all of these.

The definition of EBN has evolved from "skills of problem definition, teaching, evaluation, and the application of original research literature" (Kessenich, Guyatta, & DiCenso, 1997) to "the use of quality improvement data, other operational and evaluation data, the consensus of recognized experts, and affirmed experiences to substantiate practice" (Stetler, 2000).

Summary

As many nurses now realize, nursing needs to abandon some of the old ways and move into a new era. The linear, technical practice that was prevalent when few nurses were educated beyond the diploma and very few faculty held graduate degrees is no longer sufficient.

As nurses progress along the continuum from novices to advanced beginners and competent practitioners, they become aware that sharpening traditional intellectual skills, such as observing, questioning, and comparing and contrasting, is only one way to improve nursing practice. Developing a strong knowledge base is essential to making pertinent observations, asking crucial questions, and identifying and resolving appropriate problems. Theory and knowledge generated by research provide nurses with opportunities to raise new questions and propose new ways of improving practice. The skills of observation, questioning, comparing, and contrasting will be useful as you build a theory-based practice.

Learning Activities

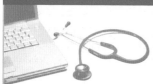

1. **Play it in threes:** Nurses and physicians frequently observe that certain events happen in threes: for example, three admissions to a busy labor and delivery department; three patient deaths in the intensive care unit; three nurses calling in sick for the night shift.

   a. What evidence would you need and how would you collect it to classify it as a phenomenon, not merely an observation?

   b. Identify at least one different observation that you would be interested in exploring at some time in the future.

2. Climbing the ladder of experience:

   a. Formulate two or more questions you would ask an expert nurse about how he or she became an expert and what it means to practice at that level.

   b. Compare your practice with a newly licensed nurse and with a nurse who has 2 or 3 years of experience in one area of practice. Before you can do this, identify two characteristics you wish to compare.

   • Characteristic one:

   • Characteristic two:

References

Baumann, S. L. (1996). Parse's research methodology and the nurse researcher-child process. *Nursing Science Quarterly, 9,* 27–32.

Benner, P. (1984). *From novice to expert: Excellence and power in clinical nursing practice.* Menlo Park, CA: Addison-Wesley.

Benner, P. (2000). Links between philosophy, theory, practice, and research. *Canadian Journal of Nursing Research, 32*(2), 7–13.

Benner, P., & Wrubel, J. (1989). *The primacy of care: Stress and coping in health and illness.* Menlo Park, CA: Addison-Wesley.

Carper, B. A. (1978). Fundamental patterns of knowing in nursing. *Advances in Nursing Science, 1,* 13–23.

Cochrane, A. L. (1979). A critical review, with particular reference to the medical profession. In *Medicine for the Year 2000* (pp. 1–11). London: Office of Health Economics.

Correnti, D. (1992). Intuition and nursing practice implications for nursing educators. *Journal of Continuing Education, 23*(2), 91–94.

Dreyfus, S. E., & Dreyfus, H. L. (1980). A five stage model of the mental activities involved in direct skill acquisition. Unpublished report supported by the Air Force Office of Scientific Research (AFSC), USAF (Contract F49620-79-0063). Berkeley, CA: University of California at Berkeley.

Ducharme, F., Ricard, N., & Duquette, A., Lavesque, L., & Lachanee, L. (1998). Empirical testing of a longitudinal model derived from Roy's Adaptation Model. *Nursing Science Quarterly, 11,* 149–159.

Fawcett, J., Watson, J., Neuman, B., Walker, P. H., & Fitzpatrick, J. J. (2001). On nursing theories and evidence. *Journal of Nursing Scholarship, 33*(2), 115–119.

Gennaro, S., Brooten, D., Roncoli, M., & Kumar S. P. (1993). Stress and health outcomes among mothers of low birth weight infants. *Western Journal of Nursing Research, 15*(1), 97–113.

Hagerty, B. M., & Patusky, K. L. (2003). Reconceptualizing the nurse-patient relationship. *Journal of Nursing Scholarship, 35*(2), 145–150.

Henderson, V. (1966). *The nature of nursing: A definition for practice, research, and education.* New York: Macmillan.

Jennings, B. M., & Loan, L. A. (2001). Misconceptions among nurses about evidence-based practice. *Journal of Nursing Scholarship, 33*(2), 121–127.

Johnson, D. (1980). The behavioral system model of nursing. In J. Riehl & C. Roy (Eds.), *Conceptual models for nursing practice* (2nd ed., pp. 207–216). New York: Appleton-Century-Crofts.

Kessenich, C. R., Guyatta, G. H., & DiCenso, A. (1997). Teaching nursing students evidence-based nursing. *Nurse Educator, 22,* 25–29.

King, I. M. (1981). *A theory for nursing: Systems, concepts, process.* New York: John Wiley & Sons.

Leininger, M. M. (1988). Leininger's theory of nursing: Cultural care diversity and universality. *Nursing Science Quarterly, 1*(4), 152–160.

Mitchell, G. J. (1999). Evidence-based practice: Critique and alternative view. *Nursing Science Quarterly, 12*(1), 30–35.

Moch, S. D. (1990). Personal knowing: Evolving research and practice. *Scholarly Inquiry for Nursing Practice: An International Journal, 4*(2), 155–170.

Murphy, J. I. (1991). Reducing the pain of intramuscular injection. *Advancing Clinical Care, 6*(4), 35.

Neuman, B. (1995). *The Neuman systems model.* Norwalk, CT: Appleton & Lange.

Nurses' Health Study History. (2002). Retrieved, from http://www.channing.harvard.edu/nhs

Orem, D. E. (1991). *Nursing: Concepts of practice* (4th ed.). St. Louis: Mosby–Year Book.

Peplau, H. E. (1952). *Interpersonal relations in nursing.* New York: G. P. Putnam.

Polit, D. F., & Beck, C. T. (2007). *Nursing Research: Generating and Assessing Evidence for Nursing Practice* (8th ed.) Philadelphia: Lippincott Williams & Wilkins.

Roy, C. (1970). Adaptation: A conceptual framework for nursing. *Nursing Outlook, 18*(3), 42–45.

Ruth-Sahd, L. A. (2003). Intuition: A critical way of knowing in a multicultural nursing curriculum. *Nursing Education Perspectives, 24,* 129–134.

Silva, M. C. (1977). Philosophy, science, theory: Interrelationships and implications for nursing research. *Image 9*(3), 59–63.

Simpson, B. (1997). Evidence-based nursing: The state of the art. *Canadian Nurse, 92,* 22–25.

Stetler, C. B. (2000). To the editor . . . Evidence-based nursing: What it is and what it is not. *Nursing Outlook, 48,* 151–152.

Watson, J. (1985). *Nursing: Human science and human caring. A theory for nursing.* Norwalk, CT: Appleton-Century-Crofts. www.rec-law.com/fen-phen/legalinfo. (2002). Retrieved.

Multidisciplinary Theory

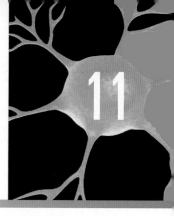

Barbara E. Chandler, PhD, OTR/L, FAOTA; Elizabeth Courts, MSN, APRN, BC, FNP; Lon McPherson, MD; Caren Wirlinger, BS, PT

Intent: This chapter provides an overview of the theoretical basis of the health-related disciplines of medicine, nursing, physical therapy, and occupational therapy. Each discipline, through an analysis of a patient story, will demonstrate how it selects and applies theory when providing care. Following the analysis, observations about the similarities and differences among the theoretical approaches are discussed.

Key Words/Concepts		
best practices	evidence-based practice	medical model
caring	Hippocrates	multidisciplinary
clinical reasoning process	KSVME framework	physical therapy
disablement model	occupational therapy	

Introduction

Each health-related discipline has theory that supports its ability to identify, relate, understand, explain, predict, influence, and control phenomena within its discipline. This theory draws from the arts, sciences, and humanities foundation that many health professions share and is designed to address discipline-specific questions.

When necessary, health care professionals share discipline-specific theory. For example, knowledge of relevant medical theory helps the nurse plan care for a stroke patient. A physician, on the other hand, may draw on relevant nursing theory to determine the best way to administer multiple medications at one time in a stroke patient experiencing difficulty swallowing. Physical therapy may have theory that supports a safer way of transferring a patient with hemiparesis from the bed to a chair that nurses and others may use. Physical therapists, in turn, may draw on nursing theory regarding the administration and timing of pain medication in order to maximize pain control during physical therapy exercises. Occupational therapy may have unique theory that helps nurses and others teach stroke patients to feed and dress themselves. In turn, occupational therapists may draw upon nursing theory to help determine the readiness of a patient to participate in rehabilitation activities.

Some health-related phenomena are too complex to be addressed simply by sharing theory; in these cases, multiple health professionals with discipline-specific expertise ideally come together as a **multidisciplinary** team and work collaboratively to provide the best patient care. For example, a physician would need to draw on his or her knowledge to determine whether a stroke was thrombotic, embolic, or hemorrhagic and then be able to prescribe appropriate treatments. Nurses would use their knowledge to design a plan of care to maintain good circulation and prevent complications in a patient immobilized by hemiparesis caused by a stroke. In addition, to rehabilitate a stroke patient to walk again and live independently, discipline-specific knowledge and expert involvement of a physical therapist and an occupational therapist are needed.

Frequently, health professionals apply theory in a multidisciplinary and collaborative manner when working with patients whose health needs cross-disciplinary boundaries. These patients, and health care in general, benefit significantly from the richness and diversity of multidisciplinary theory application and professional collaboration.

The remainder of this chapter includes an introduction to the disciplines of medicine, nursing, physical therapy, and occupational therapy and the theoretical base of each. Also included is a patient story (Nursing Story 11.1) in which each of these disciplines share how they would theoretically approach discipline-specific care. Sequencing of the discipline-specific sections is based chronologically at the point in which each discipline is needed within the context of the story and not on any type of perceived organizational or professional hierarchy. In addition, note that there are other very worthy health-related disciplines, such as speech therapy, nutrition, and social services, that would most likely be involved in the care of an actual stroke patient; however, time and space constraints prevent the inclusion of these disciplines in this analysis.

As you read this chapter, note that each discipline is unique. The authors, some of whom are clinicians and some of whom are educator-clinicians, were selected based on their expertise in providing theoretically based clinical care. Their efforts have resulted in an analysis that blends the reality, or "what is," of clinical practice with the ideal, or "what should be," which gives a more realistic view of how theory is and can be applied.

Analysis of the patient story is intended to provide you with a window into the uniqueness of each discipline's approach to providing patient care. Hopefully, looking through this window will help you recognize and understand the role and contributions of these disciplines in clinical care. It is not necessary to memorize all of the theory used in this story; however, it is important that you be able to answer the following questions:

1. What are the similarities and differences in the purpose and intent of each discipline?
2. What are the similarities and differences in the language and meanings that are used by each discipline?
3. Does each discipline view itself as theoretically based? Why or why not?
4. Are the building blocks of theory explicitly or implicitly evident within the theory presented?
5. Is it evident that the theory has been tested through research?
6. Does the theory presented enable the professionals to identify, relate, understand, explain, predict, influence, and control phenomena within their discipline?
7. Is there overlap among the disciplines in the theory applied to this story?
8. What richness does each discipline bring to the story and to other disciplines?

The Patient's Story

Hideo Yomada is a 65-year-old Japanese male who presents to the emergency department of a local medical center at 9:30 AM with right facial weakness, dysarthria, and right hemiparesis. Mr. Yomada began experiencing these symptoms at about 6:00 AM but did not notify his family until they awoke 2 hours later. Mr. Yomada is accompanied to the hospital by his wife (also 65 years old), a son (36 years old), and a daughter (30 years old).

Mr. Yomada and his family immigrated to the United States 45 years ago and have adapted to the American lifestyle with regard to work habits and diet. At home, however, they try to maintain Japanese traditions with regard to family hierarchy, customs, and social mores. Mr. Yomada has adequate health insurance. He has no known allergies and is taking no regular medications. He was diagnosed several years ago with essential hypertension and was advised by his primary care provider to institute lifestyle changes with regard to diet and exercise and come back for follow-up in 3 months. He made no lifestyle modifications and did not return for follow-up, because of his demanding work schedule. His family was aware that Mr. Yomada had started experiencing mild dizziness and right arm weakness periodically during the past 6 months but did not seek medical advice because the symptoms went away.

Mr. Yomada is president and chief executive officer of a large printing company with offices in several cities. His wife works in the home, his son is unmarried and is a junior executive with the company, and his daughter is married with children and works at home.

Clinical Course

Acute Phase

Mr. Yomada was admitted to the acute stroke unit for treatment of a left hemispheric cerebrovascular accident (CVA) with resulting right-sided facial weakness, right hemiparesis, and dysarthria. He was able to swallow but had difficulty with movement of facial muscles. Mr. Yomada was sullen and communicated little. His wife was at his side but was weepy and participated little in his care. His children visited frequently but were quiet. He was placed on bed rest, and the physician requested that an intravenous (IV) line with isotonic fluid be placed and infused at 100 mL/h. The physician also requested diagnostic imaging and laboratory studies. Once it was determined that Mr. Yomada's CVA was not hemorrhagic in nature, he was to receive IV heparin per established stroke

(continued)

NURSING STORY 11.1

The Patient's Story (Continued)

protocol, propranolol (Inderal), and a calcium channel blocker. In addition, it was requested that Mr. Yomada's ability to swallow be assessed and, if it was adequate, he could be placed on a low–saturated-fat, 2–g-sodium diet. Mr. Yomada's vital signs and neurologic assessments needed to be taken every hour until stable, and then every 2 to 4 hours as indicated by his condition. Mr. Yomada remained in the acute stroke unit until his condition stabilized and until he had been therapeutically anticoagulated.

Intermediate Phase

Mr. Yomada was transferred to the regular neurologic services floor. His symptoms remained essentially the same. Heparin was discontinued and oral warfarin sodium (Coumadin) begun. Mr. Yomada was able to serve himself soft foods in small amounts using his left hand, but intake of adequate liquids continued to be a problem. He frequently spilled fluids from his food tray, drooled heavily, and was constipated. Both his decreased ability to handle fluids and his infrequent bowel movements were a source of agitation for him. He sat in a chair three times a day at mealtime for a least 1 hour each time. He was to begin walking exercises but was resistant. He preferred doing as much for himself as possible and would become agitated when he physically could not accomplish what he wanted to do. His wife visited daily, but both were reluctant to have her participate heavily in his care. His children continued to visit daily but were reserved.

Recovery Phase

Mr. Yomada was transferred to the rehabilitation unit with similar residual symptoms. He arrived with no skin breakdown or joint contractures. However, he still struggled with fluid intake and bowel movements. His joints were mobile, but his resting position revealed mild flexion of the right elbow, external rotation of the right hip, and flexion of the right knee. He still preferred to do as much for himself as he could but readily became sullen if he could not accomplish the intended task. His wife visited daily but participated in care only when asked. His children visited daily, but participates in his care only when asked.

Application of Multidisciplinary Theory

A Medical Perspective

The Western tradition of the healing arts is rooted in the work of the ancient Greeks, particularly **Hippocrates.** Hippocrates is credited with moving society away from treating disease based on superstition and speculation and toward an objective approach that utilizes deductive and scientific reasoning. This movement also facilitated the role of the physician to evolve from sorcerer and exorcist to that of a scientist. This increased emphasis on scientific inquiry facilitated great discoveries, such as Jenner's work on developing a smallpox vaccine, Semmelweis' work on curing childbirth fever, and Fleming's discovery of penicillin. These powerful scientific advances led not only to the conquering of many diseases, but also to medicine becoming an influential and respected profession.

During this period, the interests of patients were sometimes overshadowed by the interests of the physicians and of medicine in general. In fact, the economic interests of physicians, who competed vigorously against each other, drove the development of early modern medical practice. Advocating against this trend was Dr. John Gregory, a physician at the University of Edinburgh in the mid-1700s (McCullough, 1999). He advocated that the physician was placed in the role of the fiduciary of the patient and had the responsibility of placing the care of the patient ahead of any personal and professional interests, which is foundational to today's medical practice.

Theoretical Framework

Theory and research supporting medicine and medical decision making today is very diverse, and as with other health professions, it draws heavily from the sciences (i.e., biology, chemistry, pharmacology, and systems) and the arts and humanities (i.e., sociology, psychology, philosophy, ethics, finance, and economics) (Budetti, 2008; Jonsen, 1988; Weinberg, 2001). However, medicine focuses primarily on the effective diagnosis and ethical treatment of human beings with pathophysiology. Today, medicine is seen, in part, as the practical application of ethics in the healing arts that is influenced by compassion and integrity (McCullough, 1999). These medical decisions are also tempered by patient autonomy, various types of practice constraints, and societal expectations.

Theoretical decision making in medicine is usually based on **evidence-based practice** guidelines that are developed through research and the collective determination of what constitutes "**best practices**" in medicine. These guidelines, of which thousands now exist (National Guidelines Clearinghouse, 2008), attempt to bring consistency and "best practices" to the bedside by guiding clinical decisions. These guidelines usually integrate scientific inquiry with the fiduciary interest of the patient and society. On the whole, use of these guidelines by physicians has been poor (Cabana et al., 1999; Institute of Medicine, 2008), which is resulting in recommendations for improved compliance with evidence-based clinical guidelines and computer-based clinical decision making, order entry, and medical records (Bates et al., 2003; Institute of Medicine, 2008; Jacobson, 2008) in an attempt to improve patient safety.

The reasoning process by which medical decisions are made is commonly referred to as the medical or clinical model, because of its focus on the presentation of a patient problem, the determination of a medical diagnosis, and ultimately, treatment of the pathophysiology leading to the diagnosis and its associated symptoms. The traditional medical model addresses very specific pathophysiology in relation to associated diagnostic tools, medications, and other therapeutics to provide either a cure or methods of living with the diagnosis. For example, a patient complaining of episodic dizziness and partial field blindness would most likely be ordered to have laboratory tests, such as total cholesterol, high-density lipoproteins (HDLs) (good cholesterol), low-density lipoproteins (LDLs) (bad cholesterol), triglycerides, and a serum metabolic panel to determine serum glucose, liver function, and kidney function. They may also undergo a carotid ultrasound to determine the presence of plaque in the carotid arteries. Depending of the findings of the ultrasound, a computerized axial tomography (CAT) scan, with and without contrast, may be ordered to determine the presence of old or more recent strokes. Depending on those results and the patient's symptoms, he or she may be ordered to have the gold standard exam, which is cerebral angiography, to determine if there is arterial occlusion in the arteries of the brain. If occlusion is found and the patient meets prerequisite criteria, then he or she may be a candidate for a carotid endarterectomy to remove the occluding plaque. If the patient is not a candidate for surgery, then he or she will most likely be placed on antiplatelet therapy and cholesterol-lowering agents. The patient will most likely also be advised to begin a walking regimen to improve circulation as well. All of these steps represent the use of the medical model (problem, diagnosis, and treatment) to help the patient prevent a cerebrovascular accident (CVA) or stroke.

Analysis of Mr. Yomada's Story

In the unfolding tragedy of Mr. Yomada, the immediate needs focus on the correct diagnosis, prevention of complications, determination of prognosis, and then planning for his ongoing care.

Mr. Yomada presents with hemiparesis and dysarthria, which is not an uncommon presentation with ischemic stroke. Stroke is most commonly due to thrombus formation and emboli from the heart, thoracic aorta, or carotid arteries, which account for the majority of all ischemic-based strokes (Adams et al., 2007; Caplan, 2008). In Mr. Yomada's case, his ischemic stroke appears to be originating from the occlusion of his left middle cerebral artery, which is resulting in a cortical stroke. His history of uncontrolled hypertension also raises the possibility of smaller, lacunar infarcts in the deeper brain tissues; these strokes are the result of in situ thrombosis rather than emboli (Oliveira-Filho & Kistler, 2007). Current standards of care include diagnostic imaging at the time of presentation with computed tomography (CT) of the brain (Adams et al., 2007; Caplan, 2008). While most ischemic strokes take 48 to 72 hours to become visible on CT, hemorrhages will be visible on CT immediately. Hemorrhagic stroke needs to be diagnosed promptly, because care of patients and complications associated with hemorrhagic strokes are distinctly different from ischemic-based strokes.

Unlikely possibilities for the cause of Mr. Yomada's presentation include a brain tumor or abscess. Immediate CT scanning will give some insight into whether a tumor or abscess is present, though these are best imaged with the aid of intravenous contrast (Kistler, Furie, & Hakan, 2008). Nothing in the case presentation suggests that either of these diagnoses is present.

The immediate care of Mr. Yomada focuses on the prevention of complications and on limiting further cerebral damage. Thrombolytic therapy, such as tissue plasminogen activator (tPA), could not be given because Mr. Yomada needed to present at the emergency department within 3 hours of the onset of symptoms for administration to be a viable option. While thrombolytic therapy can be dramatic because of its potential to cause a complete resolution of stroke symptoms, its benefits are more commonly seen in the months following treatment (Marler, 1995; Oliveira-Filho & Koroshetz, 2008b). In Mr. Yomada's case, heparin is administered to anticoagulate the patient's blood, presumably to reduce the chance of new emboli formation. However, while it is still common to see heparin used for ischemic stroke, this standard of care may be changing as evidenced by recent research (Adams et al., 2007; Oliveira-Filho & Koroshetz, 2008a).

Mr. Yomada is admitted to a stroke unit where close attention can be paid to his evolving neurological symptoms. There is a possibility that Mr. Yomada's condition may worsen because of secondary hemorrhage or influx of vasoactive substances into the ischemic stroke bed and the possibility of increased intracranial edema and pressure, which can lead to a progression of symptoms (Caplan, 2008; Castillo, 1999). Because stroke can also precipitate seizures, Mr. Yomada may be placed on seizure precautions and an antiseizure medication, such a Neurontin. It is also important at this time to prevent any abrupt decreases in Mr. Yomada's blood pressure because the stroke bed, or area around the stroke, will be susceptible to injury from any decrease in perfusion.

Additional studies that are commonly performed are aimed at a more precise delineation of the etiology of Mr. Yomada's stroke. An ultrasound of his carotid arteries will demonstrate the degree of atherosclerosis and, if a significant obstruction is found, a carotid endarterectomy may be needed to clear the arteries and prevent another, perhaps more catastrophic, stroke. Similarly, magnetic resonance angiography (MRA) could be used to isolate any structural abnormalities within the arteries (Adams et al., 2007; Caplan, 2008; Latchaw et al., 2003). An electrocardiogram and ongoing cardiac monitoring will be used to observe for atrial fibrillation, which is associated with mural emboli formation, and the development of cardioembolic stroke. Emboli formation associated with cardiac valvular disease may also make the patient prone to stroke. Atrial septal defects that allow communication of blood flow from venous to arterial circulation may also allow passage of venous clots to the brain. Cardiac sources of emboli, such as mural emboli and valvular disease, will be screened for by echocardiogram, and if emboli are found, it would indicate the need for prolonged anticoagulation with warfarin.

Once Mr. Yomada is shown to be stable, he will be moved to a unit that focuses specifically on stroke care. During this time, several potential complications need to be watched for and prevented. Aspiration is the most important and common complication. Mr. Yomada has some indication that he is at risk for aspiration as indicated by his cough and drooling. Nursing evaluations screen for this, and speech therapy will evaluate the degree of the risk. Mr. Yomada's ability to move both his upper and lower extremities is impaired, and occupational and physical therapy will be needed to help him retrain his extremities, regain as much function as possible, and learn compensatory strategies that will help him adapt to any residual deficits.

The optimal length of stay in an acute care facility for a patient with hemiparetic stroke and dysarthria and without complications averages 5 to 7 days (Teasell et al., 2006). Discharge options include moving the patient to an acute or subacute inpatient rehabilitation center, a skilled nursing facility, or home-based health care (InterQual Level of Care, 2008). A motivated patient with significant disability can usually be placed in an inpatient rehabilitation facility, and there is evidence to support the achievement of better outcomes for these patients (Cifu & Stewart, 1999). Patients with less motivation, stamina, and significant disabilities will be placed in subacute rehabilitation or in skilled nursing facilities.

The medical care described here is considered usual evidence-based care for acute ischemic stroke. While variations from this standard occur for a variety of reasons, the most common reason is because of patient preferences (Jonsen, 1988). Mr. Yomada has retained much of the values associated with the Japanese culture. Self-effacement, which is the suspension of one's belief in order to treat the patient as an equal, allows the physician to put aside personal preferences, values, and beliefs in order to follow Mr. Yomada's expressed wishes. It appears that Mr. Yomada is the primary decision-maker for himself, his family, and his business as well. The prognosis for full functional recovery in this situation is poor, and the expectation is that even with prolonged therapy, Mr. Yomada will continue to have significant disability for the remainder of his life. Mr. Yomada is not going to be able to run his business, his family, and most likely a significant part of his daily life. As his clinical status stabilizes and if he retains his capacity for making personal judgments, it is important that the physician have frank discussions with Mr. Yomada about his prognosis and options for care. These discussions need to be compassionate, but should be realistic and truthful. He should be encouraged to include his family in these discussions and to allow communication between the treatment team and selected family members in order to facilitate care. As long as Mr. Yomada is competent to make his own decisions, inclusion of family or others in any discussions should be limited to what Mr. Yomada allows.

Society places increasing demands on health care delivery. The current spiraling health care cost is unsustainable, so additional limitations on the type and amount of care physicians provide as dictated by payer groups and government regulation is to be expected. In Mr. Yomada's case, the insurance payer may wish to see him quickly transferred to a less expensive level of care and will need to approve transfer to a rehabilitation facility. If he does not actively participate in his rehabilitation therapy, the payer may deem his rehabilitation ineffective and stop payment. Mr. Yomada also is eligible for disability benefits through the Social Security Administration. It is probable that he will have disability coverage through his business as well.

Finally, Mr. Yomada's frustrations with his recuperation may be interpreted as evidence of depression. While major depression is common after a stroke, care must be given to interpret his behaviors in the context of his personality and culture. Side effects of antidepressants are legion and may delay or complicate his recovery. These side effects can include constipation (already a problem), urinary retention, seizures, delirium, cardiac arrhythmias, hypotension, and sedation. Antidepressant medications can be successfully used when the depressive behaviors are impeding the patient's recovery, but talking through the obstacles he faces with an appropriate professional may be just as therapeutic and significantly less problematic.

Even an otherwise healthy individual, when facing a long and major illness, presents the physician with multifaceted decision options. Medical decisions on the extent of diagnostic evaluation, treatment modalities, and prognosis must involve the patient's wishes, the limitations of practice, and the demands of society.

A Nursing Perspective

Theory is used to guide research and education and, most importantly, to identify and achieve goals of nursing practice. As a relatively young and evolving profession, nursing is still developing a body of knowledge in terms of theoretical support for practice. In actual practice, nurses do not and should not follow one particular theory in providing care. They draw from a rich and constantly evolving theoretical base that assists them in addressing diverse patient needs.

Theoretical Framework

It should be evident now that nursing knowledge is supported by diverse theory, which provides the foundation for nursing skills, helps articulate nursing values and meanings, and is influenced by nursing experiences. In Chapter 4, you learned that caring in nursing is the desire, intent, and obligation to apply relevant knowledge, skills, values, meanings, and experience (KSVME) for, with, or on behalf of those requiring or requesting assistance in achieving and maintaining their desired state of health and well-being (Bevis, 1997). By caring through the application of the **KSVME framework,** nurses are able to identify and relate significant assessment findings, understand and explain their significance to clinical situations, and predict, influence, and control clinical situations in order to bring about mutually desired patient outcomes. The KSVME framework (Webber, 2002) provides the basis for analysis of Mr. Yomada's story and incorporates many of the theories you have been reading about in previous chapters.

Analysis of Mr. Yomada's Story

Mr. Yomada's story presents the nurse with multiple opportunities to apply nursing and nonnursing theory. His is a commonly heard story in the work of the emergency department nurse, the acute neurological services nurse, and the rehabilitation nurse. Even the novice nurse identifies patterns and relationships common to patients who have experienced a left hemispheric stroke. The nurse recognizes, however, that even though Mr. Yomada has a common, disabling, medical diagnosis, he is a unique individual with unique life experiences, and his response to this diagnosis, physiologically, psychologically, and spiritually, will be unique. Nurses involved in his care, from the time he enters the emergency department through his rehabilitation, will use their collective knowledge, skills, values, meanings, and experience to identify, relate, and understand the significance of comprehensive assessment findings; explain the meaning of what is happening to Mr. Yomada and his family; and predict, influence, and possibly control various aspects of the situation in order to achieve the best possible outcome for Mr. Yomada.

Knowledge. In each clinical setting Mr. Yomada experiences, from his initial presentation in the emergency department through his rehabilitation, the nurse applies personal and professional knowledge, skills, values, meanings, and experiences to his care. The nurse uses knowledge from the sciences (e.g., anatomy, physiology, and pathophysiology) to understand the cause of the stroke and the resulting right-sided facial weakness, right hemiparesis, and dysarthria, and to explain these relationships to Mr. Yomada and his family. The nurse is also knowledgeable about theory supporting current treatment modalities for hypertension and stroke, including lifestyle changes, pharmacotherapy, nutrition therapy, physical therapy, occupational therapy, and speech therapy, because it is the nurse who implements and monitors the effect of these therapies.

The nurse uses knowledge from the arts and humanities (e.g., psychology, sociology, growth and development, religion) to understand the human response to a life-altering event that will permeate all aspects of Mr. Yomada's life and dramatically influence his roles as husband, father, grandfather, executive, and employer. It is well established that chronic illness and disability have a significant impact on physical health and psychological well-being. The nurse uses Erickson's theory of growth and development (1963, 1968, 1978), with its focus on ego integrity versus despair in the older patient, and Elizabeth Kübler-Ross' (1969) theory on loss and grieving, among others, to understand, explain, predict, and influence how Mr. Yomada will respond to his loss of function and independence and his changing roles.

Knowledge of theory associated with care and caring has a significant impact on this situation, from the perspective of the nurse, patient, and family. According to Benner and Wrubel (1989), caring establishes what is important or what matters to a person, and stress results when what matters or what is important is ignored or not considered. This is particularly important in Mr. Yomada's case. The nurse uses the Socratic method of inquiry through questioning to explore what matters in this situation. What matters to Mr. Yomada? His autonomy? His position in his family? His job? What matters to Mr. Yomada's family? Is it the possibility that he may die or be permanently disabled? What will his role within their family be? Can they provide what he needs when he leaves the hospital? How will this situation impact their daily lives? What matters to the nurse? Mr. Yomada's well-being? His recovery and ability to cope with his deficits? The prevention of complications? His, and his family's, ability to adapt to his changed health and activity status? The need to do a good job? In determining the effects of the physical and psychological stress associated with the loss of what matters to Mr. Yomada, the nurse will draw on Selye's stress adaptation theory (1956). Mr. Yomada, his family, and the nurse have to blend what matters to each of them in such a way that Mr. Yomada and his family are able to adapt effectively to these various stressors.

The nurse uses basic concepts of communication theory and Peplau's 1952 theory of developing the nurse–patient relationship to establish and subsequently maintain a therapeutic, helping relationship with Mr. Yomada and his family. In communicating with him, the nurse must also recognize the importance of the nursing law of culturally congruent care (Webber, 2008), which states that effective nursing care integrates cultural values and beliefs of diverse individuals, families, groups, communities, and global society. This law, which evolved from selected concepts of Leininger's theory of culture care diversity and universality (1984, 1991), helps you understand Mr. Yomada's and his family's verbal and nonverbal responses to the stress presented by his diagnosis, his loss of independence, and his change in roles. The nurse must be sensitive to cultural differences associated with the Yomadas' Japanese heritage and integrate those cultural values and beliefs into his care. Even though the family has incorporated many aspects of American culture into their lives, the Yomadas continue to have strong ties to their Japanese heritage. Therefore, the nurse must acquire a basic knowledge of the values and beliefs associated with the Japanese culture to better understand meanings associated with Mr. Yomada's experience and that of his family. This cultural understanding may also provide insight into why Mr. Yomada has become sullen and is not communicating during the acute phase of his hospitalization, his agitation and resistance to walking during the intermediate phase, and his continued sullenness during the recovery phase.

Awareness of theory associated with depression, loss, and grieving also gives the nurse insight into Mr. Yomada's sullenness. Does it represent depression, which, according to Kübler-Ross (1969), is a normal part of the grieving process, or does it represent a reserved stoicism that is characteristic of Japanese men (Harkreader & Hogan, 2004)? Is it also possible that the sullenness, agitation, and resistance are part of Mr. Yomada's attempt to conserve his physical and psychological energy as identified in Levine's 1969 theory of energy conservation? Does his wife's lack of participation in his care reflect a lack of caring, the desire to avoid physical contact, or respect for him as the patriarch of the family? Knowledge of Japanese culture and integration of Benner and Wrubel's 1989 work on the effects of losing what matters may help the nurse answer these questions and more, and then intervene in the most appropriate manner.

While initiating and developing the nurse–patient relationship, the nurse assesses Mr. Yomada's physiological and psychological status systematically, using von Bertalanffy's general and open system theories (1968). The nurse uses the nursing process, originally identified by Hall in 1955, to identify actual and potential problems Mr. Yomada may experience and to guide the development and implementation of a basic plan of care. The nurse also uses Maslow's theory of human motivation and hierarchy of basic human needs (1943, 1954, 1970) as a framework to guide nursing care and to assist in recognizing and prioritizing Mr. Yomada's needs that require attention and intervention. Using Maslow's theory, the nurse understands that maintaining a patent airway is of paramount importance. Because Mr. Yomada has right-sided hemiparesis and facial weakness, the nurse is concerned about his ability to swallow effectively and predicts the possibility of aspirating food and fluids, which could lead to aspiration pneumonia, a life-threatening complication of stroke. She is also concerned that inadequate fluid intake could lead to dehydration and constipation, among other things. The nurse discusses these observations and concerns with the physician who, in most cases, will order diagnostic tests to determine the adequacy of Mr. Yomada's ability to swallow. The results of these tests will then be used to guide medical and nursing management. Until the results of the tests are known, Mr. Yomada's hydration will be dependent upon the careful administration of intravenous fluids and, if necessary, the placement of an enteral feeding device, such as a nasogastric or gastroscopy tube.

It is also possible that the stroke could precipitate the occurrence of a seizure, so the nurse will most likely place Mr. Yomada on seizure precautions, ensure that there is suction and oxygen in the room and an intravenous access, and discuss with the physician the need for Ativan PRN (as needed) in case a seizure occurs and for a daily dose of antiseizure medication until the risk for seizure has subsided.

Throughout all phases of care, the nurse applies knowledge from biological and pathophysiological theory, along with theory from physics and kinesiology to prevent complications of immobility and to diminish the effects of impaired movement on all body systems. She uses specific nursing skills to prevent complications associated with immobility such as including active and passive range of motion of all joints and extremities and regular turning, coughing, deep breathing, and isometric exercises as part of Mr. Yomada's daily routine. The nurse also collaborates with physical therapy (PT) and occupational therapy (OT) to keep Mr. Yomada's body in alignment and to prevent common complications of left hemispheric stroke, such as flexion and internal rotation contractures of the affected arm, flexion and external rotation contractures of the affected hip and knee, and extension and external rotation contractures of the foot and ankle. These measures not only will help prevent complications of immobility, but will also promote Mr. Yomada's independence and potential for rehabilitation. The nurse observes techniques used by PT and OT and reinforces these techniques while participating in other aspects of care.

The nurse is also aware that immobility contributes to the development of additional complications, such as thrombophlebitis and life-threatening pulmonary emboli. She is also aware that improved mobility and isometric exercises will help minimize this possibility.

Skills. In providing nursing care for Mr. Yomada, the nurse selects and utilizes cognitive and psychomotor skills that are supported by theory. Cognitive skills include communicating therapeutically with Mr. Yomada and his family to deliver and solicit clinically relevant information. This may include asking who, what, when, where, why, and what if type questions about Mr. Yomada's situation and then connecting the answers in a way that is meaningful in the provision of his care. What matters most to Mr. Yomada? What additional health issues may be present? What complications are possible? Whom does Mr. Yomada trust? When would be the most realistic time to expect Mr. Yomada to participate in his care? Why is Mr. Yomada resistant to participate in his care? Why is Mrs. Yomada reluctant to participate in her husband's care? What if Mr. Yomada refuses to cooperate with attempts to keep him mobile and contracture free? What if Mr. Yomada's sullen demeanor is a sign of significant depression? What will be needed for Mr. Yomada's family to prepare for the eventuality of his coming home and his need for their assistance in performing his activities of daily living?

Remember, nursing is the desire, intent, and obligation to apply relevant knowledge, skills, or values, meanings, and experiences (KSVME) for, with, or on behalf of those requesting assistance in achieving and maintaining their desired state of health and well-being (Bevis, 1997). In Mr. Yomada's situation, the nurse combines knowledge and cognitive and psychomotor skills when assessing and identifying priorities of care; when moving, positioning, and helping Mr. Yomada to ambulate in order to prevent complications of immobility; when starting and maintaining an intravenous and enteral line; when safely administering medications and monitoring for adverse drug reactions; and when assisting him with activities of daily living.

The nurse also applies the nursing law of self-care throughout Mr. Yomada's hospitalization. This law, which evolved from selected concepts within Orem's theory of self-care and self-care deficit, states that effective nursing care promotes the highest level of self-care possible for individuals, families, groups, communities, and global societies (Webber, 2008). During the acute phase, Mr. Yomada is dependent on the nurse and others for his care, a phase Orem refers to as wholly compensatory. As Mr. Yomada regains some of his ability to care for himself, he moves into the partially compensatory phase, and as he and his family prepare to leave rehabilitation and go home, Mr. Yomada enters the educative-supportive phase of self-care. "An essential assumption in self-care is that when necessary, nurses will fulfill care requirements of individuals until such time that the individual or other care providers, such as family members, can assume that responsibility" (Webber, 2008).

In conjunction with Orem, the nurse may also apply Roy's adaptation model (RAM) (1970), which views the patient as an adaptive system in constant interaction with internal and external environments. The focus of RAM is that the patient is able to maintain psychological and physiological integrity in the face of a variety of internal and external environmental stimuli that threaten his unique wholeness. Application of both Orem's and Roy's theories guide the nurse in helping Mr. Yomada to progressively adapt to his changing situation and regain as much independence as possible.

Values.   While planning, implementing, and evaluating care for Mr. Yomada, the nurse is influenced by both personal and professional values. Values collectively accepted by nursing provide the standards of thought and behavior for the profession. Values shared by nurses are identified in the American Nurses Association's *Code of Ethics for Nurses with Interpretive Statements* (2005), and The International Council of Nurses' *Code for Nurses* (2006). Professional values include honesty, altruistic compassion and respect for the dignity of the patient and his family, autonomy to make necessary nursing decisions, responsibility and accountability for the planning and implementation of nursing care, and respect for Mr. Yomada's right to make his own decisions. These values are drawn primarily from philosophical theory that speaks to moral duty and obligation to do the right thing and are becoming an ever-increasing influence on nursing theory and practice (Reed, 2004). According to Kim (2004), most nursing theory is based on the "right thing to do," which means it is based on nursing values. These values guide the thoughts and behaviors of the nurses caring for Mr. Yomada and directly influence their reasoning during his care, almost to the point at which they are considered assumptions within nursing practice.

Mr. Yomada and his family also have values unique to them, both as individual men, women, and children and, collectively, as part of a family, community, and the Japanese and American society in which they live. Their values influence their health care decisions and the way they live their lives. Recognizing and respecting their values and working to integrate their values as an integral part of the plan of care are essential to successful patient care.

Meanings.   There are multiple levels of meanings and significance interacting in Mr. Yomada's story. Some of the more obvious ones are the meanings associated with Japanese American language, values, behaviors, and cultural mores; meanings unique to the relationships among him and his family members; meanings associated with the unique languages of nursing and medicine, and stroke care in particular; and the language of health care finance. In working with patients, the nurse quickly learns that behavior has multifaceted meanings and these meanings must be assessed, interpreted, and integrated therapeutically into nursing care of the patient and into communication with the family.

On a daily basis, the nurse must understand and interpret the meaning and significance of daily assessment findings, diagnostic test results, drug effects, laboratory tests, and rehabilitation potential to be able to integrate those meanings in a way that positively influences Mr. Yomada's care.

Maslow's theory of human motivation and hierarchy of needs (1943, 1954, 1970) is helpful in making this determination, because it asserts that needs drive behavior. In Mr. Yomada's situation, there are behaviors, such as his sullenness, agitation, lack of communication, and resistance to walking, that indicate there are psychological needs that are not being met. The nurse plays a significant role in assessing and interpreting the meaning of these behaviors and their underlying needs and then using that understanding to influence the delivery of care. Understanding diverse and unique meanings and how they apply in clinical situations can be a major challenge for the nurse; however, it is a challenge that must be addressed because of its significance to patient care outcomes.

Experience.   Nursing care for Mr. Yomada is influenced, in part, by the experience of the nurses involved in his care. Experience is not simply the passing of time but involves changing as a result of the experience. Learning based on experience is a valuable tool in developing expert nursing practice, and integrating experiential understanding into clinical reasoning is important in the provision of expert nursing care (Benner, 1984; Benner, Tanner, & Chesla, 1996; Benner & Wrubel, 1989). Although every patient's story, including Mr. Yomada's, is unique, the nurse recalls past experiences with patients who have had similar types of stroke and identifies similarities and differences among the experiences with them and their families. The nurse who has cared for a stroke patient who has suffered through repeated episodes of aspiration pneumonia has internalized that experience and is quick to recognize the significance of Mr. Yomada's difficulty swallowing liquids. The nurse may have also cared for a stroke patient who developed skin breakdown as a result of immobility or watched a family experience significant distress when trying to adapt after a family member had experienced a disabling stroke. Based on this knowledge and experience, the nurse predicts that Mr. Yomada and his family have the potential to experience the same thing if appropriate actions are not taken. Experience offers the opportunity to affirm theory and expand its meaning when applied to different clinical situations. In Mr. Yomada's situation, experience has a synergistic effect on the nurse's reasoning and decision making and will ultimately influence Mr. Yomada's outcomes.

Caring as the KSVME Capstone

Traditional definitions of care and caring include descriptive words and phrases, such as to have concern for, to value, to protect, to have responsibility for, and to help. All of these words and phrases are used to describe characteristic feelings and behaviors commonly associated with nursing and other human services professions (Webber, 2002); however, nursing does not have a monopoly on caring, and viewing caring in terms of vague feelings and behaviors serves neither nurses nor patients (Scotto, 2003). What distinguishes nurse caring from caring demonstrated by other human services professions? What differentiates the "what is" of caring in nursing from the "what is" of caring in other health-related professions is the intentional and purposeful application of nursing knowledge, skills, values, meanings, and experiences for, with, or on behalf of another. Having a caring intent influences nursing practice because it attaches expanded meaning and significance to everything nurses do and guides decision making in the provision of patient care. Therefore, **caring** in nursing is defined as the desire, intent, and obligation to serve through the application of nursing knowledge, skills, values, meanings, and experiences (Webber, 2002).

In the case of Mr. Yomada, nurse caring (nursing care) represents the intricate tapestry interwoven from the knowledge, skills, values, meanings, and experiences of the nurse with the knowledge, skills, values, meanings, and experiences of Mr. Yomada and his family, as well as those of other members of the health care team. This tapestry was woven in the humanistic attempt to assist Mr. Yomada and his family to adapt and recover from this life-altering event. All health care disciples care; they simply do it in different ways. The desire, intent, and obligation to serve through the application of nursing knowledge, skills, values, meanings, and experiences is what makes nurse caring unique.

Mr. Yomada's story is rich with opportunities to apply theory, and the preceding discussion is certainly not all-inclusive. While several nursing and nonnursing theories have been identified and applied in the discussion of this case, there are many others that could be used in addition to or in lieu of the ones presented. You are encouraged to continue the discussion of Mr. Yomada's experience by expanding the use of the identified theory, selecting and applying a different theory, and developing new and creative ideas about how to approach Mr. Yomada's nursing care.

A Physical Therapy Perspective

The profession of physical therapy is relatively young compared to medicine and nursing, with its roots and first organized training programs dating back to World War I (Moffat, 2004). Although the profession has continued to be heavily influenced by the rehabilitation demands of catastrophic events such as the polio epidemic and subsequent wars, **physical therapy** has grown to include a wide variety of specialties, such as orthopedic, neurological, cardiopulmonary, pediatric, industrial, and sports. Physical therapists practice at private clinics, hospitals, schools, job sites, and rehabilitation centers.

To prepare physical therapists to practice in such a variety of specialties and practice settings, their education must include a strong foundation in anatomy, kinesiology, physics, histology, pathology, statistics, and research. As in medicine, much of the "art" of physical therapy relates to the psychosocial interaction between the therapist and patient, both of whom are influenced by their life experiences, cultural influences, communication styles, motivation, and spiritual influences (Schmoll, 1995).

For decades, the efficacy of physical therapy interventions was based on anecdotal reports. Beginning in the 1960s, physical therapy, like most health professions, was challenged to build research-based theory (Myers, 1995). The response to this challenge led to a stronger research emphasis within physical therapy education programs and to the emergence of subspecialties within the profession, such as sports injury rehabilitation. In 1997, the *Guide to Physical Therapist Practice* (GPTP) was developed to better define the profession and describe the practice of physical therapy. It also provided a more uniform professional vocabulary and more clearly defined the scope of physical therapy practice as it exists currently. Perhaps most importantly, it identified evidence-based tests, measures, and treatments to be used by physical therapists (American Physical Therapy Association [APTA], 2001).

Evidence-based guidelines are even more important today because of patients' direct access to physical therapy care without a provider referral and because of increased scrutiny of physical therapy practices by third-party payers, such as Medicare and insurance companies. Physical therapists must utilize valid and appropriate treatment techniques with a strong foundation in research whether they are treating existing injuries or impairments or working with patients to maintain wellness and prevent injuries (APTA, 2001).

Theoretical Framework

The GPTP states that physical therapy practice is organized and best understood by the disablement model (APTA, 2001). Disablement, as defined by the models of Nagi; the International Classification of Impairments, Disabilities, and Handicaps (ICIDH); and the National Center for Medical Rehabilitation Research (Jette, 1994), illustrates the relationships and progression of pathophysiology that produces a physiological, psychological, and/or cognitive impairment that may result in a more long-term functional limitation or disability. Many disablement models have been developed over the years; however, Nagi's 1965 model provided the foundation for the GPTP (APTA, 2001). See Figure 11.1.

The disablement model also challenged the traditional medical model of defining disability on the basis of the original diagnosis or pathology. According to the disablement model, two patients with the same pathology and similar functional limitations may have vastly different outcomes. If one patient's environment (home, workplace, family roles, etc.) can be modified to accommodate the functional limitations, then it may be argued that there is no actual disability as compared to the other patient who is expected to function as before without the benefit of an altered environment.

INTERNATIONAL CLASSIFICATION OF IMPAIRMENTS, DISABILITIES, AND HANDICAPS (ICIDH)

"DISEASE" → IMPAIRMENT → DISABILITY → HANDICAP

NAGI SCHEME

ACTIVE PATHOLOGY → IMPAIRMENT → FUNCTIONAL LIMITATION → DISABILITY

Figure 11.1 Two models of the disablement process. (Source: Hall, C., & Brody, L. T. [1999]. *Therapeutic exercise is moving toward function.* Philadelphia: Lippincott Williams & Wilkins.)

A pathophysiological disorder may be the result of many things, including trauma, disease, or degenerative changes. Making a traditional medical diagnosis associated with pathology would typically involve identifying the disorder on a cellular or systemic level, as well as any associated disruptions of normal anatomical or physiological function. Impairments result from alterations in structure or function associated with the pathophysiological disorder. For example, a patient may have impaired mobility secondary to pain from trauma, a CVA, a fractured hip, birth trauma, and so on. Physical therapists typically would be concerned with identifying the nature of the impaired movement and then developing an appropriate diagnosis. This diagnosis may be different from the primary medical diagnosis, because the ". . . term diagnosis applies not only to diseases but also to impairments" (Norton, 1995, p. 19). For example, a physical therapist may treat a patient who has had a total hip replacement secondary to a hip fracture. The patient is now experiencing balance difficulties as the result of a prolonged period of abnormal weightbearing and attempts to compensate. It is unlikely that the orthopedic surgeon's diagnosis included balance dysfunction; however, the physical therapist would make such a diagnosis and design evidence-based treatments to address it. Functional limitations are defined as alterations in a patient's ability to perform activities the same way he or she would have prior to the onset of pathology and impairment (APTA, 2001). These limitations may involve simple physical restrictions in one's ability to bathe or dress, or may involve more complex physical or cognitive changes impacting someone's ability to operate a car or function at work. As stated earlier, the disablement model examines the concept of disability within the context of a person's ability to function within his or her physical and social environment. Disability is dependent upon the capacity of the individual, as well as the expectations imposed upon them (APTA, 2001). The disablement model continues to be revised and refined to account for more realistic scenarios such as movement in both directions along the disability continuum and other factors such as secondary complications (Jette, 2006).

Physical therapy care involves a full assessment, which includes obtaining a patient history, reviewing related medical records, and physically assessing, testing, and measuring all body systems relevant to the patient's impairment. Once the assessment is complete, the impairments are diagnosed and prioritized, and a plan of care is formulated. The plan of care specifies goals, including patient goals, and the anticipated timeframes for meeting them. The actual treatment interventions are administered and the physical therapist re-examines the patient's response to treatment and adjusts the interventions as indicated.

Analysis of Mr. Yomada's Story

During the acute phase of Mr. Yomada's post-CVA care, physical therapy's priority will be the prevention of secondary impairments while the physicians and nurses working with Mr. Yomada try to get him medically stable. The physical therapist will work closely with the nurses and occupational therapist to provide regular range of motion (ROM) to prevent contractures and help reposition him on a regular basis to avoid decubitis. A full assessment of Mr. Yomada's mobility and balance would most likely not be possible while in the intensive care unit (ICU); however, active and passive ROM exercises will provide an opportunity to minimize the effects of immobility and assess whether Mr. Yomada is exhibiting any signs of movement recovery in his right upper and lower extremities.

When Mr. Yomada is stable enough to be transferred from ICU to a regular neurological unit, a more complete assessment can be performed. This assessment would include determining his ability to sit, stand, balance, control trunk and head, and ambulate. Mr. Yomada's resistance to participating in physical therapy becomes a critical matter at this stage, especially since his eligibility for in-patient rehabilitation is dependent upon his willingness and ability to tolerate 4 to 6 hours a day of physical, occupational, and speech therapy, as well as other therapeutic activities expected of him. Medicare and other third-party insurance payers have become increasingly stringent regarding patient participation and rehab potential to justify the high cost of rehabilitation. Whether Mr. Yomada's resistance is a matter of depression or a cultural reticence to fail publicly in performing the tasks required of him, it is important that his health care providers try to help him overcome this resistance during the acute hospitalization so that he is eligible for rehabilitation services.

Once in a rehabilitation setting, application of the disablement model will focus less on the extent of Mr. Yomada's disability and more on how he is able, with accommodations, to function at home and resume his previous roles within his family, work, and social circle. Mr. Yomada's care will now involve the identification of long-term goals; however, both he and his family must be made aware of the unfavorable prognosis for significant neuromuscular return. The plan of care will be adjusted to maximize any motor function present in Mr. Yomada's affected right side and strengthening his left side in order to make safe mobility possible. In cooperation with occupational and speech therapy, Mr. Yomada will be fitted with and instructed in the use of appropriate adaptive equipment, such as a wheelchair and/or a walker or cane, and other devices that will assist him in bathing, dressing, and eating.

In analyzing Mr. Yomada's case in terms of the disablement model, the extent of his disability will be determined not so much by his residual functional limitations as by how able he is, with accommodations, to resume his previous roles.

An Occupational Therapy Perspective

Occupational therapy is a health and human service profession with a focus on assisting individuals whose ability to engage in meaningful occupations has been disrupted or delayed. Occupational therapy is wholistic in that it considers the physical, psychological, social, spiritual, and environmental aspects of caring for human beings. Occupational therapists view themselves as practicing a healing art, which has its basis in observable phenomena and scientific knowledge. The profession is evolving to a broader definition of intervention to include helping individuals to achieve greater balance and meaning in their occupations, even in the absence of identified disruption or delay. A focus on helping individuals toward wellness and a personal sense of well-being is increasingly viewed as a legitimate practice area. It is essential to understand the concept of occupation if one is to understand occupational therapy. There are many definitions of human occupation. John Dewey, an American educator, describes occupations as continuous activities that have a purpose (1916). Law et al. (1997) define occupation as activities of everyday life that are named, organized, and given value and meaning by individuals and culture. Occupation is everything people do to occupy themselves, including looking after themselves, enjoying life, and contributing to the social and economic fabric of their communities. According to the American Occupational Therapy Association (2008), disruption of occupation may lie with the individual (patient factors), it may lie within the environment (context), or it may be rooted in the interaction between the individual and the environment. Occupations are generally classified as education, work, and productive activities; play or leisure activities; activities of daily living (self-care); instrumental activities of daily living (oriented toward interacting with the environment); and social participation. The framework provides specific definitions for these areas of occupation as well as the performance skills, processes, and patterns that provide the basis for engagement in daily occupations.

The profession of occupational therapy, formally founded at the turn of the 20th century, has its roots in classical thought that activity is good for the mind and the body. Adolph Meyer (1922), an early 20th-century psychiatrist and neurobiologist at Johns Hopkins University, states that "man learns to organize time and he does it in terms of doing things" (p. 6). Meyer, an early proponent of occupational therapy (known as curative occupations at that time), recognized the value of the ability to do or to engage in meaningful occupations. An indicator of health is the ability to engage in daily occupations that are meaningful to the individual. Therapeutic expression of this thought was operationalized in the moral treatment movement for psychiatric patients in the 18th and 19th centuries. In the early part of the 20th century, individuals from nursing, psychiatry, what would later come to be known as social work, and a patient (an architect) who had experienced "curative occupation" distilled these ideas into a professional core: There is health and well-being in the ability to engage in occupations that are meaningful to the individual. The use of occupation as a therapeutic medium and a goal of intervention are intertwined. The profession as founded was reflective of its time and context, and these aspects of the field remain true today. Occupational therapy is continually evolving in its theoretical framework. However, the aspects of considering the individual in the context of his or her life and patient collaboration or participation in his or her own care remain central.

Theoretical Framework

There is no agreement among practitioners regarding which theory of occupational therapy, often called models in the professional literature, should drive practice. There is emerging consensus that occupation, rather than a focus on performance skills, processes, and patterns, should be an overarching tenet. This is seen as a return to the core principles of the profession. There is also the development of the discipline of occupational science, "an academic discipline, the purpose of which is to generate knowledge about the form, the function and the meaning of daily occupation" (Zemke & Clark, 1996, p. vii). The evolution of this discipline is fostering and has a reciprocal relationship with theoretical development in the field of occupational therapy. Many practitioners are guided by frames of reference that can be more appropriately thought of as various ways of putting theory into action. It is often much easier to discuss these frames of reference and to see them in action than to see and understand the theoretical principles underlying and guiding these actions. The line between theory and frame of reference is also blurred. Is the use of a developmental perspective a reflection of a theory of human behavior or a frame of reference to guide the timing and expectations of treatment?

There are six most commonly accepted theories of occupational therapy that consider the individual, the environment, and the interaction between them (Christiansen & Baum, 1997):

- The ecology of human performance stresses the complexity of the context in which individuals live and draws upon environmental psychology (Dunn, Brown, & McGuigan, 1994).

- The model of human occupation is a systems approach to occupational behavior, considers elements of personality theory, and originally held that human occupation was the conceptual foundation of occupational therapy (Kielhofner & Burke, 1980).

- The person-environment-occupation model is a transactive model that holds that these aspects "interact continually across time and space in ways that increase or diminish their congruence" (Christiansen & Baum, 1997, p. 93).

- The occupational adaptation model also uses a systems approach, but stresses the adaptation as a change in the functional status of the person. Occupational adaptation is seen as a "normative process, internal to the person, by which competence in occupational functioning develops" (Schkade & Schultz, 1992a, p. 836).

- The contemporary task-oriented approach combines development as both maturation and skill acquisition, motor learning and systems theory, and focuses on motor behavior as that which is seen in occupational performance (Mathiowetz & Haugen, 1994).

- The person-environment occupational performance perspective reflects "the transactional relationship between the person, occupation and environment and the influence of intrinsic and extrinsic factors on occupational performance, health and well-being" (Christiansen & Baum, 1997, p. 86).

Selecting a Theoretical Perspective. Clinical reasoning, as the process of decision making, guides occupational therapists in the selection of a theoretical perspective and the use of frames of reference. Mattingly and Fleming (1994) refer to the therapist with "the three-track mind," simultaneously using several related, but different, reasoning strategies (p. 119). Procedural reasoning is similar to the hypothesis-generating reasoning typically used in medical diagnosis. Procedural reasoning is used to identify techniques and procedures that may be therapeutic. Seeing and dealing with the patient as a person, the social being, is referred to as interactive reasoning. The therapeutic use of self is very much in evidence in this type of interaction and reasoning (Mattingly & Fleming, 1994). Conditional reasoning places the patient in the broader temporal and social contexts. Conditional reasoning is used three ways:

- The whole condition (person, illness, supports, meaning, contexts)
- How the condition could change over time depending upon variables known and unknown
- The future state of the individual (the outcome), which is conditional upon the patient's active participation in treatment and in the construction of the future image of self (Mattingly & Fleming, 1994)

These types of conditional reasoning combine to produce narrative reasoning or the construction of the patient's story (Mattingly & Fleming, 1994). Narrative is often a motivational force for patients, as well as part of the problem-solving process and motivation for the therapists. Narrative reasoning is the process therapists use to make sense of human experience, to understand, as well as a person can, the experience of another. The construction of a story helps the patient to connect to his or her life before and after a disruption in occupational engagement for whatever reason. It is important for health care professionals to remember that our interaction with a patient occurs at one point in time, and that, for most, there was a time before this interaction, and hopefully, a time after. The narrative of their life has a past, not involving health concerns; a present, involving intense concerns; and an imagined future where health concerns fade and normal life continues. Narrative reasoning helps therapists to view themselves as change agents, facilitators of change, and partners with a patient in the change process.

The future self, the reconstructed life, is immensely important. Any approach to occupational therapy intervention must consider how the patient views himself or herself. An individual patient's idiosyncratic parameters guide the occupational therapist in choosing a theoretical perspective to use. Temporal considerations are also important. Depending on the stage or focus of treatment, one theoretical perspective may come to the forefront to guide treatment and then fade in importance as the patient progresses or the focus of intervention shifts and other theoretical approaches are indicated.

Analysis of Mr. Yomada's Story

A stroke such as Mr. Yomada has experienced is a life-changing and stressful event, not only for him, but also for his family and quite possibly his employees. Reaction to illness, help seeking, help accepting, and reconstruction of a life are very closely tied to cultural and spiritual beliefs. A person's personality traits also influence this process. All practitioners in health care have worked with individuals who have the same impairment, yet experience very different levels of recovery and reconstruction of their lives. Consideration must be given to the dual cultural worlds that Mr. Yomada inhabits at work and at home. Evidence of how he reacts to his stroke and its sequelae are already evident during his acute phase of care. All of the six theoretical perspectives mentioned earlier stress the collaborative nature of the patient–therapist interaction and the importance of the patient's active participation in goal setting and intervention.

In the case of Mr. Yomada, any one of a number of theoretical perspectives could be employed. The goal would be the same, but the path to reaching it very different. During the acute phase of treatment, lasting approximately 3 days, occupational therapy services were not ordered for Mr. Yomada. During the intermediate phase of treatment, Mr. Yomada is experiencing difficulties with dysphagia, left hemiparesis, and self-care. He is most likely anticipating difficulties with his work. Potential difficulties in engaging in leisure activities and making psychosocial adjustments may not have been considered by Mr. Yomada and his family at this stage. His clinical picture, however, strongly suggests that this will be the case. Considering all of these factors, Mr. Yomada is referred for occupational therapy services during the intermediate and recovery phases of his medical treatment

The Model of Human Occupation. The model of human occupation, which draws from personality theory, occupational behavior, and system theory, considers the person as an open system and could serve as an overall theoretical perspective. This open system is seen as having three integrated subsystems: volition, habituation, and mind–brain–body performance (Kielhofner, 1995). The focus on a person's role(s) is perhaps most developed by this model. Mr. Yomada has multiple roles, which may vary in importance to him at this time. At his age of 65, he may be ready to re-evaluate which role—company president, husband, or father—is most important to him now. A focus on retirement and greater leisure may come to the forefront.

The Ecology of Human Performance. The ecology of human performance model, as a conceptual framework for intervention, stresses the person's performance of task(s) within a context (Dunn et al., 1994). Mr. Yomada, at his present stage of recovery, is having difficulty with self-care and appears especially vexed by his difficulty eating. A therapist would consider the physical, social, cultural, and temporal aspects of the environment and the expected environment after discharge from the rehabilitation facility. Intervention would focus on modification of the environment and the task (methods and media) to enable Mr. Yomada to perform self-care tasks as independently as possible. Particular attention would be paid to those tasks involved in eating as it has self-care, nutritional, and social/emotional implications. Consideration would also be given to the tasks that he will need to perform if he wishes to return to work. The environmental press of that situation would need to be evaluated.

The Person-Environment-Occupation Model. The person-environment-occupation model (Law et al., 1996) stresses multiple ways to effect change in a person's occupational performance by considering the "transactional relationship between person, occupation and environment" (Christiansen & Baum, 1997, p. 92). Intervention may focus on the person, the occupation, or the environment. Increasing a person's actual skill level; altering the environment so that the environmental press is at the level of challenge, but not frustration; or altering the occupation so that different performance components are required would be appropriate interventions under this model. Mr. Yomada's difficulties with eating may be addressed by altering the type of food he eats, timing of meals and amount of food at each meal, how food is prepared and presented, and use of adapted utensils, glasses, or cups. Interventions to help increase Mr. Yomada's actual skill in chewing, swallowing, and handling liquids would be occurring simultaneously.

The Occupational Adaptation Model. The occupational adaptation model stresses a change in the functional state of the person, hopefully to occupational competency. It views adaptation as a developmentally normal process that is most likely to be seen in times of transition. As such, it appears to have ready applicability in the rehabilitative area. The focus is on increasing the individual's ability to adapt to environmental demands and to integrate those adaptive responses into a repertoire of behavior. The occupational adaptation process (self-initiation, generalization, and mastery) (Schkade & Schultz, 1992a, 1992b) may be well suited to Mr. Yomada's personality but probably would not provide enough guidance in the very early stages of treatment. A focus on skill acquisition in the early stages would probably be necessary to gain and maintain Mr. Yomada's motivation and investment in the therapeutic process.

The Contemporary Task-Oriented Approach. The contemporary task-oriented approach uses contemporary motor theories as the basis for intervention, which focuses on occupational performance (Mathiowetz & Haugen, 1994). Functional tasks are used to facilitate and organize motor behavior. More organized motor behavior leads to increased task and occupational performance. An occupational therapist using this theoretical perspective with Mr. Yomada would focus on enhancing the efficiency of Mr. Yomada's movements through participation in daily tasks that are familiar to him and for which he is motivated.

The Person-Environment-Occupational Performance. Finally, the person-environment-occupational performance model stresses the interaction between the individual and the environment as the point of occupational performance or engagement. The therapist is seen as a "teacher-facilitator" in this problem-asset model. The development of life performance skills and an increased sense of health and well-being are the expected outcomes. Intervention would focus on treatment activities similar to those in the person-environment-occupation model, but would also include family education and identification of social supports and networks (Christiansen & Baum, 1997). Mr. Yomada's family is viewed as an integral part of the therapeutic relationship and as central to his recovery and occupational well-being. This involvement would have to occur in a manner acceptable to Mr. Yomada, which would necessitate understanding and respecting his views on help seeking and help accepting.

Comparison of Perspectives

The reader may have surmised by now that there is a great deal of similarity and overlap in these theoretical approaches. All have their basis, at least in part, on observed phenomena and each theory is at a different point of research testing. It is expected that these theories will evolve over time as they continue to be applied clinically.

All of these theories view the therapist–patient relationship as collaborative and an interactive process. Occupational therapists view themselves as working with people, not doing things to them. All of these theories of occupational therapy have, in some manner, the performance of occupations that are important to the individual and that allow the individual to fulfill the roles he or she values as the central tenet of a desired outcome. The use of a theory to guide treatment often has a temporal component to it. Certain theories are more applicable at certain stages of a patient occupational dysfunction experience or, in other words, along the function–dysfunction continuum. Similar to the concept of zones of proximal development used in pediatric practice, certain theories just fit better at different times in a "patient's story." Whether the clinical situation calls for a focus on initial skill acquisition (habilitation), remediation, compensation, or adaptation also guides one to certain theoretical approaches.

There is perhaps more variability in the frames of reference used to treat underlying performance components of occupational (dys)function than in the theoretical approaches to the therapeutic process. Biomechanical, developmental, coping, acquisitional, visual-perceptual, cognitive, sensory integrative, behavioral, psychosocial, and other frames of reference are used in occupational therapy treatment. It is important to remember that these frames of reference may be viewed as theories of phenomena other than occupation. They provide the "what" and "how" of treatment, while the theoretical perspectives provide the "why."

Mr. Yomada presents challenges to those working with him. Without an understanding of who he was, what he did, what he valued, how he viewed himself, who he loved, and who loved him, any intervention will not connect his past life with his present and with the future he hopes to have.

General Observations

The multidisciplinary approach to this story clearly demonstrates the uniqueness and commonalities among the disciplines in their approach to patient care. In analyzing each of these sections, the following observations were made.

Observation 1

It is clearly evident that all of the disciplines that were discussed use theory to identify, relate, understand, explain, predict, influence, and control phenomena. A significant amount of the theoretical base for each discipline is drawn from the arts, sciences, and humanities, with the remainder representing discipline-specific theory. While some disciplines prefer the language of models and frameworks to theory, all of the disciplines have a theoretical base that is both established and speculative in nature.

It is also evident that each discipline uses preselected reasoning processes to guide the application of theory. These processes include medical decision making or the medical model, the nursing process, the disablement process in physical therapy, and the clinical reasoning process in occupational therapy. In actuality, and regardless of what they are called, they are all processes that provide structure for basic reasoning. That is not to say that these processes do not have theoretical support associated with them; however, their primary purpose is to facilitate the application of theory, not to be the theory. It is also interesting to note that when discussing Mr. Yomada's story and the approach to his care, the step-by-step use of these reasoning processes was not readily apparent. This could mean several things, including the fact that they were using the reasoning process tacitly. It could also mean that professionals with more education and experience think faster and at a higher level than these reasoning processes reflect.

Does the fact that these disciplines do not use the same theoretical language in the same way mean they are not theoretically based? No. More than likely, there is a rich theoretical base underlying these models and frameworks. However, the obvious variations may be one reason why theory and its use remain vague to so many students and practitioners alike. The variations in language and use may also reflect the chronological and theoretical maturity of each of the individual disciplines. Although the uniqueness of each discipline is important, the inconsistency in the language and reasoning processes may actually be a contributing factor to problems communicating across disciplines.

Observation 2

Another particularly valuable observation is that although all of the disciplines spoke to multidisciplinary collaboration, how this collaboration would be operationalized was not made clear. In actuality, what is observed is more like multidisciplinary referral or cooperation instead of collaboration. All of the disciplines work with the same patient, but they may not be working together for the same patient. This has implications for all disciplines, not the least of which is to specifically define what multidisciplinary collaboration means and to determine what approach best serves the patient. The challenge will be to reconcile the issue in a way that makes collaboration effective and desirable to implement, not just trendy to speak of.

Observation 3

Some of the disciplinary parallels that were revealed are also interesting to focus on. Medicine and physical therapy were closely aligned in that they were acute problem-oriented disciplines that focused on physical pathophysiology when addressing patient care issues. Nursing and occupational therapy, on the other hand, appeared more holistic in their approach, focusing on the experiences and including nonphysical patient and family issues, such as quality of life, role confusion, and lifestyle adjustments; both spoke of doing things with or on behalf of the patient.

These differences among the disciplines do not imply a "better than" or a "less than" situation; they simply imply varied focuses and approaches—differences that may lie in the very nature of these professions, the models and theories that support them, and the personal characteristics of people who are drawn to them. It is important that you understand these differences so that you can develop a sincere respect for what each discipline offers and identify ways that you can best work in a collaborative manner.

Summary

Mr. Yomada's story is rich with opportunities for multidisciplinary collaboration. As he navigates the health care system, his care is multifaceted. Nurses, physicians, physical therapists, occupational therapists, speech therapists, social workers, recreational therapists, dieticians, pharmacists, and other professionals participate in his care. Collaboration among the disciplines is essential to prevent fragmentation of Mr. Yomada's care. In rehabilitation settings, the importance given to collaboration is evident in the multidisciplinary conferences held weekly (or more frequently) in which the patient's needs are discussed from the perspective of each discipline. Each member of the health care team provides input about the patient. It is truly a team effort focused on achieving the best outcome.

It is evident that all of these disciplines have a common, as well as a discipline-specific, foundation. It is also just as evident that there is theoretical and conceptual overlap among the disciplines that provides a basis for cooperation and collaboration if practitioners will take the time to recognize and utilize them. Table 11.1 provides a summary of these observations.

Table 11.1   Summary of Interdisciplinary Observations

Discipline	Primary Theoretical Base	Reasoning Processes	Focus of Care
Medicine (point of entry into the acute health care system[a])	Arts and sciences— emphasis on biologic and pharmacologic theory Diagnostic/ Therapeutic modalities	Medical/Clinical model	Diagnosis and treatment of pathophysiology
Nursing	Arts and sciences— emphasis on biologic, psychological, and sociologic theory Caring through application of discipline-specific (KSVME)	Nursing process— basic level Clinical reasoning— upper level	Identification of patient's and family's holistic needs and selection of appropriate intervention or appropriate referral
Physical therapy	Arts and sciences base—emphasis on biologic, physics, and kinetic theory Discipline-specific, conceptually based processes and guidelines centered on movement	Disablement framework	Maintaining or improving motor movement and motor control
Occupational therapy	Arts and sciences base—emphasis on biologic, psychological, and sociologic theory Theoretically based models centered on occupation	Clinical reasoning process	Maximizing participation in occupational (work, play, daily living) activities that are meaningful to the patient and enhance quality of life

[a]Nurse practitioners may be the point of entry into acute care in some situations.

The quality and cost effectiveness of health care is significantly enhanced when there is understanding and appreciation for what each discipline brings to patient care. The common goal for all health-related disciplines is to provide the best possible care for patients. When looking at the benefits of multidisciplinary collaboration, the old adage of the whole being greater than the sum of the parts, again, has significant relevance. Ultimately, the beneficiary will be the patient.

Learning Activities

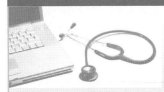

1. Discuss with your nursing faculty the possibility of spending time with a physician, physical therapist, occupational therapist, or other health-related professional. Look at how this professional approaches patient care and the theoretical basis for his or her actions.

2. Read additional patient stories, and identify differences and similarities between each discipline's involved theoretical focus.

3. When caring for patients, identify needs that might best be met by the theory, knowledge, and skill of another health professional. How would you approach involving other professionals in your patients' care?

4. Participate in multidisciplinary collaborative conferences. Identify the theoretical basis for discussion used by each of the participants.

References

Medicine

Adams, H. P., del Zoppo, G., & Alberts, M. J., et al. (2007). Guidelines for the early management of patients with ischemic stroke: A scientific statement from the Stroke Council of the American Stroke Association. *Stroke: A Journal of Cerebral Circulation, 115*, e478–e534.

Bates, D. W., Kuperman, G. J., Wang, S., Gandhi, T., Kittler, A., & Volk, L. (2003). Ten commandments for effective clinical decision support: Making the practice of evidence-based medicine a reality. *Journal of the American Medical Informatics Association, 10*(6), 523–530.

Budetti, P. P. (2008). Market justice and US health care. *Journal of the American Medical Association, 299*(1), 92–94.

Cabana, M. D., Rand, C. S., Powe, N. R., Wu, A. W., Wilson, M. H., & Abboud, P. A. (1999). Why don't physicians follow clinical practice guidelines? A framework for improvement. *Journal of the American Medical Association, 282*(15), 1458–1465.

Caplan, L. R. (2008). Overview of the evaluation of stroke. *Uptodate.* Retrieved May 21, 2008, from http://www.uptodate.com/online/content/topic.do?topicKey=cva_dise/11962&selectedTitle=1-150&source=search_result

Castillo, J. (1999). Deteriorating stroke: Diagnostic criteria, predictors, mechanisms and treatment. *Cerebrovascular Disease (Basel Switzerland), 9*[Suppl 3], 1–8.

Cifu, D. X., & Stewart, D. G. (1999). Factors affecting functional outcome after stroke: A critical review of rehabilitation interventions. *Archives of Physical Medicine and Rehabilitation, 80*(5).

Institute of Medicine. (2008). *Knowing what works in health care: A roadmap for the nation.* Washington, DC: Author.

InterQual Level of Care. (2008). *Level of care.* Retrieved May 22, 2008, from http://www.mckesson.com/en_us/McKesson.com/For+Payors/Private+Sector/InterQual+Criteria+Products/InterQual+Level+of+Care+Criteria.html

Jacobson, P. (2008). Transforming clinical practice guidelines into legislative mandates: Proceed with abundant caution. *Journal of the American Medical Association, 299*(2), 208–210.

Jonsen, A. R. (1988). Ethics in the practice of medicine. In R. L. Cecil & J. B. Wyngaarden (Eds.), *Cecil textbook of medicine* (pp. 12–15). Philadelphia: W. B. Saunders.

Kistler, J. P., Furie, K. L., & Hakan, A. Y. (2008). Initial evaluation and management of ischemic attack and minor stroke. *Uptodate.* Retrieved May 22, 2008, from http://www.uptodate.com/online/content/topic.do?topicKey=cva_dise/6023&selectedTitle=2-150&source=search_result

Latchaw, R. E., Yonas, H., & Hunter, G. J., et al. (2003). Guidelines and recommendations for perfusion imaging in cerebral ischemia: A scientific statement for healthcare professionals by the writing group on perfusion imaging, from the Council on Cardiovascular Radiology of the American Heart Association. *Stroke: A Journal of Cerebral Circulation, 34*(4), 1084–1104.

Marler, J. (1995). Tissue plasminogen activator for acute ischemia. *New England Journal of Medicine, 333*(24), 58–59.

McCullough, L. B. (1999). *A primer on bioethics.* Houston: Baylor College of Medicine.

National Guidelines Clearinghouse. (2008). Retrieved May 22, 2008, from http://www.guideline.gov/

Oliveira-Filho, J., & Kistler, J. P. (2007) Lacunar infarcts. *Uptodate.* Retrieved May 22, 2008, from http://www.uptodate.com/online/content/topic. do?topicKey=cva_dise/9393&selectedTitle=7 ~150&source=search_result

Oliveira-Filho, J., & Koroshetz, W. J. (2008a). Antithrombotic treatment of acute ischemic stroke. *Uptodate.* Retrieved May 22, 2008, from http://www.uptodate.com/online/content/topic. do?topicKey=cva_dise/10615&selectedTitle= 1~150&source=search_result

Oliveira-Filho, J., & Koroshetz, W. J. (2008b). Fibrolytic (thrombolytic) therapy for acute ischemic stroke. *Uptodate.* Retrieved May 22, 2008, from http://www.uptodate. com/online/ content/topic.do?topicKey=cva_dise/6308& selectedTitle=8~150&source=search_result

Teasell, R., Foley, N., Saltel, K., Bhogal, S., Jutai, J., & Speechly, M. (2006). *Evidence-based review of stroke rehabilitation.* Retrieved May 22, 2008, from http://www. ebrsr.com/modules/appendix9.pdf

Weinberg, G. M. (2001). *An introduction to general systems thinking.* New York: Dorset House.

Nursing

American Nurses Association. (2005). *Code of ethics for nurses with interpretive statements.* Washington, DC: American Nurses Publishing.

Benner, P. (1984). *From novice to expert: Excellence and power in clinical nursing practice.* Menlo Park, CA: Addison-Wesley.

Benner, P., Tanner, C. A., & Chesla, C. A. (1996). *Expertise in nursing practice: Caring, clinical judgment, and ethics.* New York: Springer.

Benner, P., & Wrubel, J. (1989). *The primacy of care: Stress and coping in health and illness.* Menlo Park, CA: Addison-Wesley.

Bevis, E. O. (1997). *Caring, expertise, and fire in the belly.* Unpublished manuscript.

Erickson, E. H. (1963). *Childhood and society* (2nd ed.). New York: W. W. Norton.

Erickson, E. H. (1968). *Identity: Youth in crisis.* New York: W. W. Norton.

Erickson, E. H. (1978). *Adulthood.* New York: W. W. Norton.

Hall, L. E. (1955, June). Quality of nursing care. *Public Health News.* Newark, NJ: State Department of Health.

Harkreader, H., & Hogan, M. A. (2004). *Fundamentals of nursing: Caring and clinical judgment* (2nd ed.). Philadelphia: W. B. Saunders.

International Council of Nurses. (2006). *ICN code for nurses: Ethical concept applied to nursing.* Retrieved May 22, 2008, from http://www.icn. ch/icncode.pdf

Kim, H. S. (2004). Theoretical thinking in nursing: Problems and prospects. In P. G. Reed, N. B. Crawford, & L. H. Nicoll (Eds.), *Perspectives on nursing theory,* (pp. 63–74). Philadelphia: Lippincott Williams & Wilkins.

Kübler-Ross, E. (1969). *On death and dying.* New York: Macmillan.

Leininger, M. (Ed.). (1984). *Care: The essence of nursing and health.* Thorofare, NJ: Charles B. Slack.

Leininger, M. (1991). *Culture care diversity and universality: A theory of nursing.* New York: National League for Nursing.

Levine, M. E. (1969). *Introduction to clinical nursing.* Philadelphia: F. A. Davis.

Maslow, A. H. (1943). A theory of human motivation. *Psychology Review, 50,* 370–339.

Maslow, A. H. (1954). *Motivation and personality.* New York: Harper & Brothers.

Maslow, A. H. (1970). *Motivation and personality* (2nd ed.). New York: Harper & Row.

Orem, D. (1971). *Concepts of practice.* New York: McGraw-Hill.

Orem, D. (1991). *Nursing: Concepts of practice* (4th ed.). St. Louis: Mosby.

Peplau, H. E. (1952). *Interpersonal relations in nursing.* New York: G. P. Putnam.

Scotto, C. J. (2003). A new view of caring. *Journal of nursing education, 142*(7), 289–291.

Reed, P. (2004). Nursing theorizing as an ethical endeavor. In P. G. Reed, N. C. Shearer, & L. H. Nicoll (Eds.), *Perspectives on nursing theory* (4th ed., pp. 247–354). Philadelphia: Lippincott Williams & Wilkins.

Physical Therapy

American Physical Therapy Association. (2001). *Guide to physical therapist practice.* Alexandria, VA: Author.

Jette, A. M. (1994). Physical disablement concepts for physical therapy research and practice. *Physical Therapy, 74,* 380–386.

Jette, A. M. (2006). Toward a common language for function, disability and health. *Physical Therapy, 86,* 726–734.

Moffat, M. (2004). The history of physical therapy practice in the United States. *Journal of Physical Therapy Education, 17*(3), 15–25.

Occupational Therapy

American Occupational Therapy Association. (2008). *The occupational therapy practice framework: Domain and process* (2nd ed.). Bethesda, MD: AOTA Press.

Christiansen, C., & Baum, C. (1997). Person-environment occupational performance: A conceptual model for practice. In C. Christiansen & C. Baum (Eds.), *Occupational therapy: Enabling function and well-being.* Thorofare, NJ: Slack Incorporated.

Dewey, J. (1916). *Democracy and education. An introduction to the philosophy of education* (1966 ed.). New York: Free Press.

Dunn, W., Brown, C., & McGuigan, A. (1994). The ecology of human performance: A framework for considering the effect of context. *American Journal of Occupational Therapy, 48,* 595–607.

Kielhofner, G. (1995). *A model of human occupation: Theory and application* (2nd ed.). Baltimore: Williams & Wilkins.

Roy, C. (1970). Adaptation: A conceptual framework in nursing. *Nursing Outlook, 18,* 42–45.

Selye, H. (1956). *The stress of life.* New York: McGraw-Hill.

Von Bertalanffy, L. (1968). *General system theory: Foundations, development, applications.* New York: Braziller.

Webber, P. (2002). A curriculum framework for nursing. *Journal of Nursing Education, 41*(1), 15–24.

Webber, P. B. (2008). Yes Virginia, nursing does have laws. *Nursing Science Quarterly, 21*(1), 68–73.

Myers, R. S. (1995). Historical perspective, assumptions and ethical considerations for physical therapy practice. In R. S. Myers (Ed.), *Saunder's manual of physical therapy practice.* Philadelphia: W. B. Saunders.

Norton, B. J. (1995). Clinical decision making in physical therapy practice. In R. S. Myers (Ed.), *Saunders manual of physical therapy practice* (pp. 17–36). Philadelphia: W. B. Saunders.

Schmoll, B. J. (1995). Behavioral and social science: Considerations for current practice. In R. S. Myers (Ed.), *Saunders manual of physical therapy practice* (pp. 37–61). Philadelphia: W. B. Saunders.

Kielhofner, G., & Burke, J. (1980). A model of human occupation, part I: Conceptual framework and content. *American Journal of Occupational Therapy, 34,* 572–581.

Law, M., Cooper, B., Strong, S., Stewart, D., Rigby P., & Letts, L. (1996). The person-environment-occupation model: A transactive approach to occupational performance. *Canadian Journal of Occupational Therapy, 63,* 9–23.

Law, M., Cooper, B., Strong, S., Stewart, D., Rigby, P., & Letts, L. (1997). Theoretical contexts for the practice of occupational therapy. In C. Christiansen & C. Baum (Eds.), *Occupational therapy: Enabling function and well-being.* Thorofare, NJ: Slack Incorporated.

Mathiowetz, V., & Haugen, J. (1994). Motor behavior research: Implications for therapeutic approaches to central nervous system dysfunction. *American Journal of Occupational Therapy, 48,* 733–745.

Mattingly, C., & Fleming, M. (1994). *Clinical reasoning: Forms of inquiry in a therapeutic practice.* Philadelphia: F. A. Davis.

Meyer, A. (1922). The philosophy of occupational therapy. *Archives of Occupational Therapy, 1*(I), 1–10.

Schkade, J. K., & Schultz, S. (1992a). Occupational adaptation: Toward a holistic approach for contemporary practice, part I. *American Journal of Occupational Therapy, 46,* 829–837.

Schkade, J. K., & Schultz, S. (1992b). Occupational adaptation: Toward a holistic approach for contemporary practice, part II. *American Journal of Occupational Therapy, 46,* 917–925.

Zemke, R., & Clark, F. (1996). *Occupational science: The evolving discipline.* Philadelphia: F. A. Davis.

The Future

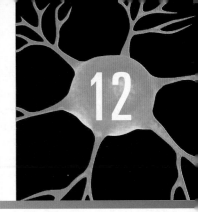

12

Intent: An examination of the status of nursing theory and research in the health care community, the university, and the scientific world helps identify future challenges and potential changes in nursing as a profession, a discipline, and a science.

Key Words/Concepts		
discipline	profession	science
knowledge	scholarship	scientist

Introduction

The future of theory and research in nursing will affect the application and use of **knowledge** in nursing practice as well as knowledge development. For example, since the original publication of this book in 2001, nursing has adopted evidence-based practice. This has led to a change in the role of research as well as the approaches that faculty use in teaching.

This final chapter views nursing from the standpoint of a profession, an academic discipline, and a science. Profession refers to the practice arm of nursing, discipline to the educational arm, and science to theoretical knowledge and research as they are applied to practice and education. An examination of profession, discipline, and science will exercise your reasoning skills to identify and consider alternative responses to the questions posed about these concepts.

Nursing as a Profession

Nurses have debated for a long time whether or not they are members of a vocation, an occupation, or a profession. While you may believe you are entering a profession, some nurses and other health care workers may question whether nursing really is a profession. Answers to the following three questions will help you understand what a profession is and its relationship to theory and research: What is a profession? Is nursing a profession? Why is the development of theory and research important for the recognition of nursing as a profession?

What Is a Profession?

You may believe that because you are called a professional nurse, you belong to a profession. Before accepting that assumption, you need to explore the definition of profession. In Table 12.1, we compare basic dimensions of the definitions of profession from Flexner (1915), Bixler and Bixler (1959), and Pavalko (1971). We compare these dimensions to find commonalities between them and nursing, not necessarily to identify differences. The differences in the statements in many instances merely reflect changes of language between 1915, 1954, 1971, and even today. For example, Pavalko uses the phrase theoretical framework, which has been used only recently in nursing. If Flexner or the Bixlers were writing today, they would probably use that language, too.

Abraham Flexner is well known for evaluating medical schools in the early 1900s. The status of medicine came under question during his review of the 155 schools of medicine in the United States at that time. After publishing his report, medicine changed its educational identity and redefined itself as a profession (Flexner, 1910). Flexner's (1915) eight dimensions of a profession continue to be useful in examining the concept of profession. The Bixlers, a husband and wife team who both were sociologists, wrote at length about nursing and its professional status (Bixler & Bixler, 1959). Their elaboration of Flexner's dimensions helped interpret the application to nursing. A more recent definition of profession comes from Pavalko, another sociologist (1971). Pavalko's definition attracted the attention of nurses, who used it as a more modern approach. The definition of profession below uses elements from each of the above definitions:

> A **profession** is a vocation or occupation that requires specialized knowledge, skills, scientific methods, and values based on research and is taught in an institution of higher education. A profession advocates high ethical standards of its members and engages in expanding its body of knowledge through research. Members of a profession function autonomously, are committed to advanced study, and are motivated by service to society.

Is Nursing a Profession?

The following discussion focuses on the above definition, although you may use the definition of Flexner, Bixler and Bixler, or Pavalko as you proceed to answer the question: Is nursing a profession?

The first sentence of the definition states: *A profession is a vocation or occupation that requires specialized knowledge, skills, scientific methods, and values based on research and is taught in an institution of higher education.* Most nurses agree that nursing is a vocation or occupation and that nurses need specialized knowledge, skills, scientific methods, and values based on research to carry out an effective practice. Although theory frequently plays a hidden role in defining the scientific knowledge and principles you use in your practice, the use of a theoretical framework upon which to base research verifies that the principles are within the body of knowledge we call nursing.

Table 12.1   Dimensions of Flexner, Bixler and Bixler, and Pavalko Definitions of a Profession

Abraham Flexner (1915)	G.K. Bixler & R.W. Bixler (1959)	R. Pavalko (1971)
Intellectual action	Intellectual level of higher learning Attracts individuals of intellectual qualities	An educational period
Personal responsibility	Functions autonomously Controls professional activity Freedom of action	Elements of self-motivation
Practice based on knowledge	Well-defined, well-organized body of specialized knowledge	Theoretical framework
Practical application	Applies body of knowledge in practical services	Professional practice based on theoretical framework
Theorizing	Enlarges body of knowledge using scientific method	Theoretical framework
Teachable techniques	Entrusts education to institutions of higher education Opportunities for professional growth	Training or educational
Organized internally	Well-organized body of knowledge	Theoretical framework
Motivated by altruism	Formulates professional policy Attracts individuals who exalt personal gain Views occupation as a life work	Code of ethics Commitment to lifelong learning
Motivated by societal good	Vital to human and social welfare Economic security	Relevance to social values Member is in control of the profession

The phrase *taught in an institution of higher education* is especially important to nurses because of our unusual educational history. Remember, American nursing education began and continued for many years in hospitals, not in recognized educational institutions. The first schools of nursing in this country were established in hospitals in 1873; however, it was not until

1916 that the first baccalaureate programs were established in universities. Unfortunately, early university programs resembled hospital programs rather than other fields of study in the university. At first, many institutions awarded a diploma, not a degree. These programs focused on procedures, training, and learning by apprenticeship. As university and 4-year college nursing programs developed, they gradually adopted characteristics of the institution, such as a liberal education core and a regular schedule of academic terms. In 1952, a major shift from hospital-based education to community college-based education for nurses began with the establishment of the associate degree in nursing (Montag, 1959).

In 2003, the nursing workforce was composed of 25% diploma-prepared nurses, 34% associate degrees, and 31% baccalaureates. The remaining 10% held graduate degrees and probably only 1% or less held doctorates. Most nurses receive their basic nursing education in community colleges, 4-year colleges, or universities (Kalisch & Kalisch, 2004). In general, professional status is not awarded to occupations on the basis of the beginning level of education, but on the highest level. Remember that only five programs leading to a doctorate in nursing were in existence in 1970 (McBride, 1999). That number increased to 90 by January 2004. By 2007, there were 51 Doctor of Nursing Practice (DNP) programs.

Although nursing prepares the majority of its members at the associate degree level, the first professional degree required for most health care professions is at the graduate level. Graduates of these professions are prepared to provide a high level of care and to think creatively about their practice and how it can be improved. In many cases, they contribute to the growing body of knowledge (McBride, 1999). They are eligible to enter doctoral programs to pursue a research career. You probably agree that nursing meets the initial dimension in the definition of profession. If you consider only the total number of nurses obtaining their basic education in colleges and universities, you could come to the conclusion that nursing is a profession, but there are two additional elements to consider.

The second sentence in the definition states: *A profession advocates high ethical standards of its members and engages in expanding its body of knowledge through research.* Nursing has advocated high ethical standards through the American Nurses Association (ANA) Code of Ethics and the International Council of Nurses (ICN) Code for Nurses (ANA, 2001; ICN, 1973). Nurses are regularly involved in discussions about ethical dilemmas both as students in educational programs and graduates in practice settings. Nursing appears to meet the dimension of ethical standards.

In earlier chapters, you became acquainted with the idea that nursing has a body of knowledge and that the body of knowledge is expanded through scientific research. Nurses have engaged in expanding the body of knowledge in recent years, but this has been a minor effort compared to the size of the nursing workforce and to the responsibilities nurses have for health care. The effort has been limited for two reasons: the small number of nurses holding doctoral degrees and the lack of significant funds for conducting nursing research. Although some master's-prepared nurses participate in research, the small number of nurses with doctoral degrees are responsible for conducting the research. The number is increasing slowly, but what about funds to support this research?

Before the National Institute of Nursing Research (NINR) and its predecessor were established (see Chapter 6), funds to study nursing and health care problems were very limited. Nurses were not viewed as researchers, and nursing was not viewed as a formal body of scientific knowledge. Even though NINR funds have increased markedly in recent years, the NINR continues to have the smallest budget in the National Institutes of Health (NIH). These limited funds and the small number of nurses with research preparation raise too many concerns to accept this section of the definition of profession as describing the current status of nursing.

The final sentence in the definition states: *Members of a profession function autonomously, are committed to advanced study, and are motivated by service to society.* Most individuals enter nursing to serve society, and they do so regardless of where they work—at the bedside, in the community, in management, in the classroom, or in a laboratory. They focus on improving the health and well-being of others and on teaching people to prevent illness and accidents. They model healthy behaviors, care for the sick and injured, and help rehabilitate the disabled. They work extra hours when needed and staff free clinics and homeless shelters during their free time. Some travel to third-world countries to offer care that is not available there. Although there are exceptions, when you look at the nurses you know and work with, you will realize that most nurses help others. They indeed are motivated to serve others and, through them, society.

On the other hand, few nurses are committed to continue either informal or formal education. In 2000, only about 16% of associate degree–prepared nurses continued to the baccalaureate (Kalisch & Kalisch, 2004). There is no universal requirement for continuing education for nurses, and less than half of the states require validation of education for renewal of licensure (Yoder-Wise, 2000). This is different from many other health care professions that support mandatory continuing education. Less than 200,000 of more than 2.5 million nurses in the country hold graduate degrees, and only 12,500 of those have doctoral degrees; this demonstrates how low the commitment of nurses is to formal advanced education. Until the number of nurses holding advanced degrees increases, it is impossible to support that nursing meets this dimension of a profession.

The final dimension is whether nurses function autonomously. As a student, much of your practice relies on policy, procedures, physicians' orders, and faculty direction. As a licensed nurse, your responsibility increases, and as you gain experience in clinical reasoning, you will function more autonomously. As nurses move from the hospital to the community setting, their autonomy increases again. Still another step is taken as increasing numbers of nurses become prepared as advanced practitioners.

Nursing has made significant strides to position itself in higher education, expand the body of nursing knowledge, increase the opportunities for graduate education, and increase the autonomy of practicing nurses. Most nurses are effective, committed caregivers and are designated as professional by licensure even though they do not fully meet full professional status.

Why Is the Development of Theory and Research Important for the Recognition of Nursing as a Profession?

The areas in which nursing fails to meet the definition of a profession relate primarily to expanding its body of knowledge, committing itself to advanced education, and functioning at an autonomous level. Most basic nursing education is located in higher education, but larger numbers of nurses must continue their study through doctoral and postdoctoral levels. A specialized body of nursing knowledge guides practice in some instances, but the majority of nursing knowledge still needs to be tested, verified, expanded, and linked to current nursing theory. The autonomy of nursing increases as individuals sharpen their critical thinking and clinical reasoning skills, but nurses with less than a baccalaureate will not be able to function autonomously.

As nursing theory shifts to testing and expanding knowledge, there will be increased recognition of nursing as a profession. Increasing the number of nurses prepared at the master's and doctoral levels will bring increased potential for actual professional practice. Through the development of clinical reasoning and decision-making skills, the nurse will understand the value of advanced education.

The development of nursing theory and research will affect what nursing is and how it is perceived. As nursing meets the criteria for professional status, it stimulates further theoretical and research development. Theory and research courses initially were limited to graduate study. The language of theory, research, and science stimulated an understanding of the body of knowledge and the ability to integrate it into practice. Introducing theory and research into baccalaureate education not only affects professional practice, but also upgrades the content of graduate programs.

As nurses turn their attention to the theoretical body of knowledge, they will increase their recognition of nursing as a profession. Whether nursing is ultimately recognized as a profession will depend on its research and its theoretical development and their effect on practice.

Nursing as a Discipline

The nursing community generally supports the idea that nursing is a profession; however, few nurses view nursing as a discipline. Even nurses who are members of interdisciplinary and multidisciplinary teams may not think of nursing as an academic discipline. In your college or university classes, you study many disciplines, such as anatomy, biology, history, mathematics, and psychology, but few apply the label of discipline to nursing.

Using questions about nursing as a discipline as we did about nursing as a profession results in the following: What is a discipline? Is nursing a discipline? Why is the development of theory important for the recognition of nursing as a discipline? As you explore the concept of discipline, keep in mind what you have learned about professions and how the development of theory and research affects nursing as a profession.

What Is a Discipline?

A discipline is a branch of knowledge or a field of study. This is illustrated in college and university departments that reflect various fields of study. Each department has its own body of knowledge and offers one or more majors within the boundaries of that body of knowledge. You might say that a department owns the knowledge in a particular discipline and, as the owner, exercises certain rights and responsibilities about the majors, the courses that it offers, and the focus of research conducted by its faculty.

Let's look at an example of ownership. If you attended a college before entering the nursing major, you expected to transfer the credits you earned at that institution to the one in which you are now enrolled. If these credits are in psychology, for example, the psychology department decides whether the credits are comparable to its course offerings and, therefore, acceptable for transfer. Likewise, the mathematics department has the right to decide the math courses that are transferable and the history department the history courses. That is one way each discipline—psychology, mathematics, and history—exercises ownership of its body of knowledge. Because the nursing department owns the disciplinary rights of nursing courses, it is also responsible to decide the nursing credits that are transferable. This simple example of ownership should help you understand how ownership boundaries are monitored and disputes are resolved.

A discipline is a branch of knowledge or a field of study with the purpose to pursue, develop, and disseminate its distinct body of knowledge (Doheny, Cook, & Stopper, 1997). The body of knowledge helps distinguish one discipline from others and sets boundaries between them. Sometimes setting disciplinary boundaries is difficult in education, practice, and research. In the university, for example, several departments may teach courses in research. In the practice setting, nurses and social workers may debate who is responsible for discharge planning or case management, with different institutions arriving at conflicting decisions. In the research laboratory, scientists from various disciplines may seek grants related to health care. For example, a governmental agency or private foundation may call for grant proposals to design methods of measuring health status in preschool children. Unless they specifically focus the request on one or more disciplines, they may receive viable proposals from nursing as well as medicine, public health, dentistry, social work, education, and others. In this case, many groups possess some "ownership" related to children's health status. By considering the above ideas, let's propose the following definition of discipline:

> A **discipline** is a field of study with a distinct theoretical body of knowledge and defined boundaries whose purpose is to guide the pursuit, development, and dissemination of knowledge, research, and practice.

Is Nursing a Discipline?

Nursing is a field of study in over 700 four-year colleges and universities. Although nursing education is recognized for its rigorous curriculum, excellent students, and teaching competence, these characteristics are insufficient to meet the definition of a discipline. Disciplinary curricula are based on a distinct theoretical body of knowledge that is recognized by other, more traditional disciplines in higher education. As you know, the development of a body of knowledge depends not only on theory, but also on research to test and verify relationships between concepts and propositions.

The above definition recognizes that the body of knowledge is developed within designated boundaries and guides the pursuit, development, and dissemination of that knowledge. There are many commonalities between disciplines, so the definition does not declare that the boundaries are impervious.

Various efforts can be used to set boundaries for the body of nursing knowledge. At the lowest level, the outline of content in a course syllabus is selected within certain boundaries determined by the school, the faculty, and individual professors. These boundaries may be influenced by prior course outlines, textbooks, and periodical literature; the professor's education and experience; state board and national accreditation standards; and the school's undergraduate curriculum committee. Members of the curriculum committee are responsible for ensuring that certain nursing content is taught, that it is organized appropriately, and that unnecessary repetition is avoided. Although nursing courses in one university may vary from those in another university, state and national standards may help decide the direction for setting course and curricular boundaries.

The boundaries alluded to in the definition speak primarily to research, when it refers to the pursuit, development, and dissemination of knowledge. The number of universities in which faculty members receive funding to conduct research is growing. In some universities, faculty members adopt a specific focus to guide faculty and doctoral students in selecting projects to study. For example, faculty in one university may select chronic pain as an area of inquiry. Individuals and groups of faculty members focus their efforts to obtain funds for research in that area. This concentration of dollars and research effort on a particular health problem, such as chronic pain, not only encourages collaboration in finding and testing alternatives, but also may accelerate resolution of the problem.

Large schools of nursing may divide nursing knowledge into specialty areas and establish several departments. For example, there may be a department of physiological nursing, psychiatric and mental health nursing, or community health nursing. These departments may each design distinct bodies of knowledge that provide the focus for teaching, practice, and research. The dissemination of knowledge is important, and faculty members publish articles and books about their research and make presentations at professional meetings.

Nursing is increasingly recognized as a discipline in higher education. Within the academic setting, nursing meets the dimensions of the definition. The label of academic discipline serves a more useful purpose in the university than the label of profession.

Why Is the Development of Theory and Research Important for the Recognition of Nursing as a Discipline?

Since the 1970s, nursing education and practice have changed markedly with the development and expansion of theory and research, the specialization of nursing, and the rise of advanced practice nursing.

In 1900, nursing was absent from higher education, but 100 years later, it is a viable field of study, including doctoral and postdoctoral education in increasing numbers of universities. Nursing has established boundaries for scientific investigation in some educational and practice settings, and nurse scientists are receiving highly competitive federal research funds. These awards contribute to the verification of existing knowledge and to the addition of new nursing knowledge. They also increase nursing eligibility for recognition as an academic discipline.

In the 1950s, nurses such as Johnson (1959) were involved in identifying the content to teach in graduate nursing courses. In essence, faculty members were setting boundaries for what we now know as the academic discipline of nursing. It was many years later before these boundaries became instrumental in defining research efforts of individuals and groups. The development of theory and the expansion of research will continue to be important in stimulating the further development of nursing as a discipline, as it sets the stage for what nursing is and how it is defined.

To become members of a fully recognized discipline, nurses must develop a stubborn skepticism about practice as well as a pervasive passion for inquiry. You must prove that nursing has an impact on health and health care, and you must believe that nursing practice can be improved. Anyone who thinks that nursing practice is as good as it is ever going to get or is unwilling to consider change will be unable to identify phenomena to study, to add to the body of knowledge, to improve practice, or to stimulate theoretical development. **Scholarship** requires relentless questioning that pushes the edge of knowledge and integrates sources of knowledge into practice and teaching. Every current and future nurse must respond to change and help to decide the direction that change should take.

Changes in the nursing discipline have decreased the isolation of nursing in 4-year colleges and universities. Educational isolation negatively affects students, faculty, curricula, and research. The more extensions faculty and students can make across the campus, the better acquainted they become with the culture of higher education and the disciplines that make up that culture. Faculty and students in all disciplines benefit when they acclimate to interdisciplinary and multidisciplinary experiences and the expanded environments available in higher education.

The organizational structure and naming of nursing in higher education have not always been consistent with the rest of the university. One might surmise that differences occurred because of the unusual history of nursing education that was described in Chapter 6. After nursing education spent 80 years in the hospital setting, Esther Lucile Brown (1954) urged nurses to move to the university campus and organize themselves in a manner similar to other schools and departments, such as engineering. Some nursing programs made the physical move to the campus but failed to become integrated into the university culture, thereby slowing the acceptance of nursing as an academic discipline. The development of theory and the expansion of research have changed the position of nursing in the academic setting from profession to discipline, but the body of knowledge and its boundaries as defined by theory and research must be strengthened before nursing meets the full definition of a discipline.

Meeting the criteria for professional status provides recognition in the practice field, and being recognized as an academic discipline enhances the place of nursing in the university. Both of these are crucial to the growth of nursing and its ultimate acceptance as a science.

Nursing as a Science

The nursing literature regularly refers to the nursing profession and, at times, the nursing discipline, but until recently, the phrase nursing science was seldom found. In 1988, a journal called *Nursing Science Quarterly* began publication. At least informally, that permitted nurses to use science to describe nursing.

When nursing is recognized as a profession and nursing education establishes itself firmly as a discipline in higher education, practice and education will support the development of nursing as a science. The evidence of progress in this effort will be a growing intellectual reputation based on a scientific body of knowledge and research that verifies, corrects, and adds to that body of knowledge. The transition from profession to discipline to science is clear. Each step builds on those that precede it.

For many years, nursing was viewed as not meeting the qualifications for consideration as a field of study in higher education and, therefore, was isolated from the scientific community. The scientific environment that enhanced the life of students, faculty members, scientists, and researchers in other disciplines had little or no effect on nursing education or practice. It was well into the 1980s before the number of nurses prepared to conduct scientific investigations was adequate to merit recognition by the NIH, a primary source of federal funds for health care research in this country. As nurse faculty in universities shifted from being teachers to professors with multiple responsibilities of education, research, practice, and service, they found themselves slowly integrated into the scientific community.

In the nursing major, you achieve graduation requirements by completing science courses, such as anatomy, physiology, psychology, sociology, and microbiology. Although you may identify these as science courses, you may not be aware why they are called sciences. If you do not know the distinguishing characteristics of a science, you will not be able to assess the scientific attributes of nursing.

What Is a Science?

As a student nurse, you are familiar with natural and biological sciences, such as anatomy and physiology, and may have also studied biology, chemistry, and physics. You may have also enrolled in courses in the social sciences, such as psychology, sociology, anthropology, and political science. As you think about those courses, try to identify similarities about them, including an organized body of knowledge, identifying and explaining actions and events, and the boundaries that separate these disciplines. Using these ideas should facilitate your understanding of the following definition:

> A **science** is a unified body of knowledge in which phenomena are observed, identified, described, and investigated. The results of such investigations yield evidence and theoretical explanation of ideas central to a specific discipline and potential resolution of its problems.

Scientific investigation in the health care disciplines focuses on the health and well-being of individuals, groups, and communities. The definition of science contains ideas you will recognize from earlier discussions about profession and discipline. It follows, then, that individuals who have accumulated expert knowledge in a science and who are involved in scientific work are called **scientists.** Table 12.2 depicts some of the similarities between the components of profession, discipline, and science. As you shift from profession to discipline to science, however, there is increasing specificity in a number of components. For example, the second component goes from specified knowledge in a profession to defined boundaries of the body of knowledge in a discipline, and finally to a unified body of knowledge in science. The fifth component provides a second example: high ethical standards for professionals, academic freedom for professors and students in the discipline, and

Table 12.2 Comparison of Profession, Discipline, and Science

Profession	Discipline	Science
Vocation/occupation	Education, research, service	Research experimental investigation
Specialized knowledge and skills	Defined knowledge boundaries	Unified body of knowledge
Methods based on scientific principles	Evidence-based practice	Experimental investigation
Institution of higher learning	Pursuit, development, dissemination of knowledge	Observation, identification, and description of phenomena
High ethical standards	Academic freedom for faculty and students	Assurance of human rights
Expanding body of knowledge	Distinct theoretical body of knowledge	Unified body of knowledge
Autonomous functioning	The classroom and the laboratory	The laboratory
Continuous study	Pursuit of knowledge	Pursuit of solutions and answers
Service to society	For the betterment of society	Health needs of society

assurance of human rights for subjects of research in science. Some components are more difficult to follow until you gain a broader understanding of knowledge and theory.

Is Nursing a Science?

Nurses hesitate to call their colleagues scientists unless they hold advanced degrees in a science, such as physiology or psychology. As with the concepts of profession and discipline, nursing is moving toward increasing acceptance as a scientific field. Increasing the number of nurse scientists and using titles and language consistent with those used in other university departments and disciplines help substantiate that progress. Let's look at nursing for the answer of whether nursing is a science.

Nursing has a body of knowledge that encompasses a large, diverse practice arena. You may care for infants and children as well as the elderly. You practice in homes, schools, free clinics, health departments, and critical care units in hospitals. You may choose to be a nurse practitioner, a vice president of nursing, a nurse attorney, an editor of a nursing journal, a legislator, a professor, or a dean. Although you are responsible for the patient's activities of daily living and his or her environment in one case, in other cases, you are monitoring life and death. Although you may agree that nursing has a body of knowledge, it is easy to see why there is little unity about what that body of knowledge should encompass. In Chapter 6, we enumerated the priorities for research funding that the NINR sets every 5 years. Although these priorities speak to only part of the body of nursing knowledge, there is unity in setting this agenda at the national level.

In a number of universities and academic health centers, nursing has built a firm base of research for expanding scientific knowledge and implementing the findings into practice. Faculty strive to provide theoretical explanations for central ideas in nursing. What are some of these central ideas and where do they come from? Central ideas in nursing come from the practice setting and vary considerably depending on the goals and outcomes of care. In the home health care setting, a central idea may relate to how family members can be trained to be observers and historians between the visits of the nurse. In the rehabilitation center, a central idea may relate to stimulating behavioral change consistent with a disability. These are only beginning ideas, but they provide a base for adopting these and other ideas as a part of the science of nursing.

Why Is the Development of Theory and Research Important for the Recognition of Nursing as a Science?

Nursing theory is closely tied to the professional, disciplinary, and scientific status of nursing. An important link, however, is the one between theory and the effects of the findings of research on health care. Nursing has taken major steps to establish itself as a credible scientific field through the expansion of doctoral and postdoctoral education in nursing. Educational programs for undergraduate and graduate nursing students have gained a reputation of being innovative, stimulating, and challenging. However, major changes still must take place in higher education and the health care community before nursing can achieve a position in the scientific world that is significant and fully accepted as a contributor to health care advancements.

You may hear or read about medical breakthroughs reported in the *New England Journal of Medicine* and the *Journal of the American Medical Association* on the evening news or the daily paper. How often do you hear about health care breakthroughs attributed to the research of nurses in the news media? Although breakthroughs may not occur as frequently in nursing as in medicine, why are they seldom part of the evening news? It may be as simple as the lack of a copy of a scientific nursing journal or it may be the reputation of nursing as an occupation, rather than a science.

The future of nursing as a science is related to the continuing development and use of relevant, practice-based knowledge. To generate the most useful propositions and phenomena for nursing investigation, nurse researchers and scientists must rely on expert advanced practice nurses. The future of nursing scholarship depends on an expanding knowledge base and a clear understanding of the effect of nursing care on patient outcomes (Anonymous, 1997). In the practice environment, clinical scholarship is paramount and will become more valued and rewarded in the future as the need increases to demonstrate nurses' contributions to health care (Lindsay, 1997). There are still many questions to answer: How will the future of nursing scholarship overcome the small proportion of nurses prepared at the doctoral and postdoctoral levels? Will the separation between the technical nurse and the nurse scientist strengthen nursing practice or make it more divisive? How will the bedside nurse, prepared in the community college, be affected by increasing the emphasis on an intellectual approach to resolve health problems and dilemmas? What impact will health care changes have on nursing's goal for advanced scholarship? In 1997, Cody predicted that the application of scientific findings in nursing would be the thing of the future, but he did not set a date when he thought that might occur.

Summary

This book's preface highlights the importance of baccalaureate-prepared nurses, whether newly graduated or experienced, being familiar with nursing and non-nursing theory, understanding and using theory in practice, and understanding relationships between theory, knowledge, reasoning, and research. The master's-prepared nurse needs to be aware of advances in nursing knowledge, able to analyze and test major contemporary nursing theories, and able to identify and explore practice-based phenomena and hypotheses. At each level, nurses with baccalaureate and master's degrees may assist in furthering the body of nursing knowledge; however, the leadership, theoretical thinking, and significant research come from nurses with doctorates and postdoctorates.

Nurses have made huge strides since the 1980s in cultivating a place among the health professions and the scholarly disciplines. Nurses have expanded their influence in academic health science centers and are recognized by private philanthropy and funding bodies in the federal government as serious contenders for research grants. The future of nursing and nursing education relies heavily on nursing theory and research for improving the profession, the discipline, and nursing as a science.

In 1997, Sister Callista Roy wrote: "This century challenges leaders to direct the greatest growth period nursing scholarship will ever know with boldness, courage, and vision. Nursing knowledge provides the basis for redesigning the world of nursing. A quiet revolution in nursing knowledge development provides a solid basis for creating solutions" (Lindsay, 1997, p. 225).

Nursing knowledge results when scientists test ideas and concepts and then accept or discard those ideas. In the 15th century, scientists declared that the world was flat. Obviously, they were wrong. When nurses accept research before the results are validated, they may also be wrong. For example, at one time, incubators for premature infants were flooded with high levels of oxygen. Later scientists discovered that this hyperoxygenation caused blindness. At one time, postoperative patients were confined to bed for days and weeks, and that later proved to lead to thrombophlebitis and pulmonary emboli. Now patients are walking out of the hospital the day of surgery in many instances and are involved in productive activities within days or weeks.

Tomorrow's nurses must anticipate that the practices of today will be cast aside when research demonstrates that there are more effective ways to meet health care needs. In the bold, courageous days of tomorrow, it will be the pattern, not the exception, for the baccalaureate-prepared nurse to continue into graduate study. The measurement of the profession, discipline, and science of nursing will be at the highest level of educational preparation.

We complete this chapter and this book with a challenge: Continue learning about theory and its impact on what you know and are able to practice. Use what you have learned to redesign your world, and be bold and courageous in shaping your practice of nursing. Consider that your education is only beginning and strive toward further formal education.

Learning Activities

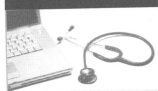

1. One giant step for health care: Gather into groups of two or three students and adopt roles of other health professionals—physicians, pharmacists, dentists, physical therapists—as well as nurses. Propose theoretical ideas that bring these professions together in advancing health care.

2. The crystal ball of nursing theory: Compose a theoretical model from the theories you have studied. Identify gaps and inadequacies, and design a model that helps close these gaps and correct the inadequacies.

3. Looking to the future: Many of you will practice until well into the 21st century. Write a short paper on your perception of nursing as a profession, a discipline, and a science in the year 2040. Share your ideas in class to see how similar they are.

4. Story-telling: Write a story about your experience as a college or university student enrolled in courses with students from other majors; include how you have handled questions and comments from faculty and students about the place of nursing in higher education.

References

American Nurses Association. (2001). *Code of ethics for nurses with interpretive statements.* Washington, DC: Author.

Anonymous. (1997). Future of nursing scholarship. *Image—Journal of Nursing Scholarship, 29,* 117–121.

Bixler, G. K., & Bixler, R. W. (1959). The professional status of nursing. *American Journal of Nursing, 59,* 1142–1146.

Brown, E. L. (1954). *Nursing for the future.* New York: Russell Sage Foundation.

Cody, W. K. (1997). Of tombstones, milestones, and gemstones: A retrospective and prospective on nursing theory. *Nursing Science Quarterly, 10,* 3–5.

Doheny, M. O., Cook, C. B., & Stopper, M. C. (1997). *The discipline of nursing: An introduction.* Stamford, CT: Appleton & Lange.

Flexner, A. (1910). *Medical education in the United States and Canada: A report to the Carnegie Foundation for the Advancement of Teaching* (Bulletin No. 4). New York: Carnegie Foundation for the Advancement of Teaching.

Flexner, A. (1915). Is social work a profession? *School and Society, 1*(26), 901–911.

International Council of Nurses. (1973). *Code for nurses: Ethical concepts applied to nursing.* Geneva: Author.

Johnson, D. E. (1959). The nature of science in nursing. *Nursing Outlook, 7,* 292–294.

Kalisch, P. K., & Kalisch, B. J. (2004). *American nursing: A history.* Philadelphia: Lippincott William & Wilkins.

Lindsay, A. M. (Ed). (1997). Future of nursing scholarship. *Image—Journal of Nursing Scholarship, 29,* 224–228.

McBride, A. B. (1999). Breakthroughs in nursing education: Looking back, looking forward. *Nursing Outlook, 47*(3), 114–119.

Montag, M. (1959). *Community college education for nursing: An experiment in technical education for nursing.* New York: Columbia University, Teachers College.

Pavalko, R. (1971). *Sociology of occupations and professions.* Itasca, IL: Peacock.

Yoder-Wise, P. (2000). State and Association/Certifying Boards CE Requirements Annual Survey. *Journal of Continuing Education in Nursing, 31,* 4–12.

Searching the Internet for Nursing Theory, Nurse Theorists, and Related Information

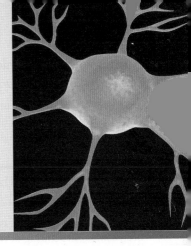

By now you are familiar with how to locate information for class preparation and assignments. There are many books, articles, and Internet sites about nursing theory that will help you as you seek information about theories and theorists. There are new sites being developed, so don't limit yourself to the ones mentioned here. The following Internet sites were identified and selected for inclusion on this list in 2008. They represent only some of the sites that were available at the time and should be used as examples of what you may find.

Always check when the last upgrade of the information was done, although not all sites indicate when they are updated. Also, be aware that some information may not be accurate. For example, Florence Nightingale was born on May 12, 1820, although one site listed the date of her birth as May 15, 1820, for many years. In another site, the title of Myra Levine's theory on conservation is incorrect. Most of the sites listed below are one or two pages in length. For sites that are longer, the actual number of pages is listed.

General Information

The first five listings below are general sources that provide links to many nursing theories and theorists. We have not listed the names of the nurse theorists for each site, since the author of the site does that. If you have difficulty accessing a site, try the links on one or more of the other listings. There are many duplicates among the sites. After the first five listings, there are three sites of international organizations that provide broader information about theory, science, and systems. Although you may not wish to use these now, remember they are here for future use.

The Clayton College and State University Department of Nursing
http://www.healthsci.clayton.edu/eichelberger/nursing.htm (12 pages)

This site provides links to 37 nurse theorists including 18 of the ones included in Chapter 7 and a few international ones. It also provides a brief list of nursing theory books. Updated: 1/1/07.

NurseScribe
http://www.enursescribe.com/nurse_theorists.htm (6 pages)

This site was initially labeled Nurses Station; now it is called NurseScribe. The site provides links to 20 well-known theorists/theories as well as other models and middle-range theories. Updated: 7/20/07.

Nursing Theories—Middle Range
http://www.nurses.info/nursing_theory_midrange_theories.htm

This new listing provides information about 41 theorists, some of which are already presented in Chapter 7, including Evelyn Adam, Ida Jean Orlando, Madeleine Leininger, and Hildegarde Peplau. You might want to check these theories and identify why they are listed as midrange theories.

San Diego University Hahn School of Nursing and Health Sciences
http://www.lib.newpaltz.edu/databases/handouts/nursing/nursing_theory.html

This site has over 25 links to nurse theorists including some international ones. There has been some restructuring of the site to include midrange theories and nursing models as well as some theories that have not been classified as yet. Updated: 6/6/08.

American Association for the Advancement of Science (AAAS)
http://www.aaas.org

This is the general web site for the AAAS and provides an overview of the history of the organization and its emphasis. The AAAS was the parent organization for the International Society for Systems Sciences, formerly known as the Society for General Systems Research.

International Society for Systems Sciences (ISSS)
http://www.isss.org

The ISSS web site is for international audiences interested in multiple aspects of systems theory and research. It originally was known as the Society for General Systems Research and was part of the AAAS.

Sigma Theta Tau International
http://www.nursingsociety.org (10 pages)

Sigma Theta Tau International provides general information about registering and searching for research. The site allows researchers to link to other researchers working in the same areas of study. Margaret Newman's health model is used to illustrate the Knowledge Net. Other information on this site that may be helpful includes discussions about using key words, quantitative and qualitative data sections, and access to the library and on-site journals.

International Web Sites

As the interest in global nursing rises, the number of Internet sites being developed increases.

Greece
Sharon L. Van Sell and Ioannis A. Kalofissudis

See the Clayton College and State University Department of Nursing and San Diego University Hahn School of Nursing and Health Sciences sites listed earlier.

United Kingdom
England
Brian E. Hodges and Dr. Phil Baker

See the Clayton College and State University Department of Nursing, NurseScribe, and San Diego University Hahn School of Nursing and Health Sciences sites listed earlier.

Scotland
Nancy Roper, Winifred W. Logan, and Alison T. Tierney

See the Clayton College and State University Department of Nursing and San Diego University Hahn School of Nursing and Health Sciences sites listed earlier.

Other Nurse Theorist Sites

Most of the nursing theorists/theories discussed in Chapter 7 are listed in one or more of the four general Internet sites related to nursing. The sites for each of the following theorists are repeated below. You will want to check those sources first, but may search other sites as well. In addition to the general sites, some other examples are included.

Additional Information

In this section, we have selected sites listed as nurse theorists but that present either a unique approach to the presentation or provide other information related to theory, research, or related topics.

A Creative Beginning

http://nursing.jbpub.com/sitzman/artGallery.cfm

The Jones and Bartlett Nursing Theory Art Gallery displays creative works of nursing students. There are four categories: theories that define nursing in a general sense, or philosophies; theories about broad nursing practice, or grand theories; theories about specific nursing actions, or middle-range theories; and theories that defy classification.

If you have made artistic impressions of nursing theory or wish to do so, there is an e-mail address where you can send them for consideration.

Online Exhibit of Margaret A. Newman: Nurse Theorist

http://library.utmem.edu/exhibits/newman/

The University of Tennessee Health Sciences Library announces the opening of the professional papers of Margaret Newman. A group of pictures starting with her graduation class in 1962 and featuring other high points in her career such as admission to the American Academy of Nursing in 1976 and the publication of the 1994 edition of *Health as Expanding Consciousness* document her evolution as a professional (revised 4/18/06).

Hildegard Peplau and the Nurse–Client Relationship

http://en.wikipedia.org/wiki/Hildegard_Peplau

Many nurses recognize Peplau's work as revolutionary in her approach to the relationship between the patient and the nurse. Her model continues to be useful to nurse scientists as they seek
new approaches to more sophisticated and therapeutic interventions. While we may tout
Nightingale's *Notes on Nursing* (1859/1992) as an early contribution to nursing literature, Peplau's seminal work *Interpersonal Relations in Nursing*, published in 1952, brought nursing literature into the mid-20th century.

Nightingale Knew More than she Thought . . .

http://www.nihe.org

The Nightingale Institute for Health & the Environment incorporates many of today's nurse theorists into the ideas of Nightingale about environment. Remember her emphasis on cleanliness
of houses, rooms, floors, and even the patient? Some say that she did not have a theory, when, in
fact, she focused on many of today's issues.

This paper speaks to Sister Callista Roy's adaptation model, which might better focus on
adapting the environment for the patient rather than enabling the patient to adapt to the environment. Madeline Leininger and her sensitivity to culture and its role in health and healing recognize the environment, while Parse views the influence of severe weather conditions on human
thoughts, feelings, and decisions. Even Benner, with her focus on the evolution of nursing competency, benefits from Nightingale's interpretation of basic fundamentals for nursing practice.
This seven-page paper is a stimulus to examine the environment in many important ways.

Evaluating your Nursing Collection

http://www.pubmedcentral.nih.gov/articlerender.fcgi?artid=1924961

This 4½-page document about a working history collection from the *Journal of the Medical Library Association* (JMLA) has an 11-item Weeding Checklist and an additional 2½-page reference
list. It may help you understand the need for libraries to conduct periodic weeding, and also may
help individuals make some difficult decisions.

C-BaCR Worksheet

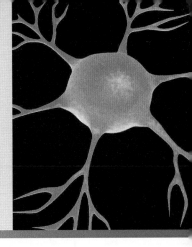

- List reference information (is the article in a refereed journal?)
- Has the study undergone review by a human subjects review board and is there evidence that the rights of subjects were protected?
- Is the language understandable and is there minimal use of jargon?

PHASE I: Intent						PHASE II: Relationships					PHASE III: Usefulness	
What is the intent of the study and phenomenon of interest?	What is the research question and is it within the boundaries of nursing practice?	Is the literature review adequate and reflective of the current knowledge?	Internal concepts/variables within the research question are identified and defined. What are the IV and DV?		Relevant external variables (EV) and assumptions (A) are identified and defined	Research Design and Rules of Evidence					Findings/Conclusions/Relevance to Nursing	Future Research
			IV	DV	EV	A	Method	Theoretical Framework	Population Study Sample	Measurement Method	Limitations		

Glossary

Abductive reasoning: The formation of potential propositions based on personal and nursing knowledge, skills, values, meanings, and experience and not on empirically based evidence or facts.

Academic degree: An academic title conferred by a college or university upon completion of a program of study.

Acceleration: A change in speed, either increase or decrease, or in the direction of an object.

Adaptation: Changes or adjustments made in response to new or unresolved conditions.

Analyze: The process of determining the nature of the whole; appraising and evaluating the value and significance of theory.

Appraise: To estimate the quality, use, and other features of the whole; to judge.

Aristotle: Ancient Greek philosopher and scientist. Student of Plato.

Arts: The study of human and social phenomena, such as language, art, music, and history. See also *humanities* and *science.*

Assess: To evaluate or appraise the value of.

Assumption: A concept in the form of an assumed truth that influences or has the potential to influence other concepts or propositions.

Axiom: A proposition asserted to be true.

Body of knowledge: The entire substance of what has been perceived, discovered, or learned about in a field of study, including its structure.

Boundary: The border or limit of an area of concern. In nursing theory, this may be the setting in which nursing takes place, the type of recipients receiving care, or the role of the nurse.

Cause: That which produces an effect or result.

C-BaC: A criterion-based critique model designed to increase understanding of theory and its usefulness in nursing practice.

C-BaCR: A criterion-based critique model designed to increase understanding of research and its usefulness in nursing practice.

Change: To make or become different.

Chaos: The perception of disorder and confusion.

Cognitive: Having to do with thinking or thought.

Communication: Intentional sharing of information.

Compare: To identify similarities or common features of two or more entities.

Complexity: The degree of complication.

Concept: Words or phrases that identify, define, and establish structure and boundaries for ideas generated about phenomena.

Conceptual definition: Broad definition of a concept.

Conceptual framework: A framework of concepts used to organize curriculum, theory, and research.

Construct: Concepts with measurable specificity.

Contrast: To identify differences between two or more entities.

Control: To take charge of. In nursing, controlling involves altering or changing one or more concepts or variables within a situation to bring about a desirable outcome.

Criterion [pl., criteria]: A standard, rule, or test on which a judgment or decision is based.

Criterion based: A type of standard used to assess objectively specific components of intellectual work and to make judgments.

Critical thinking: Utilizing scientific facts, principles, and laws to identify, relate, understand, explain, predict, influence, and control actual and potential concepts and propositions.

Criticism: An evaluation that tends to focus on weaknesses and limitations.

Critique: A broad objective evaluation used to judge strengths and limitations of intellectual work.

Deductive reasoning: Using broad facts, principles, laws, or theories to address narrower yet related phenomena, concepts, and propositions.

Dependent variable: A variable (concept) that has been influenced or changed by another variable.

Developmental stages: Categories of physiological and psychological growth.

Discipline: A field of study with a distinct theoretical body of knowledge within defined boundaries whose purpose is to guide the pursuit, development, and dissemination of knowledge.

Discipline-specific theory: Theory developed within a particular discipline to address discipline-specific phenomena.

Driving Forces: Behaviors that encourage change.

Effect: A result or consequence.

Emerita/Emeritus: One who has honorably retired from a faculty, but is retained on the roll.

Entropy: Adapting to changes within the environment in order to maintain homeostasis.

Environment: Surroundings or conditions in which something exists or operates.

Epistemology: The study of knowledge; examination of the origin, history, nature, scope, functions, processes, and limitations of knowledge.

Equifinality: Having more than one way to accomplish a goal.

Established theory: The collective culmination of facts, principles, and laws that have been repeatedly tested through research and over time and found to be consistently valid and reliable.

Evaluate: To ascertain the value or worth; to examine and judge carefully.

Evidence: The data on which a judgment or conclusion may be based; that which may furnish proof.

Evidence-based nursing: "The use of quality improvement data, other operational and evaluation data, the consensus of recognized experts, and affirmed experiences to substantiate [nursing] practice" (Stetler, 2000).

Experience: Defining, refining, and changing knowledge, skills, values, and meanings as a result of actively engaging in nursing situations over time.

Explain: To interpret information, its components, and its significance, to others.

Fact: An observation consistently proven true over time.

Feedback: Energy, information, or matter that is received as a response to a stimulus.

Force field: The environment in which opposing forces exist and interact.

General adaptation syndrome: Systemic response to stress.

Gravity: The natural phenomenon of attraction between two massive bodies.

Grounded: Based in reality.

Hermeneutics: The science of interpreting words and their evolving meanings.

Hierarchy: Classification according to importance, power, size, etc.

Historicism: The development of knowledge using experience, beliefs, and empirical evidence to make conceptual leaps at an educated guess or speculative theory.

Holistic: Referring to wholeness.

Honorary degree: An academic title conferred by a college or university in recognition of an achievement or distinguished activity.

Human needs: Those physiological (air, food, water) and psychological (love, belonging, self-esteem) factors that motivate human behavior.

Humanities: The study of literature, philosophy, and the arts as opposed to science. See also *arts*.

Hypothesis [pl., hypotheses]: Formal statement describing an anticipated and measurable relationship(s) between two or more concepts or variables.

Idea: The product of organized thought about the origin, nature, boundaries, and significance of phenomena.

Identify: To recognize or distinguish.

Independent variable: Variable (concept) that influences or causes something to happen to another variable.

Inductive reasoning: Using concepts or variables to develop new propositions.

Inertia: The tendency of a body at rest to remain at rest or a body in motion to remain in motion unless affected by an external force.

Interaction: Exchange of energy, information, or matter.

Influence: To have an effect on. In nursing, influencing involves persuading someone to alter or change one or more concepts or variables in a situation to bring about a desirable outcome.

Intuition: The act of knowing something without a conscious awareness of what or how it was observed.

Jargon: The specialized or technical language of a trade, profession, or similar group.

Know(ing): To be aware of.

Knowledge: Culmination of the integration of what is known and understood through learning and experience.

Law: An absolute truth that guides thought and behavior.

Law of culturally congruent care: Effective nursing care integrates cultural values, mores, and beliefs of diverse individuals, families, groups, communities, and global society.

Law of self-care: Effective nursing care promotes the highest level of self-care possible for individuals, families, groups, communities, and global society.

Local adaptation syndrome: Localized response to stress.

Logical adequacy: A method of explaining and validating theory, facts, principles, and laws that includes, but goes beyond, empirical testing. Logical adequacy is dependent upon teleologic, practical usefulness, and universality.

Logical empiricism: Reasoning through experimentation and statistics.

Meaning: Define the context, purpose, and intent of language.

Model: Diagrams used to demonstrate relationships.

Modernism: A philosophy of knowledge development that focuses on the discovery of facts, objectivity, logic, technology, physicality, linear cause and effect, and belief in universal principles and laws. See *postmodernism.*

Motivation: The reason for actions or behaviors.

Moving: A stage during the change process when the actual change is planned and initiated.

Observation: The process of watching, listening, and being aware of individuals, events, and relationships. See *purposeful observation* and *intuition.*

Open system: A system in constant integration with its environment and other systems and subsystems.

Operational definition: A definition that is very specific and measurable.

Operationalize: To make it ready for use.

Phenomenon [pl., phenomena]: Observable connection or relationship between objects, events, or ideas.

Philosophy: Broad, connected statements about beliefs and values that have the potential to guide thinking and behavior of individuals, disciplines, and societies.

Plato: Ancient Greek philosopher and teacher. Student of Socrates.

Postmodernism: A movement toward knowledge discovery that does not rely exclusively on empirical evidence of phenomena but that also focuses on the discovery of the meaning of phenomena. See *modernism.*

Predict(ing): Explaining what may happen in the future based on existing information

Principle: A truth that is foundational to other truths.

Profession: A vocation or occupation that requires specialized knowledge, skills, and scientific methods based on research and is taught in an institution of higher education. A profession advocates high ethical standards of its members and engages in expanding its body of knowledge. Members of a profession function autonomously, are committed to advanced study, and are motivated by service to society.

Proposition: A statement that describes a directional relationship between two or more concepts or variables.

Purposeful observation: The intent to collect information for the purpose of making judgments.

Qualitative research: Research that focuses on the meaning of phenomena as they occur naturally.

Quantitative research: Research that focuses on interpretation of phenomena through experimentation and statistical data.

Questioning: An expression of inquiry that invites or calls for a reply.

Reason(ing): Utilizing scientific facts, principles, laws, and phenomenological and experiential information to identify, relate, understand, explain, predict, influence, and control actual, potential, or perceived concepts and propositions.

Refreezing: A stage in the change process where change has been accomplished and is becoming established.

Research: The diligent, systematic inquiry or investigation of phenomena that assists in validating and refining established theory and knowledge and generating new theory and knowledge.

Restraining forces: Behaviors that oppose change. Also known as static forces.

Scholarship: Research or study that requires relentless questioning that pushes the edge of knowledge and integrates sources of knowledge into practice.

Science: A unified body of knowledge in which phenomena are observed, identified, described, and investigated. The results of investigations yield evidence and theoretical explanations of ideas central to that discipline.

Sciences: The study of the physical and natural world and behavior, such as biology, chemistry, physics, and psychology.

Significance: The meaning and importance of something.

Skills: Acts or activities in the cognitive and psychomotor domain that are selected, performed, and evaluated for, with, or on behalf of those for whom nurses care.

Socrates: Ancient Greek philosopher, scientist, and teacher. Teacher of Plato.

Socratic method: A method of investigative inquiry used by Socrates.

Speculative theory: Theory that has yet to be tested through research and found to be consistently true, valid, and reliable.

Stress: The body's physiological and psychological response to situations it considers threatening.

Subsystem: Connected, interdependent, interacting elements that are part of a larger system.

Support theory: Theory from the arts, sciences, humanities, and related disciplines that support nursing practice and the development of nursing theory.

System: Connected, interdependent, interacting elements (components, people, etc.) that are hierarchically organized into a single entity for the purposes of maintaining homeostasis and achieving a common goal.

Theorem: A proposition that has been deduced from an axiom and is either true or needs to be proven as true.

Theorist: The individual or group that develops, disseminates, and refines a theory.

Theory: Organized information intended to explain phenomena.

Theoretical DNA: A phrase representing concepts and theory from the arts, sciences, and humanities that are foundational to a significant part of nursing theory.

Triangulation research: Research that uses more than one methodology, such as qualitative and quantitative methods.

Unfreezing: A stage of the change process where the need for change becomes apparent.

Understand: To comprehend or grasp the significance of.

Values: Enduring beliefs, attributes, or ideals that establish moral and ethical boundaries.

Variable: Concepts or constructs whose characteristics vary.

Whole: All of something.

Wholeness: A whole that is more than the sum of its parts.

Reference

Stetler, C. B. (2000). To the editor . . . evidence-based nursing: What it is and what it isn't. *Nursing Outlook, 48,* 151–152.

Index

Page numbers followed by *b* indicate boxes; those followed by *f* indicate figures; and those followed by *t* indicate tables.